AF529652

PHARMACEUTICAL RESEARCH AND DEVELOPMENT

ENCYCLOPAEDIA OF BIOPHARMACEUTICAL - I

PHARMACEUTICAL RESEARCH AND DEVELOPMENT

By

Dr. Shiv Kant Prasad

School of Studies of Zoology & Biotechnology
Vikram University
Ujjain (M.P.)
(India)

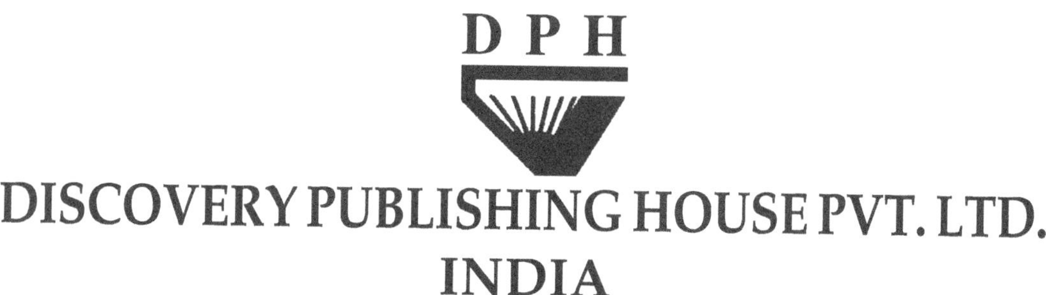

Published by:

DISCOVERY PUBLISHING HOUSE PVT. LTD.
4383/4B, Ansari Road, Darya Ganj
New Delhi-110 002 (India)
Phone : +91-11-23279245; 23253475; 43596065
E-mail : discoverybooksindia@gmail.com
discoverypublishinghouse@gmail.com
namitwasan9@gmail.com
web : www.discoverypublishinggroup.com

First Edition: **2011**

Reprinted: **2022**

ISBN: 978-81-8356-594-3(Set)
ISBN: 978-81-8356-733-6

Pharmaceutical Research and Development

Printed at:
Infinity Imaging Systems
Delhi

Preface

The present title "Encyclopaedia of Biopharmaceutical" has been written for those in the pharmaceutical research and those responsible for the education and training in pharmaceutical science and technology of graduate and undergraduate students. Medicine is an ever changing science. As new research and clinical experience broaden our knowledge, changes in treatment and drug therapy are required. This branch of life science has progressed enormously in recent years and the significant advances in therapeutics and an understanding of the need to optimize during delivery in the body have brought about an increased awareness of the valuable role played by the dosage forms. This statement is as true as it was back in ninteenth century and perhaps more so, given the increasing emphasis being placed on discovery, development, and use of large molecular entities as therapeutic and diagnostic agents. Development of these abilities requires an integration of knowledge, skills, attitudes, and values that can be acquired only through structured learning process including independent study, hands on practice and the availability of advanced literature. This tittle has designed to meet such needs of learners in the health professions.

In the last two decades, the pharmaceutical industry has experimented and successfully adopted several integrated and multidisciplinary approaches in the research areas of dring compound screening, toxicological evaluation, and pharmaceutical product development. The book is written in a concise style that facilitates an in-depth level of understanding of the essential concepts. The objectives of the present title are three folds: (i) to serve as a useful tool to help guide scientists in research and development by out-lining the theory and successful practice of in vitro - in vivo correlation, (ii) to help formulators apply the tool in designing and developing prototypes that enable selection of clinical formulations, and (iii) to help formulate strategy(ies) for product life-cycle management.

To make the work more comprehensive and informative, the author has consulted many authoritative books, research journals, abstracts, monographs etc., so there can be no claim to originality except in the manner of treatment.

The author expresses his thanks to his friends and colleagues whose continue inspirations have initiated him to bring out this book.

The author expresses his gratitude to Mr. Wasan and staff of M/s Discovery Publishing House Pvt. Ltd. for their whole hearted co-operation in the publication of this book.

Author

CONTENTS

1

INTRODUCTION

To deny that advances in health delivery and research, including therapeutic medicines during the past sixty years, have not been of significant benefit to mankind is to deny reality. Equally, few will be prepared to deny that the future will be one of at least equal promise. Children will be born with their genes profiled, 'personalized' medicines will be a reality, gene and stem cell therapies will be mature disciplines with major implications for the degenerative disorders of an aging world. This new world will be one of artificial cells and machines, many specifically created de novo with an expanded genetic code and that will execute unique tasks ranging from the site- and disease-specific delivery of drugs, genes, and gene repair instructions to neuronal- and DNA-based computers. These advances will have been made possible by a remarkable several generations of scientific research, culminating in the reading of multiple genomes, including the human genome.

The promise of Ehrlich, written ironically enough on the eve of World War 1, remains unfulfilled. Indeed, the world now faces challenges at least as large as those that existed at the turn of the 20th century. Two thirds of the world – the 'poor world' – still lives without adequate education, food, health care, sanitation and water, whilst the 'rich world' follows policies that largely ensure the continuation of this division, despite the spectacular advances in science and technology over the past one hundred years. Nowhere have these advances been as dramatic, spectacular or promising as in medicine and the pharmaceutical sciences, yet nowhere is there greater inequity of application, distribution, or benefits.

Indeed, in many important respects, the material gap between the rich and the poor worlds has increased rather than decreased. Some 11 million children die every year from starvation and other largely preventable diseases, almost 2 billion people live on less than one dollar a day, some 1.5 billion people routinely lack clean drinking water and sanitation, and malaria and other tropical diseases affect almost one billion people and account for some 5 million annual deaths. And this year, worldwide deaths from AIDS reach 3 million. The United Nations Human Development Report for 2003 notes that the 1990s, far from being a decade of progress, have actually seen remarkable reversals: 54 out of 175 countries are poorer in 2001 than in 1991; in 14 out of 175 countries, more children are dying before the age of five; in 21 out of 175 countries, more people are starving; and in 12 out of 175 countries, fewer children are being educated. The gap between the rich and the poor worlds has actually increased in several areas of the world. Science has delivered for the rich world, but party and politics have blinded our eyes and have limited the participation of the poor world. Progress will not be possible until we break their cycle of poor health driving poverty: this is not likely to occur in the present Washington-driven 'free market Darwinism' model of economic development. Indeed, in the

United States, where this policy is most slavishly advocated and followed, there has been a remarkable increase in income inequality between the richest and the poorest segments together with a considerable weakening of the social infrastructure of the country. Such market-driven ideologies provide little or no incentive for the development of drugs for the diseases of the poor world, and alternative models must be adopted.

The challenges for the poor world in the 21st century are many. In particular, the absence of an adequate scientific and educational infrastructure confers an enormous disadvantage in an environment dominated increasingly by trade and intellectual property imbalance. The ongoing efforts to impose the existing standards of patent and copyright protection on the poor world are, in fact, likely to exacerbate the cycle of poor health and poverty. The selfish discussions over the past several years on making AIDS and other drugs available to the poor world provide adequate, and offensive, testimony to this point. Furthermore, the increasing enclosure of the scientific commons, to which aim universities that have always been the major contributor to this commons are now enthusiastic partners, will only exacerbate the problems of the poor world by diminishing their access to scientific and technological knowledge.

A recent issue of The Economist observed, 'That the mental landscape today is almost unrecognizable from that of, say two centuries ago, is due almost entirely to the work of two groups of thinkers – scientists and economists. Add engineers to that and you have an explanation of why the physical, commercial and political landscapes have changed just as radically'. This is true: science is mankind's greatest intellectual achievement, but its full realization will come only when it is placed fully in the service of man. We are a long way from that goal and in the absence of that achievement, particularly in the delivery of critical medicines and health services, our science will be naught for our comfort – physically or spiritually.

Drug Discovery Process

The traditional process of drug discovery has been directed by target generation from observations of the biological activity of a natural product or synthetic entity on a physiological or pathological process. Typically, the identification of a lead active structure was followed by iterative structural modification and biological testing. This process, essentially a 'one molecule at a time' approach relying heavily on trial and error, serendipity, scientific intuition, genius, and luck has achieved many notable therapeutic successes. Prominent examples include the development of antibiotics, β-adrenoceptor blockers, histamine H_2 receptor antagonists, ACE inhibitors, calcium blockers, and angiotensin II receptor blockers. The essential mechanism of action or the structure of the underlying target not being a necessary prerequisite, the characteristics of this process are that the target is phenotypically defined and validated – blood pressure, acid secretion, smooth muscle relaxation or contraction etc. In contrast, the advent of genomics has led to the development of genotypically defined targets with defined structure, but frequently with undefined or only hypothetical phenotypical function.

It has been estimated that currently available drugs are directed towards some five hundred molecular targets with membrane receptors, notably G protein coupled entities, constituting almost 50% of the total. The heady promise of the genome project was that the human genome would be composed of perhaps as many as 150,000 genes generating on a 'one gene = one protein' rationale a ca. 300-fold increase in the number of possible drug targets. This number, together with the targets potentially realizable from bacterial and parasite genomes, was predicted to change dramatically the scale of the drug discovery enterprise. Simultaneously, the development of the new technologies of combinatorial chemistry, high-throughput screening, and informatics generated the *Viagra*-fueled 'bigger is better' model of drug development – the larger the company and the greater the throughput from chemistry and screening, the greater would be the output.

That the human genome expresses only some 30,000 genes (more than, but not dramatically so, our less complex fly, worm, and mouse relatives) means necessarily that the complexity of human organization is defined by multiple use of the same gene - splice variants, alleles in the population, post-translational modification etc. - and by the combinatorial diversification of regulatory and signaling pathways. From this relatively limited gene catalog, the human probably expresses in spatially and temporally limited manner as many as 100,000 proteins. A protein target may not be druggable because of its intrinsic properties or expression, but also because of a role it may play in regulatory networks other than the one of pathological interest. The elucidation of the cellular signaling network is therefore a critical component of the target validation problem. Increasingly, a systems biology based approach is needed whereby an integrated approach, rather than a reductionist component analysis, is employed to understand the relationship between the overall function of a biological system and the effects of perturbations such as disease or small molecules. Additionally, for a protein target to be druggable, there must be certain characteristics of the protein binding site: if one member of a gene family can bind a drug then it is assumed that other members will likely share this property. Using this approach, it has been estimated that ca. 10% of the proteins expressed by the human genome will fall into the druggable category. Three to four thousand targets is a far cry from the in excess of one hundred thousand targets originally claimed, although the former number may well increase as the roles of genes of previously unknown function are discovered.

The power of genomics to generate targets of well-defined proteins - receptors, channels, enzymes, etc. - to use in high-throughput screening has been extremely useful for generating 'hits' of appropriate affinity and, in a number of systems, to generate functional activity also. However, since these same systems usually, if not invariably, lack the complex signaling characteristics of 'real' cells and the integrated functional physiological properties of organ systems, they remain limited in their predictive properties and have probably served to consume very large amounts of research capital investment to the satisfaction of narrowly focused basic science without increasing the productivity of drug discovery.

Thus, critical to genomics-based target discovery is the issue of target validation - the determination of the actual role(s) of any potential gene target - the linkage between gene and phenotype. The technologies involved are several and include the analysis of gene and protein expression in normal and diseased tissues, knockout, conditional knockout, and knock-in animals, the creation of mutant (ethyl-nitrosourea-induced) mice, the use of model organisms including *Drosophila melanogaster* and *Caenorhabditis elegans*, and most recently the use of small interfering RNA. The elucidation of the mouse genome will place increased emphasis on this animal for target validation, the modeling of human diseases and drug discovery platforms. However, a too facile assumption of identity between animal and human models may be exceedingly counterproductive to therapy discovery and advancement. In any event, much human disease is almost certainly due to the influence of multiple genes, and, for those relatively few human diseases that are single gene failures, we do not need animal models with which to understand the problem.

The transition from phenotype-based to genotype-based drug discovery has brought with it the realization that biology is governed by a set of basic themes - *diversity*, *replication*, *evolution*, and *self-organization* - that are now recognized as generally applicable to disciplines from anthropology to zoology, including engineering and synthetic chemistry, and that are intimately linked through the process of biological recognition. These themes have had a major impact on chemistry, a discipline that remains fundamental to the drug-discovery process.

Chemical Diversity

A simplistic view of combinatorial chemistry suggests that by synthesizing all possible molecules and screening against all possible targets all possible drugs will be discovered. This view, expressed here in grossly exaggerated fashion, has yielded to a much more nuanced view of combinatorial chemistry, whereby the real issue is generating the maximum possible diversity within chemical libraries that encompass both the structural prerequisites for biological activity and for the appropriate pharmacokinetic and toxicological properties.

Nature is, of course, the ultimate combinatorial chemist. A limited repertoire of 20 amino acids and a rather larger number of protein folds has generated the several thousand catalytic, regulatory, immune, and structural proteins that constitute the existing cellular repertoire. Combinatorial chemistry in its various guises has proven to be extremely useful both in generating 'hits' and in exploiting molecular space around a 'lead' structure. In principle, outside of considerations of the amount of matter in the universe and of the database problems of tracking and compiling compounds made, there are few limitations to the number of molecules that can be made by combinatorial chemistry techniques. It has been estimated that the number of potential small drug molecules that could be made lies between 10^{62} and 10^{63}. To attempt such a synthesis would be a mindless effort, and in practice, very careful consideration is required to ensure that an appropriate diversity of chemical space is explored and that this space is focused around 'drug-like' or pharmacophoric structures. The existence of such pharmacophoric or 'privileged' structures derives from the repeated presence in proteins of folds and domains that recognize generic structural skeletons. Intuitively, this has been recognized by medicinal chemists for decades as with the repeated presence of the diphenylmethyl and related hydrophobic double ring systems in many active drugs. Nature has, of course, linked combinatorial peptide and protein chemistry with biological selection to generate the most biologically fit molecules. The cone snails of the *Conus* genus with some 500 species generating as many as 50,000 toxins provide a potent example of this strategy played out in Nature: these venomous snails produce disulfide-bridged toxins of rigid three dimensional structure that exhibit both high affinity and selectivity for a variety of ion channels and neurotransmitter receptors. *Conus* appears to follow a combinatorial approach whereby the peptides are biosynthesized as larger precursors with a stable N-terminus and a hypervariable C-terminus region, the latter permitting amino acid change in discrete regions to tailor pharmacological specificity from ion channels to neurotransmitter receptors. This strategy presumably permits Conus to match its venom production with its prey preference.

Self-Organization

The fundamental importance of template-guided reactions in biological systems is well known. Now, template-guided synthesis – '*click chemistry*' – is achieving significance in drug design. The use of an enzyme active site to guide selectively molecular building blocks to a target structure and then permit them to link covalently has been described to yield an inhibitor of the enzyme acetylcholinesterase with femtomolar affinity – several hundred times more potent than existing inhibitors. The use of a biological macromolecule as a template to both select and synthesize potent and specific ligands would appear to offer significant opportunity for the self-synthesis and targeting of new and active drug molecules.

Evolution

One of the major achievements of chemistry over the past decade has been the translation to the test tube of biological (Darwinian) evolution. Darwinian evolution exhibits three fundamental processes – selection, amplification, and mutation – regardless of whether it takes place in molecules or organisms. The in vitro evolution of DNA, RNA, and proteins to generate molecules of altered and desired properties has met with considerable success: the process is ideal for the optimization of protein therapeutic molecules where de novo design is difficult [20]. The process is now being applied to small molecules by the strategy termed 'Dynamic Combinatorial Chemistry'. Dynamic combinatorial chemistry provides for the synthesis of molecules under reversible conditions – thermodynamic control vs. the kinetic control of conventional combinatorial chemistry – in the presence of a selection mechanism, a template for which some molecules will have enhanced affinity, thus shifting the equilibrium to favor production of this molecular species. In principle, an appropriate supply of elementary small molecule building blocks and the presence of the appropriate template will serve as a chemical factory for the production of 'lead', 'candidate', and 'drug' molecules.

Replication

The genesis of molecular replication is a phenomenon of epochal significance and is classically embodied in nucleotide sequences. Outside of DNA, an increasing number of self-replicating systems exist that permit the replication of both peptides and small molecules. Self-replication demands that a molecule be able to serve as a template to pre-organize molecular fragments for reaction – '*template-guided synthesis*'. When the molecule produced is identical to the template then an auto-catalytic cascade can be initiated. Increasingly complex self-reproducing molecules are being described. A number of systems of small-molecule replication are known based on the self-complementarity of base-pairing mechanisms analogous to those that occur in nucleic acid replication. These systems can also show a behavior that incorporates '*evolution*' and '*mutation*' into the generation of enhanced replication processes. Self-replicating peptides are of particular importance because of their relationship to prebiotic conditions. The description by Lee et al. that a helically structured 32-residue peptide can autocatalyze its own synthesis provides proof of the concept that in vitro replicating systems are not limited to small molecules only.

Shape of Things to Come

Since the time of Paul Ehrlich, a principal goal of medicine has been the development of the '*magic bullet*' targeted only to those specific cells or pathways that are defective or are expressed only in disease states. Such a magic bullet would be without undesirable side effects since it would target only the component unique to the disease state. Although substantial selectivity of action has been obtained for a number of drugs, it is exceedingly rare that complete specificity is achieved. However, progress is being made through an increased understanding of the principles of biological recognition processes, processes that typically occur with uniquely defined specificity as revealed, for example, in the immune system and demonstrated with therapeutic antibodies. Molecules such as Gleevec and Herceptin that target a tyrosine kinase overactive in chronic myelogenous leukemia and the overexpressed growth factor receptor Her2 in breast cancer, respectively, provide contemporary examples of such targeted molecular specificity.

Recent developments in '*viraceuticals*' exploit the tools of molecular biology to ensure that engineered viruses interact only with cells expressing a specific pathology. The tumor suppressor gene that encodes the protein p53, often described as a '*guardian of the genome*' is defective in over 50% of human cancers. Hence, approaches to restore its function are an attractive form of chemotherapy. The E1B gene of the adenovirus encodes a protein that inactivates p53: a virus lacking this protein can replicate in and destroy p53-deficient cells present in tumors, but cannot do so in cells with functional p53. Similarly, an engineered vesicular stomatitis virus (VSV) that expresses CD4 and CXCR4 chemokine receptors, the coreceptors for HIV cell fusion and entry, will fuse and lyse only those cells – HIV-infected cells – that express the viral protein gp120 as the indicator of infection. The clinical limitations to this approach are real, but they derive not from lack of specificity of action, but rather from the use of replication-competent viruses and the potential detrimental consequences of such replication.

Engineered viruses can be thought of as '*nano-factories*' capable of replicating in specific environments to produce specific therapeutic effects. There are clearly serious limitations to any consideration of their clinical use at the present time, but the concept of a nano-factory for drug synthesis and delivery remains an attractive one. Already genetically engineered bacteria are employed as 'factories' for the production of novel polyketide antibiotics and nonribosomal peptides, and yeast has been engineered to synthesize hydrocortisone. It is not difficult to contemplate such '*bacteria*' or '*yeast*' cells being constructed de novo with the sole designed functions of synthesizing specific drugs and targeting diseased or infected cells and tissues.

The influence of the genome project and the paradigms of biology will be profound indeed on virtually all aspects of the human enterprise. Nowhere are they perhaps larger than in medicine and the pharmaceutical sciences. Not just in the prospects and promises of gene and stem-cell therapy, but in the application of new diagnostic procedures, new and more-selective and more-efficacious medicines, the generation of personalized medicine, and the actual elimination of diseases. The recent reporting of the genome of the malaria parasite and mosquito will ultimately be very bad news for the disease of malaria since we now have the genomes from all three participants in this most costly disease – man, the mosquito, and the parasite. From this knowledge should emerge a cure. Whether this is so will now depend critically on public policy: science counts for naught in the absence of public and political will and the integrity to use it to beneficial ends.

Balancing the Promises and the Problems

The postgenomic era has brought with it the promise of both dramatically increased productivity of drug discovery, of increased creativity of exploitation of novel targets and mechanisms, and the introduction of personalized medicine that better matched disease, patient, and drug. It is difficult to believe that from our knowledge of the human, bacterial, and parasitic genomes, from the increasingly sophisticated technologies of structure-based design, combinatorial chemistry, and screening approaches plus the arrival of human-genome databases that can be mined for genetic links to individual variants of disease, that the predicted success will not ultimately arrive. However, the path will be longer and more expensive than was originally advocated: to date and for a number of reasons, this promise has not been fulfilled either quantitatively or qualitatively.

The original anticipation that the new technologies of combinatorial chemistry, high-throughput screening, and structure-based design would, together with the more than 100,000 new targets anticipated from the human-genome project, generate an arsenal of new and more-efficacious drugs has not been realized. Indeed, the recognition that the human genome perhaps codes as few as 30,000 genes means that the complexity of the human is not determined by numbers alone, but rather by multiple use of the same gene and by the signaling networks. Thus, the issue of target validation – the linkage between the gene and the phenotypic and disease states–assumes critical significance. There is also no evidence that the series of mergers of companies has yielded either efficiencies of operation or enhanced creativity. Indeed, with the introduction of new technologies and the increased search for new targets, global research and development costs have more than doubled over the past decade (it is claimed that the cost of introducing a new drug now exceeds $800 million) whilst the number of new molecular entities introduced has decreased by ca. 50%. Part of the problem is that each newly introduced technology, from structure-based design, to combinatorial chemistry, to high- throughput screening, and genomics, has been regarded as the savior of the discovery process. The reality is, of course, that all of these technologies are useful, but only to the extent of the creativity of the minds employing them. There are, in fact, several likely contributors to the increased cost and decreasing productivity currently seen. First, the time line for payoff by the new technologies is going to be significantly longer than was originally assumed; second, many of the 'easy' diseases have already been tackled with the consequence that there are many useful drugs available for such diseases. A case in point is hypertension with in excess of one hundred drugs in some ten mechanistic categories. In contrast, the neurodegenerative disorders, increasingly common in aging societies are far more difficult to study both clinically and preclinically. Third, the industry has been self-seduced with the goal of ever increasing returns on investment with the consequence that many potential areas with medical need have been neglected because they will not produce such levels of profit.

A combination of increasing costs, decreased productivity together with a decreased level of innovation in newly introduced drugs are all indications of an industry in major trouble. However, at 18%, the profits of the pharmaceutical industry remain amongst the highest, if not the highest, of any industry, whilst the costs of drugs to the public has escalated in the United States, the largest single market, at rates significantly in excess of the general rate of inflation. These issues have been subject to extensive discussion. At the same time, the pharmaceutical industry has fallen from grace in the public eye and it is too frequently regarded by large segments of the public, because of its ill-conceived efforts to preserve its intellectual property rights at virtually any cost, to be just another greedy multinational concern. This was particularly clear to the world in 2001 when thirty nine multinational pharmaceutical companies sued the government of South Africa headed by President Nelson Mandela over the protection of their intellectual property rights for AIDS drugs.

Finally, the statements from Alan Roses of GlaxoSmithKline that 'The vast majority of drugs – more than 90% – only work in 30 or 50% of the people', 'I wouldn't say most drugs don't work. I would say that most drugs work in 30 to 50% ofpeople. Drugs out there on the market work, but they don't work on everybody'. This is an unsurprising clinical statement, but one that is significantly at odds with the general marketing messages of major pharmaceutical companies.

In the face of decreasing productivity and the desire to maintain the very high profit levels to which this business-oriented industry is now accustomed, the major pharmaceutical companies have adopted an approach that emphasizes the following general strategies:

1. Focus on so-called 'blockbuster' drugs – drugs that have market sales in excess of $1 billion per year.
2. Focus on chronically vs. acutely used drugs – HMGCoA inhibitors vs. antibiotics.
3. Focus on the United States market.
4. De-emphasize drugs that are primarily applicable in the 'poor world'.
5. Emphasize marketing – including direct-to-consumer advertising on a mass scale – to spur consumer-based demand with the message that a 'pill-a-day' is the route to the pursuit of happiness.
6. Emphasize drug use over acceptance of life changes.
7. Increase efforts to maintain and extent patent life.
8. Emphasize 'life-style' diseases – hair loss, erectile dysfunction, etc.
9. Enlarge the role of drugs in existing disorders and/or exaggerate the seriousness of existing disorders – attention deficit disorder, irritable bowel syndrome, mild depression, etc.
10. Invent new diseases – 'social phobia', 'female sexual dysfunction', etc.
11. Work closely with Congress to ensure favorable legislation is passed.
12. Ensure that intellectual property rights are maintained worldwide.

To be sure, the industry has received some bad publicity, most notably from its wrong-headed approach to the availability of drugs in the poor world. However, overall, this has been an extremely successful approach for the major pharmaceutical industry. The US market now constitutes ca. 50% of the world market and increasingly major pharmaceutical companies have shifted more of their research development and marketing to the United States where the drug prices are the highest in the world. To maintain this position and high profitability, the industry employs more than 650 Washington lobbyists and is a major and enthusiastic contributor of 'campaign funds' to largely Republican members: total expenditures on political activities since 1997 are in excess of $600 million. Recent successes of the industry in the USA include a provision in the new Medicare prescription bill that prohibits the Federal government from negotiating lower drug prices and the prevention of imports of cheaper drugs from other countries, notably Canada. Nothing in the present political climate suggests that significant change in this approach is likely to occur or to be resisted by Congress. Indeed, it is probable that there will be increased pressure from the US government to ensure that drug prices in countries that are currently regulated as part of their comprehensive health care systems be allowed to rise to unregulated levels as part of 'free trade' agreements.

For Whom, for What?

The delivery of and access to health care and medicines is deficient and defective in both the rich and the poor worlds. For all of its scientific promise, the current model of pharmaceutical development is flawed, probably fatally, and needs major surgery. There are two principal issues. First, recognition that ill-health and disease is a driving force for the economic and physical inequality that characterizes at least 50% of the world population. Second, recognition that the benefits of science, including medicines development, must be more equitably shared and that the current Western trend towards the privatization of science makes this goal progressively less attainable.

Health and Inequalities

The former President of the United States, Jimmy Carter, observed on receiving the Nobel Peace Prize in November2002, 'I was asked to discuss, here in Oslo, the greatest challenge that the world faces. I decided that the most serious and universal problem is the growing chasm between the richest and the poorest people on earth'. This chasm is, of course, not new but it is much to the shame of the rich world that the promises of economic coprosperity implicit in the globalization imperative have been too often hollow indeed. The most-recent data from the Food and Agricultural Organization of the United Nations reveal that, even in a time of worldwide food availability, the number of undernourished actually increased from 1995–1997 to 1999–2001: 'Bluntly stated, the problem is not so much a lack of food as a lack of political will'. A significant contributor to this food insecurity is the increase in the AIDS population in the developing world: in 2003 an estimated 40 million people are afflicted with the virus, some 5 million contracted the virus and a record 3 million died form AIDS. In the absence of far greater public health, scientific and financial resources, it is estimated that there will be 100 million cases of AIDS worldwide by the end of this decade. Efforts by the United States to ban the use of the phrase '*reproductive health*' in reports from the United Nations Population Fund and to advocate 'abstinence only' policies in the developing world should, together with the most- recent statements from the Vatican arguing against condom use in AIDS- inflicted countries, be treated with the contempt that such primitive philosophies deserve.

In fact, the relationship between health, poverty, and economic development is well recognized with the following consequences:

1. Poor health reduces healthy life expectancy and educational achievements.
2. Poor health reduces investments and returns on investment.
3. Poor health reduces parental investment in children.
4. Poor health reduces social and political stability.

Once established, the cycle of poor health–poverty–economic deprivation becomes difficult to break, in significant part because efforts to break the cycle have focused principally on providing economic aid (and this too frequently in 'tied' form), rather than the creation and provision of health services that could break the cycle at its inception. The relationship between health and poverty is, of course, long established, it being generally well recognized that increased wealth brings, within limits, greater health. This relationship extends both between countries and regions of the world, but also between regions and populations of a given country. Two principles appear to operate. First, the absolute level of wealth, and second, the relative distribution of wealth. As expected, with increased societal wealth, expressed as gross domestic product per capita (GDPc), life expectancy increases: this relationship plateaus above GDPc levels of $10,000–20,000. This relationship is scarcely surprising since wealth generates at both societal and personal levels the infrastructure of education, sanitation, and public health, and transportation that form critical components of a contemporary society. Nonetheless, GDPc is a blunt instrument in assessing national wealth as Paul Krugman has observed in a trenchant comparison of health outcomes, poverty, and living standards between Sweden and the United States. Thus, the second component of the relationship between wealth and health is the distribution of wealth within and between societies: societies that have significant relative differences in wealth have lower life expectancies than societies with a more-egalitarian wealth distribution. This appears to hold regardless of absolute wealth levels. The relationship between income inequality and health has been described by a number of workers and likely has a number of origins. These include the underinvestment by society in health and physical infrastructure in discrete regions, and the fragmentation of psychosocial relationships with increasingly hierarchical social structure.

These observations are of considerable significance to considerations of the future of health care in both the rich and the poor worlds. Clearly, there is the need for a necessary investment to provide the necessary health infrastructure including medicines, hospitals, and public health. However, there is also a significant 'fine tuning' effect on health outcomes that appears to originate from relative wealth distribution within a society. How to ensure both the absolute increases in wealth necessary for health care in the poor world without increasing further the distribution gap is a major issue in an era of galloping globalization and the attendant maldistribution of intellectual property rights.

An additional contributing factor to the infrastructure gap between the rich and the poor worlds is the relative production and availability of scientists, engineers, and health personnel. The United States, Europe, and Japan have some 70 engineers and scientists per 100,000 population: sub- Saharan Africa has less than one. There are, for example, more African engineers and scientists working in the United States than in the entire continent of Africa. Of even greater immediate significance is the equally large disparity in the distribution of health personnel across the rich and poor worlds. The United States has some 300 physicians per 100,000 population, and in excess of 900 nurses; in contrast, Botswana has fewer than 20 physicians and 200 nurses per 100,000 population and Chad is even worse off. These numbers represent significant global problems that, when coupled with the increasing privatization of knowledge, will serve to exacerbate the already dangerous levels of worldwide inequality. Compounding this problem is the ongoing and increasing ability of the rich world to attract scientists, engineers, and health personnel from the poor world. Thus, ca. 50% of the graduate students in the United States and postdoctoral fellows are of nondomestic origin, principally from the so-called 'developing countries'. Similarly, the aggressive recruitment of health personnel, notably nurses and physicians from the poor world, represents a brain drain that impacts immediately the already fragile health-care infrastructure of the poor world. Absent a significant return by these individuals to their country of origin, the net result is a continued impoverishment of the country of origin, and, not coincidentally, a significant benefit to the recipient country which, thus, spared the cost of developing its own adequate scientific and health personnel. These issues of inequality are not, of course new, and were noted admirably by Anatole France (1844–1924) in his famous irony, 'The law in its majestic equality, forbids the rich as well as the poor to sleep under bridges.'

Science and the Social Order

Over half a century ago, Robert Merton defined an ethos of science based on the following values: the free and open exchange of knowledge, an unrestricted pursuit of this knowledge independent of self-interest and an acceptance that science is a product of nature and not of politics, religion, or culture in general. Accordingly, Merton defined four sets of norms that define science: '*universalism*', '*communalism*', '*disinterestedness*', and '*organized skepticism*'. These norms contribute to what may be defined as an 'intellectual commons' of science – a freely generated and freely available pool of 'certified knowledge'. It has been a particular role of universities and similar institutions to contribute to and maintain this commons. However, Merton also recognized that science as an organized social activity interacts with society itself: science and society are thus interdependent entities and the conduct of science is influenced by the imperatives of society.

These norms are, in fact, subject to continual societal challenge. The imposition of 'Aryan' and 'Marxist' dogma are major examples from the 20th century, and the United States remains prominent for efforts to impose fundamentalist religious values on the teaching of biology. Additionally, the norms are challenged from within as the traditional role of the universities is altered through the impact of commercial funding sources and priorities on communalism and disinterestedness.

Intellectual Property and the Commons of Science

Two principal actions in 1980 served to define new boundaries of patentable knowledge and have dramatically impacted both the pharmaceutical sciences and the intellectual commons and are simultaneously serving to redefine the nature of the university. First, the United States Supreme Court decision in Diamond vs. Chakrabarty has enabled the patenting of living things from bacteria to DNA sequences and genes and transgenic animals: in principle, the ruling permits the patenting of human clones, and, in the United States, legislative action will be necessary to ban this. Second, the passage of the Bayh–Dole act permitted universities (and their faculty members) to obtain title to inventions from research supported by Federal funds. This latter action, together with a variety of legislative actions designed to foster university–industrial cooperation, initiated a significant increase in industry-sponsored university research, particularly in the biological and biomedical (life) sciences. In the year 2002, American universities collected ca. $1 billion in royalty income, filed 6500 patents, executed some 3700 licensing deals and created over 400 companies. Universities now own in excess of 5% of U.S. patents, and the majority of this activity has occurred in the life sciences area. The issues of intellectual property policy on the openness of science have been discussed in detail from a general perspective by the Royal Society of London and by the Nuffield Council on Bioethics from the perspective of patents on genes. A recent report from the Federal Trade Commission of the United States appears to recognize that the patent process has become too easy and that, in fact, too many patents are issued: once issued, a patent is extremely expensive to refute.

There are at least three important consequences to this transformation of university research activity in the life sciences:

1. Knowledge that would have entered the science commons is now being patented and available only through licensing mechanisms – exclusive or nonexclusive. We run the very real danger of creating a scientific 'anti-commons' whereby information is not freely available or available only at an unaffordable price. Furthermore, in the life sciences arena, patenting activity has moved increasingly 'upstream' from the chemical composition of the actual drug molecule to the gene sequence of the drug target. Thus, patents have become increasingly enclosing of the scientific commons and can actually restrict rather than advance progress in a field – the very antithesis of the purpose of a patent. This has a dual impact: it prevents new therapies from being developed because they will infringe the gene patent and it prevents the use of genes and gene products as research and diagnostic tools.
2. The poor world is doubly impacted by this. First, the knowledge is locked away and may require unaffordable access. Second, the tools and technologies necessary to develop such knowledge and

obtain the patents are less-available (or unavailable) in the poor world, which thus falls further behind in the knowledge economy. This issue was well recognized by the Commission on Intellectual Property Rights, which advocated that the developing world should accept an international intellectual property system, but one that is crafted and nuanced to the needs of the developing countries and that is modifiable with increasing economic development.

3. Universities may be hoist with their own petard. It has been generally assumed that there is a legitimate 'research and educational' exclusion for the use of patented material. Recent court cases in the United States indicate that this is not so, a reasoning based at least partially on the grounds that universities are avid patent seekers and engaged in commercial activities. If this ruling is upheld, university research will become progressively encumbered by the necessity to navigate financially and intellectually around patents that cover components of ongoing research.

Finally, for universities that are progressively embracing the industrial model of research, the traditional role of 'free and unencumbered inquiry' that has generally been thought to define academic work will be lost if faculty and students are unable to have such intercourse when the academic commons have been enclosed. Furthermore, organizations that choose to impose on themselves restrictions on freedom and openness of inquiry should not be surprised if outside influences, including legislatures, act similarly: universities may, in fact, be 'hoist with their own petard'. We have forgotten the words of Thomas Jefferson who wrote in 1813, 'The exclusive right to invention is given not of natural right, but for the benefit of society.'

Ethical Issues

Although the commercial support of university research is not new, the past decade has seen increasing concern over conflict-of-interest issues, bias in research, and loss of public confidence of the public-interest role of the university. Typical examples include industry sponsors refusing publication of unfavorable research results, research publications that report more-favorably on particular drugs or drug classes when support is provided by industry, conflicts when scientists and clinical investigators have financial ties to the companies whose drugs or protocols they are investigating, and data withholding by investigators to avoid information access. Most recently, a series of conflicts have been reported for senior clinical scientists from the National Institutes of Health some of whom consulted for the very firms over whose drugs they exerted regulatory approval.

Collectively, these ethical problems represent a major challenge to the integrity of the core values of the university and to the biomedical sciences in particular and they further diminish the role of the university as a venue of public intellectualism and public-interest science.

There are several obvious conclusions that may be drawn from this brief survey of current pharmaceutical research. First, the current business model of 'big' pharmaceutical research is broken. It is too expensive and not productive enough. Second, despite the promise of genomics, it is probably true that many of the 'easy' targets – hypertension, hyperacidity etc. – have largely been satisfied. No one doubts that genomics will generate new targets and that it will also generate 'personalized' medicine to make more-effective use of existing medicines and to facilitate the development of new ones. However, these approaches will take time, and a longer time than we had so confidently predicted a decade ago. Third, society needs to see medicines as only one component of total health care.

Many of the disorders for which we use or seek drugs are essentially completely or largely man-made and could be better and more cheaply approached by public health and environmental approaches. Prominent examples here include lung cancer, obesity, and an increasing number of behavioral disorders. Finally, the pharmaceutical industry is an easy target to criticize – it is profitable, arrogant, and its products are indispensable. Nonetheless, many of us, or our family members, may owe our lives to a particular drug: this should not be forgotten. The tragedy is that more than 50% of the world population does not have that choice: that is unacceptable. For the latter population new methods must be found to deliver medicines and health care, since it is quite evident that, in its present form, the market-driven pharmaceutical industry intent on preserving its intellectual property rights has neither the motive nor the intention to do so. Charity is not the answer, since that does not guarantee sustainable relief and it breeds both resentment in the recipient and hubris in the donor.

Ideally perhaps, individual countries would have the scientific ability and the infrastructure to generate their own medicines by cost-effective processes. This is not now possible save for a few countries in the poor world, including Brazil, China, and India. Clearly, the sub-Saharan African countries that are being devastated by AIDS fall completely outside of this possibility. Although the WTO has now agreed on the principle of compulsory licensing to permit import of needed drugs into countries that lack manufacturing infrastructure from countries that are making them under compulsory licensing conditions. Given the reluctance of the rich world to give up these intellectual property rights, it will be of interest to see how well this process will actually work in practice. An alternative for existing drugs, notably AIDS drugs, would be for an organization such as the World Health Organization to 'buy out' the patent holders thus providing the patent holder with a 'market return' and simplifying the issue of drug availability in the poor world. For new drugs - against tropical and parasitic diseases - several possibilities exist accepting that these diseases will not be a major priority of the existing pharmaceutical industry. Such possibilities include efforts by nongovernmental organizations such as the 'Drugs for Neglected Diseases' sponsored by Medecins sans Frontieres, the Global Alliance for TB Development, the Medicines for Malaria Venture, and the Institute for One World Health. These will not be simple ventures to run, and in the meantime millions of significantly avoidable deaths will occur. The rich world can take little comfort from this.

2

STEM AND ARTIFICIAL CELLS

Research on stem cells allows us to get the information about how an organism grows and develops from a single cell and how healthy normal cells replace damaged cells in adult organisms. This promising area of stem cell studies is fascinating scientists to investigate the possibility of cell-based therapies to treat a wide range of diseases, which is referred to as regenerative medicine. Stem cells have two important characteristics that distinguish them from other types of cells. First, they are capable of renewing themselves for long periods through cell division. Second, under some experimental conditions, the cells can be induced to be the functional cells, such as the beating cells of the heart muscle, the albumin-producing cells of the liver, or the insulin-secreting cells of the pancreas. Thus, it is now hypothesized by researchers that stem cells may, in the near future, play a basic role in treating diseases such as heart disease, liver disease, and diabetes. Toward that goal, it is important to understand stem cell biology and its therapeutics. Eventually, control of the growth and differentiation of stem cells will be a big tool in the fields of regenerative medicine, tissue engineering, drug discovery, and toxicity testing.

Although normal human cells are ideal to develop cell therapy, it is unlikely that human cells can be isolated on a scale sufficient to treat many patients. The use of animal cells results in the concerns related to the transmission of infectious pathogens and immunologic and physiologic incompatibilities between the donor and humans. Human embryonic stem cells and bone marrow multipotent adult progenitor cells have receive much attention as a possible source for such cell therapy and drug discovery. It is unlikely that perfect control of differentiation of these multipotent cells will be achieved in very near future. Another attractive cell source is human-derived cell lines. In particular, the use of tightly regulated clonal human cell lines are of value. Such cell lines grow economically in tissue culture and provide the advantage of uniformity, sterility, and freedom of pathogens. Reversible immortalization mediated by Cre/loxP site recombination seems to be the most reliable approach to construct human cells for the clinical setting.

EMBRYONIC STEM CELLS

Embryonic stem cells have become a very important source for basic research and possible clinical applications since more than 20 years ago when the establishment of mouse embryonic stem cells (ES cells) was achieved by Evans and Kaufman and Martin. They established the pluripotent cells from the inner cell mass of the blastocyst, mouse ES cells, and developed the culture conditions for the cells *in vitro*. The achievement evolved the studies on teratocarcinomas, tumors that arise in the gonads of several inbred strains and consist of an array of somatic tissues juxtaposed together in a disorganized fashion, and gave the origins of the concept of embryonal carcinoma (EC). As teratocarcinomas could also induced by grafting the blastocyst to ectopic sites, it was likely that pluripotent cell lines could be derived directly from the blastocyst. As expected, a stable diploid cell line that could differentiate into all embryonic cell types was established and formed functional germ cells after transplantation into chimeric mice. Testicular teratocarcinomas occur spontaneously in humans, and pluripotent cell lines were derived from the teratocarcinomas. In 1998, human ES cell lines were established from pre-implanted embryos by Thomson et al. Frozen human embryos that were produced by *in vitro* fertilization at an early stage were thawed and cultured to the blastocyst stage. Fourteen inner cell masses were isolated, and five ES cell lines were established. During the first 8 months of culture, no period of replicative crisis was observed in any cell lines. The principal characteristics of the established cells were that the cells expressed high levels of telomerase activity, which suggests that their life span exceeds that of somatic cells. These cells also expressed surface markers that are typical of human embryonic carcinoma cells, such stage-specific embryonic antigen (SSEA)-3, SSEA-4, TRA-1-60, TRA-1-81, and alkaline phosphatase. The cells also expressed the Transcription Factor Octamer binding protein 4 (Oct-4) to undergo somatic differentiation. ES cells could be used for many different purposes, including early development research, toxicology and drug screening, and gene and protein screening. One of the most important uses is for regenerative medicine and cell therapy, which involves the transplantation of healthy, functional, and propagating cells to restore the viability or function of deficient tissues and organs. The availability of reliable cells is essential for the toxicology and drug discovery process. The primary cells, immortalized cells, and genetically modified cells have been used for drug discovery; however, the inconsistent availability of the primary cells and the genetic abnormalities of transformed cells are the current problems with such application. ES cells could offer considerable advantages due to their plasticity, proliferative capacity, and the ability to undergo homologous recombination at relatively high frequency. In conclusion, ES cells may offer several important advantages in the field of basic biology, drug dis covery, and the future cell therapies in various human diseases.

Properties of Embryonic Stem Cells

Pluripotency

Mouse ES cells. Culturing mouse ES cells from the inner cell mass of the preimplanted blastocyst were first reported more than 20 years ago. To date only three species of mammals have yielded long-term cultures of self-renewing ES cells: mice, monkeys, and humans. Mouse ES cells lines have shown an unlimited capacity of proliferation and ability to contribute to all cell lineages, which are defined as pluripotency to all definitive tissues: ectoderm, mesoderm, and endoderm. Leukemia inhibitory factor (LIF), a cytokine belonging to the IL-6 family, has been identified as an exogenous signal to maintain ES self-renewal. LIF was initially identified by its activity to induce differentiation of M1 leukemia cells, whereas it mediates the opposite cellular responses in ES cells. The signal transduction of LIF consists in the LIF-specific receptor subunit LIFRβ and the common signal transducer gp130, which is shared between the members of the IL-6 cytokine family; the gp130 signaling regulates several cell functions through signal transduction and activation of transcription factor STAT3 that may interact and affect the function of common target genes. Cytokines, including IL-6, IL-11, oncostatin M, ciliary neurotrophic factor, and cardiotrophin-1, show similar properties maintaining the pluripotency of mES cells. A coculture of mouse ES cells on an inactivated mouse embryonic fibroblast layer is also required to maintain the undifferentiated stage. Thus, production of some critical factors of the fibroblast layer is required either to promote self-renewal of mouse ES cells or to suppress their differentiation. The activation of STAT3 is essential to the LIF signaling pathway, but it plays an accessory role to maintain ES cell identity. Moreover, there are two major pathways of intracellular signal transduction downstream of gp130; the Jak-Stat pathway and the Shp2-Erk pathway. As Jak and Shp2 interact with separate subdomains of the intracellular domain of gp-130, it has been demonstrated that the activation of Jak but not Shp2 is sufficient to preserve an undifferentiated status of mouse ES cells. The finding means that the LIF signal is mainly transmitted to the nuclei by the Jak-STAT signal pathway and the Shp2-Erk pathway does not contribute directly to stem cell renewal as demonstrated when adding Erk kinase inhibitor PD98059 in the medium resulting in self-renewal. Although STAT3 acts as a transcription factor to activate target genes, there is only one gene whose specific function in pluripotent cell population is confirmed, that is, the POU-family transcription factor octamer-3/4 (Oct-3/4) encoded by Pou5f1. The essential role of Oct-3/4 in mouse development has been revealed by targeting gene deletion. Oct-3/4-deficient embryos fail to initiate fetal development because the prospective founder cells of the ICM do not require pluripotency and become diverted into the trophoectoderm lineage, which indicates that Oct-3/4 is essential to establish a pluripotent cell population in preimplantation development. ES cells require a critical level of Oct-3/4 to maintain stem cell renewal, and at least a twofold increase in the expression of Oct-3/4 causes differentiation of mouse ES cells into the endoderm and mesoderm, whereas reduction to less than 50% of the normal expression level of Oct-3/4 triggers de-differentiation of mouse ES cells into the trophectoderm. Recently identification of the homeodomain protein Nanog as another key regulator of pluripotentiality has opened another door of the complicated system of pluripotency; the dosage of Nanog is a critical determinant of cytokine-independent colony formation, and the forced expression of this protein confers constitutive self-renewal in ES cells without gp-130 stimulation; Nanog may act to restrict the differentiation-inducing potential of Oct-3/4. Other investigators have reported that the induction of the expression of Inhibitor of differentiation (Id) by addition of TGF-β1/bone morphogenetic protein (BMP) in combination with LIF sustains self-renewal via the Smad pathway. Recent studies have implicated the importance of Wnt-signaling pathways in the maintenance of ES cell pluripotency. Components of the β catenin Wnt-signaling pathway are expressed in ES cells, and it is likely that activation of the Wnt-signaling pathway using a glycogen synthase kinase (GSK)-3-specific inhibitor (BIO) that maintains the pluripotent state of human ES and mouse ES cells.

The pluripotency of ES cells depends on the balance of various signaling molecules, and thus, such imbalance causes differentiation of ES cells. Many other molecules, such as Genesis, Rex-1, Sox2, GBX2, and UTF1, have been identified with a potential role in defining pluripotency.

Human ES cells

The murine models of isolation, derivation, culture, and characterization in ES cells have provided valuable information to the generation of human ES (hES) cell lines derived from the embryos at the preimplantation stage, which involves culturing embryos to the morula or blastocyst stage. These embryos are donated for research to establish hES cell lines. Thomson et al. isolated from the ICM of human blastocysts, placed on inactivated murine feeder cells, and successfully performed initial derivations of hES cell lines. Since that time, many laboratories have applied the same techniques to derivate hES cell lines. hES cells have been currently characterized by a set of markers and their differentiation capacity. These criteria include the expression of several surface markers and transcription factors that associated with an undifferentiated state. In addition, maintenance of extended proliferating capacity, pluripotency, and normal euploid karyotype without marked change in the epigenetic status of hES cells is a crucial issue for the future use of the cells in clinical trials. Several surface markers have been identified to characterize hES cells, in which glycolipids and glycoproteins, such as SSEA-4, TRA-1-60, and TRA-1-81, that are expressed in human embryocarcinoma cells are present in hES cells. Some surface antigens initially described in other stem cells are AC133, CD-9, CD-117, and CD-135, which are also expressed in hES cells. The stability of the expression of these surface markers in hES cells after culture for prolonged periods of time has been maintained.

Several critical transcription factors that play a critical role in maintaining self-renewal of stem cells have now been identified, and these analyses are also useful for characterization of hES cells.

One of these transcriptional factors is Oct-3/4, and several Oct-3/4-targeting genes have been identified in hES cells, which are Utf-1, Rex-1, PDGFαR, Otx-2, Lefty-1, and Nanog. However, their specific roles have not been identified, and their expression has been retained in hES cells for over a year in culture. Additionally, all hES cell lines express high levels of telomerase, an enzyme that helps to maintain telomeres that protect the end of the chromosomes. Telomerase activity and long telomeres are characteristics of proliferating cells in embryonic tissue and germ cells. As cells divide and differentiate throughout the life span of an organism or cell line, the telomeres become progressively shortened and lose the ability to maintain their length. The functions of telomeres and telomerase seem to be important in the cell division, normal development, and aging [26]. Mouse ES cells have shown to require activation of the gp-130/STAT3 pathway to maintain the cells in the undifferentiated stage. This activation is generally achieved by the addition of LIF to the culture medium. In contrast, it has been demonstrated that the addition of exogenous LIF to hES cell culture does not maintain the pluripotent capacity of hES cells. However, common intracellular signaling pathways exist between mES cells and hES cells to regulate self-renewal and to maintain an undifferentiated state. These signaling pathways have not yet been clarified, although transcriptional profiling or gene expression technology has identified several genes, transcription factors, ligand/receptor pairs, and secreted inhibitors of signaling pathways. hES cells can be maintained in several different conditions by the use of growth factors belonging to the TGF-β1/BMP superfamily, fibroblast growth factor (FGF) family, and Wnt family.

Previous studies have demonstrated that prolonged propagation of undifferentiated hES cells requires culture of the cells on embryonic fibroblast feeder layers. The use of bFGF has become a common thread in the culture medium formulas, which have been recently developed by using feeder-free conditions. hES cells can be maintained in serum replacement-containing medium that has been supplemented with 36–40 ng/mL of bFGF, in which culture condition the cells can retain the expression of surface markers, transcription factors, normal karyotype, telomerase activity, and pluripotency of hES cells conventionally cultured on embryonic fibroblast feeder layers. The mechanism of bFGF activity in hES cell culture remains unclear, but it has been demonstrated that treatment with 40–100 ng/mL of bFGF inhibits BMP signaling in hES cells. A further role of bFGF in hES cells to maintain pluripotentiality is activation of the phosphatidylinositol 3-kinase (P13K/Akt, PKB) pathway, which subsequently enhances the expression of extracellular matrix molecules (ECMs). Removal of bFGF in hES cell culture or the treatment of the cells with chemical inhibitors of the PKB pathway results in down-regulation of the expression of hES cell markers as well as a decrease in ECM components.

Differentiation

Pluripotency is one of the defining features of ES cells. The most definitive test of pluripotency of the cells is the formation of chimeras in mice in which the mES cells are injected into the blastocyst. The approach cannot be applied to assess pluripotency of hES cells, therefore, and teratoma formation after injection of embryonic bodies (EBs) of hES cells *in vitro* into immunocompromised mice is currently used to validate the pluripotency of the established hES cell lines in culture. In the case of mES cells, once differentiation of ES cells has started, the cells representing the primary germ layers spontaneously develop *in vitro* in the absence of LIF. The culture conditions to form EBs include hanging drops, suspension mass culture, or the use of methylcellulose. Initially, an outer layer of endoderm-like cells forms within ESs, followed by the development of an ectodermal layer and subsequent specification of mesodermal cells over a period of a few days. The generation of specific functional cell types from hES cells has been demonstrated both *in vitro* and *in vivo*. In fact, with the rapid interest in gene targeting for the development of genetically modified mice, most of the efforts directed toward ES cells have been made in the maintenance of ES cells in an undifferentiated state. Although research on *in vitro* differentiation of ES cells has been limited. investigators have demonstrated differentiation protocols, which assess the differentiated cells via expression analysis of cell-specific markers. However, very few markers are specific for one cell type, and for that reason, panels of markers must be used in these experiments. Understanding of cellular differentiation during embryogenesis has led to methods for enriching populations of specific cell types: First, genetic manipulation of ES cells facilitates differentiation and serves as a framework for genetic engineering of ES cells by key transcription factors to regulate their cell fate. Second, culture conditions supplemented with established growth factors can be used. Several samples of clinically and pharmacologically relevancy have been proposed, including almost any kind of cells, such as chondrocytes, atrial and ventricular cardiomyocytes, hepatocytes, pancreatic islet cells, and motor neurons. Third, coculture conditions have been reported to facilitate and produce differentiated cells. Fourth, ectopic implantation of ES cells into syngenic or immune-compromised mice produces specific cell types. Although such transplantation is a powerful approach, this is not a practical method for deriving cells to be evaluated in clinical experiment. Currently the desired cells cannot be developed on a stable large scale. Inductive differentiation protocols have generated many cell types to further enrich *in vitro* differentiated populations by the use of selective methods that are based on the expression of specific marker proteins. Such selective protocols can include promoter-based recovering strategies, based on GFP-dependent cell sorting, or antibiotic selection, and have allowed the enrichment of increasingly defined phenotypes from ES cells. Cell sorters have been applied to enrich the populations by using specific cell surface markers of ES cell derivatives.

Investigators have used the forced gene expression to influence *in vitro* differentiation of ES cells. For example, constitutive overexpression of murine *Pax 4* in ES cells combined with an inductive protocol has resulted in an enrichment of nestin-positive progenitors and insulin-producing cells among other cells found in pancreatic islets. Finally, the next step in developing clinical trials and drug discovery is the use of internal bioimplants using bioactive materials that provide biological signals at the site of damaged tissues *in vivo*. This next generation of implantable bioartificial devices can permit the evaluation of the potential of ES cell derivatives *in vivo* without having direct contact with the blood circulation. Such an approach allows researchers to avoid a risk of tumor formation of ES cell derivatives and to examine the fate of such cells in an isolation manner from the body.

Endodermal differentiation. The pancreas and liver are the derivatives of the definitive endoderm; hepatic and pancreatic cells are of special therapeutic interest for the treatment of diabetes mellitus and hepatic failure. Theoretically, both cells can be generated from ES cells. Researchers have demonstrated different strategies *in vitro* to differentiated mES cells in hepatocyte-like cells; these cells have shown specific transcription factors and proteins of normal hepatocytes; they also have been shown the presence of the two lineages of the liver cells, bile duct epithelial cells and oval cells. Once the cells are transplanted, these cells can integrate into the hepatic parenchyma and function in the host liver. It has been previously demonstrated that ES cells can differentiate into hepatocyte-like cells through *in vivo* differentiation of mES cells in the damaged host liver and subsequent recovery of mES cell-derived hepatocytes by the use of an albumin-promoter-derived GFP expression system. Briefly, mES cells in which an albumin-promoter-derived GFP expression cassette was externally introduced were injected into the spleen of the hepatic-injured mice and tumors were developed after 3 weeks. Examination of the tumors showed the presence of hepatocytes derived from mES cells. These hepatocytes were positive for hepatic markers for at least 3 weeks and were capable of proliferating. The cells were highly characterized by revealing correspondence in 98% of gene expression profiles compared with primary mouse hepatocytes. It is known that the formation of EBs itself can raise the cell population expressing hepatocyte phenotype, but such a population in EBs is estimated to be considerably small. Differentiation and isolation of hepatocyte-like cells from hES cells has been demonstrated by using hES cells that are stably transfected with the reporter gene of GFP fused to an albumin-promoter. The generation of ES-derived insulin-producing cells may represent a critical cell source for the treatment of diabetes. In this field, ES cells hold a great hope as a source of β-cells, but unfortunately this has proven to be more complicated than expected. Both mouse and human ES cells can be manipulated to contain insulin and even to regulate insulin secretion. Several methods have been used to obtain enriched populations by the stable transfection with a cDNA construct containing a neomycin-resistance gene under the control of the insulin or Nkx6.1 promoter, by the selection with nestin-positive cells, or induction of critical transcription factors, such as pax4 and pdx-1. Although these reports have encouraged that ES cells can generate cells containing insulin and pancreatic β-cell markers, a recent report has demonstrated that insulin-positivity of ES cell derivatives was considerable due to insulin uptake from culture media by apoptotic cells. Measurement of C-peptide, which is excised from proinsulin in the process of maturation of insulin, has been strongly recommended when demonstrating differentiation of ES cells to pancreatic beta cells. Differentiation protocols have to clarify that ES cells are directed to definitive endoderm, not to visceral endoderm, which has similar markers of gene expression but different pathways from pancreatic beta cell lineage. According to the latest research, the differentiation ratio of insulin-positive cells from ES cell populations is about 2.7% compared with less than 1% in undifferentiated controls.

Ectodermal differentiation. Epithelial cell differentiation from ES cells has been identified by the presence of cytokeratines and specific keratinocyte markers. Enrichment of keratinocytes *in vitro* from ES cells has been achieved by seeding the cells on various extracellular matrices in the presence of bone morphoprotein (BMP-4) and/or ascorbate; such protocols promote the formation of epidermal equivalents. It has been reported that the resulting tissue displays patterns similar to the embryonic skin. The cells express the late differentiation markers of fibroblasts, which suggests that ES cells have the capacity to reconstitute fully differentiated skin *in vitro*. Researchers have reported a differentiation capacity of ES cells into neurons and glial cells. The neural differentiation ratios have significantly improved by the introduction of numerous strategies, including lineage selections (dopaminergic, serotonergic, or γ-aminobutyric acid (GABA)-ergic neurons), astrocytes, oligodendrocytes, glutamatergic and cholinergic neurons, and growth factors. The possibility of producing dopaminergic neurons from ES cells has been demonstrated by the use of both fibroblast growth factor 8 (FGF8) and sonic hedgehog, which were implicated as tandem initiators of dopaminergic neurogenesis. Later, the enrichment of dopaminergic neurons has been acheived by mimicking the oxygen tension of the developing midbrain.

When such cells were implanted into 6-OHDA-lesioned rats, where nigrostrial dopaminergics afferents are largely lost, the brain function restored normalcy to the dopamine-depleted animals. Similar results were observed in animal experiments by the transplantation of monkey ES cell-derived dopaminergic neurons into 1-methyl-4-phenyl-1,2,3,6-tetrahydropyridine (MPTP)-lesioned adult cymolgus monkeys, in which treatment-associated behavioral improvement was noted by 10 weeks after transplantation. In general, proliferation of neural precursor cells is induced by the addition of FGF and epidermal growth factor (EGF) into the culture medium. Thereafter, neural differentiation can be facilitated by the addition of neural differentiation factors, such as glial cell line-derived neurotrophic factors (GDNFs), neurturin (NT), TGF-β3, and IL-1β. Although the ability of hES cells to generate derivatives of the neural ephitelium has been demonstrated, the selective derivation of neuron subtypes has been difficult to achieve until now. Therefore, long-term survival of the grafted cells has not been successful in experimental models, and a potential risk of teratoma formation by undifferentiated cell populations after implantation should be carefully studied before any therapeutic clinical trials can be considered.

Mesodermal differentiation. The mesodermal germ layer has the capacity to differentiate into muscle, bone, cartilage, blood, and connective tissues. ES cells also have been successfully used to reconstitute mesodermal developmetal processes *in vitro* by generating several mesodermal cell types, such as adipogenic cells, chondrogenic cells, osteoblasts, and myogenic cells. One of the mostly studied cell lineages in ES cells is cardiomyocytes. Similar to other differentiation protocols, the generation of cardiomyocytes from ES cells requires an initial aggregation step to form EBs. Within EBs, cardiomyocytes are located between an epithelial layer and a basal layer of mesenchymal cells. Cardiomyocytes are easy to identify *in vitro*, because they spontaneously contract after 3–4 days of culture. The number of spontaneously beating cells can be increased by adding differentiation-inducing factors, such as dimethyl sulfoxide (DMSO), retinoic acid, Dynorphin B, and cardiogenol derivatives. Developmental changes of cardiomyocytes can be correlated with the length of time in culture and divided into three stages: early (pacemaker-like cells), intermediate, and terminal (atrail-, ventricular-, nodal-, His-, and purkinje-like cells). hES cell-derived cardiomyocytes have showed the expected molecular, structural, electrophysiologic, and contractile properties of nascent embryonic myocardium. hES cell-derived cardiomyocytes differ from those of mouse in an important and potencially exploitable capacity, that is, proliferation. In contrast to the limited proliferation of mouse ES cell-derived cardiomyocytes, human ES cell-derived cardiomyocytes show sustained cell cycle activity both *in vitro* and *in vivo* (in the heart of the nude rats). *In vivo* studies with hES cell-derived cardiomyocytes have increased lately and suggested that hES cell-resulting cardiomyocytes engraft and integrate into the host myocardium in experimental immunosuppressed animals. These data represent an exciting proof-of-concept evidence for the potential application of hES cell-derived cardiomyocytes in the formation of biological pacemakers. Several important challenges include long-term follow-up of the grafts to confirm whether such cells maintain their pace-making ability over time and development of efficient protocols for large-scale production of highly purified cells without any risks of teratoma formation of the cells *in vivo*.

Hematopoietic cells and blood vessels are believed to arise from common progenitor cells, hemangioblasts. Cystic EBs increase the generation of blood islands containing erythrocytes and macrophages, and differentiation of the cells on semi-solid medium is efficient for the formation of neutrophils, mast cells, macrophages, and erythrocytes. Application of fetal calf serum (FCS), cytokines such as IL-1 and IL-3, or granulocyte–macrophage colony stimulating factor (GM–CSF) in ES cell culture generates early hematopoietic precursor cells expressing both embryonic z globin (βH1) and adult β major globin RNAs. Experiments to identify potential inducers of the hematopoietic lineage indicate that Wnt3 is one of the most important signaling molecules that play a significant role in enhancing hematopoietic commitment during *in vitro* differentiation of ES cells.

Use and Applications of ES Cells

One of the uses of mES cells is the development of genetically modified mice. Researchers have conducted genetic modifications in mES cells to generate genetically modified mice to evaluate specific functions of the targeted genes. These engineered mice have selectively inactivated specific genes to evaluate their target functions and toxicity. This technology can be applied to *in vivo* assays to test for clinical conditions of the central nervous system, cardiovascular diseases, tumors, and metabolic changes in muscle, fat, and bone. The approach has become a crucial method for the utility of different targets in toxicology. Another significant use of ES cells is achieved by a homologous recombination that allows the preplanned replacement of mutations in endogenous murine alleles. Base changes allow an inactivation of specific domains or an alteration of binding sites of a specific protein. For example, single-base changes allow the expression of conserved human mutations. An allelic variant in presenilin 1 is associated with early onset of Alzheimer's disease.

Undifferentiated ES cells

The use of undifferentiated ES cells has been rapidly facilitated to gain functional information and to generate and evaluate knockout mice. An example was the development and evaluation of a nuclear factor-κβ precursor p105 in ES cells. The genetically modified ES cells had specific deletions in the C-terminal region of the p105 gene. These cells demonstrated that p105 was important in the control of NF-κβ-binding activity, detailing the role of NF-κβ in inflammatory responses. Researchers have also used ES cells deficient in specific genes in the undifferentiated state to evaluate the gene function in the cell development *in vitro*.

Differentiated ES cells

Researchers have demonstrated that cells derived from ES cells *in vitro* reflect the cellular physiology of relevant to primary cells. Gene inactivation has been applied to study events in signaling pathways that could be relevant in specific cell types. For example, there is the role of mitogen-activated protein kinase kinase-1 (MEKK1) in a cellular model of postischemic reperfusion injury using ES cell-derived cardiomyocytes. This approach clearly allows time- and cost-saving evaluation of target genes. In addition, results from knockout cells derived from ES cells can provide clues as to the developmental cause of embryonic lethality.

Teratoma formation has been used to evaluate the role of target gene expression on the cell proliferation and differentiation of the resulting tumor formation. This kind of strategy was applied to demonstrate a reduced proliferative capacity of ES cells null for cyclooxygenase 2 compared with cyclooxygenase 1-deficient or wild-type ES cells. The strategy can be used to evaluate the role of potential cancer-inducing targets on cell proliferation. Reproductive toxicity is a target where ES cells could be applied to *in vitro* teratology assays. Such a procedure could reduce the use of animal procedures. It has been reported that 78% of correlation exists between the data of *in vivo* and *in vitro* experiments using ES cells as an alternative to animal testing in teratology and embryo-toxicity testing. The aim is to overcome the limitation of availability of primary cells or the genetic abnormality of immortalized cell lines. Generation of specific cell and tissue types is necessary rather than heterogeneous populations that can result from spontaneous differentiation of ES cells. For this reason, ES cell lines expressing GFP selectively in the specific differentiation to cardiomyocytes or hepatocytes have been designed [84]. Finally, therapeutic concepts of ES cells must be well argued. Some difficulties can be identified in the application of adult stem cells or embryonic stem cells, in order to develop stem cell-replacement therapy. We need to meticulously select the best candidates of cells in terms of the facilities to propagate, manipulate, and select the most purified population of the desired cell type. We need to produce immune tolerance when allogenic cells are used for stem cell-based cell therapy. In addition, ES cells bring certain advantages against the rest of stem cells.

Firstly, adult stem cells are difficult to isolate and hard to propagate in culture; in contrast, ES cells are derived easily once an embryo has been obtained and they can grow indefinitely in culture. ES cells can be manipulated genetically by homologous recombination to correct a genetic defect. On the other hand, adult stem cells can be genetically manipulated only by the introduction of retroviral gene delivery, which overexpress the transduced genes and could happen in an insertional mutagenesis. ES cells have the capacity to differentiate into any kind of tissue of the body, that is, pluripotent, but adult stem cells are multipotent and their differentiation capacity seems to be restricted. Protocols must be well developed in ES cells to generate an enrichment population of cells of a specific lineage or cell type. Furthermore, if therapeutic application is the final goal of ES cells, culturing techniques need to be scaled up for mass production of clinically relevant quantities of the specified cells. Finally, immunological barriers must be overcome. Regarding this issue some promising alternatives have been suggested lately. Nuclear transplantation denotes the introduction of a nucleus from an adult donor cell into an enucleated oocyte to generate a cloned embryo. When transferred to the uterus of a female, this embryo has the potential to become an infant that is a clone of the adult donor cell; this process is referred as to "*reproductive cloning*". When explanted in culture, this embryo can give rise to ES cells that have the potential to become almost any type of cells present in the adult body. The resulting ES cells by nuclear transfer are genetically identical to the donor and thus potentially useful for therapeutic applications; this process is called "*therapeutic cloning*". Therapeutic cloning may substantially improve the treatment for neurodegenerative diseases, blood disorders, or diabetes, because the therapy for such diseases is currently limited by the availability or immunocompatibility of tissue transplants. Indeed, experiments in animals have shown that nuclear cloning combined with gene and cell therapy represents a valid strategy for treating genetic disorders.

Considerable progress has been made toward the generation of more defined culture conditions of ES cells since the initial isolation and growth conditions were described. There have been many modifications of the procedures, including growth of ES cells, differentiation potential, and cell lines establishment. The availability of hES cells represents an extraordinary opportunity for cell transplantation that may be applicable to humans in the future. Despite exciting advantages and advances in the field of hES cell research, many challenges have to be addressed in the near future. The culture conditions have to improved and be humanized. The cells cultured in xenogeneic conditions are likely to be considered and regulated. Concerns about the infection from nonhuman pathogens are the most discussed issues for the clinical application. Although ES cells offer great promise for regenerative medicine, the near-term applications could be in drug discovery. Researchers might have a store of stem cells lines derived from many human populations from different ethnicities and gene variations. These cells can be of extreme importance in the development of effective and safe therapeutics.

Adult Somatic Stem Cells or Postnatal Stem Cells

In the past few decades, a true revolution has been occurring in a spectacular way in the field of medicine and biology. Regenerative medicine with the intention of tissue regeneration, and thus the curative treatment of diseases, has awoken maximum interest from scientific communities all over the world. The likelihood that the human body contains the cells capable of regenerating and repairing the damaged or disease tissues has turned from an implausible subject to a virtual belief. It has been well known that stem cells with differentiating potential to replenish progeny are present in postnatal tissues of mammals. Recently many studies have demonstrated the abilities of stem cells to form multiple types of cells and the presence of such cells in an increasing number of tissues. We attempt here to provide an overview of adult stem cells in terms of possible mechanisms of their differentiation and their potential in therapeutic use. The presence of adult somatic stem cell or cell progenitor has been clearly identified in several tissues. It has primarily been easily identified in tissues with high cell replication. These cells contribute to repair and regeneration throughout the life span in adult tissues, which also have the capacity of cell renewal. Recently, the concept of stem cell niches was proposed, in which stem cells exist in small numbers in silence under normal conditions but become activated after tissue injury or other pathological conditions. Some stem cells possess enormous plasticity to differentiate into any cell types derived from the germinal layers (mesoderm, ectoderm, and endoderm). In contrast, other stem cells can only terminally differentiate into the same germinal layer from which they originated. Several factors, which are not clearly understood, are involved in the regulation of stem cells in terms of their potential of differentiation, tissue repair, and regeneration. On the other hand, the tragedy includes the development and progression of malignancy due to their longevity with respect to the body life span and their ability to give rise to multiple cell phenotypes. Based on the nature of stem cells, there is a worldwide interest in stem cell research to understand the natural growth and senescence of the cells and to balance tissue repair and regeneration through the life span.

Studies on the mechanism that controls the maintenance of stem cells and differentiation signals is useful to understand how external (toxins, radiation, etc.) and internal injuries (cytogenetic alterations, mutation, etc.) potentially modify the fate of stem cells and eventually lead them to malignant transformation. Stem cells can withstand over stressful environmental events associated with tissue damage after surgical procedures, exposure to toxics agents, and extreme cold and then repopulate and repair adult tissues. Although such *in vivo* environments seem to be transient and hostile against host cells and mature cells are easily destroyed, stem cells can survive, differentiate, and regenerate the tissue. Their differentiation capacities investigated under a variable controlled environment may allow us a window into the regenerative process of adult tissues. To facilitate stem cell research, *in vitro* culture should mimic native niches of stem cells *in vivo* by application of matrices, growth factors, and drug delivery systems.

General Concepts of Stem Cells

The name *stem cells* is commonly used to refer the cells that are relatively undifferentiated while retaining the ability to divide and proliferate throughout postnatal life, providing progenitor cells that can differentiate into tissue-specific cells. The ability of stem or progenitor cells to give rise to different populations of terminally differentiated cells is referred to as plasticity. Thus, their potential is called totipotent, pluripotent, or multipotent. The term *totipotent* should be strictly reserved for the unique stem cells that can form embryonic and extra-embryonic membranes, which are the most primitive about 4 days after fecundation. The term *pluripotent* is used to refer to the stem cells' ability to form all cell types of the proper embryo, except for the extra-embryonic membranes and their tissues. In contrast, the term *multipotent* is used to name those that give rise to a subset of cell lineages. During the development process, the totipotent stem cells originate and pluripotent stem cells come out of the germ layers. Afterward multipotent stem cells are generated. These cells, in turn, form the oligopotent progenitor cells in the developing organs. Moreover, intestinal progenitor cells are considered to be quadripotent; they can form progeny that become mucous, absorptive, neuroendocrine, or Paneth cells. In the case of bronchiallining cells, the progenitors are tripotent: Progenyturninto neuroendocrine, mucous, or ciliated cells. The oval cells of the liver are bipotent; they can derivate into duct cells and hepatocytes. Other type of cells, such as epidermal progenitors, are unipotent to produce only a single progeny.

Tissue homeostasis and stem cell renewal

Physiological tissue renewal is accomplished by a delicate balance among specialized cells, young progeny, and their tissue-specific stem cells. They perpetually renew, which is evident in many tissues, such as, blood, skin, gastrointestinal tract, respiratory tract, and testis. In contrast, other tissues, including cardiac and neural tissues, seem to have a limited response under regenerative circumstances. Thus, it was considered that cardiac and neural tissues had no regenerative capacities. Asynchronous division is a typical *in vivo* pattern of stem cells; it is defined by the division of one stem cell to give rise to one daughter cell that remains as a stem cell while another undergoes the process of differentiation. The transiently amplifying cells provide an expanded population that differentiates into more mature cells, which can no longer proliferate and eventually die. Such phenomenon is observed in most tissues, however, others, such as the liver and pancreas, are mainly driven by replication of mature cells rather than stem cell division and differentiation under normal conditions. Occasionally, in those tissues under toxic DNA-damage conditions when replication of mature cells is compromised, facultative stem cells accomplish the tissue regeneration.

Stem cells and their niches

The microenvironment or the stem cell niche tightly regulates the behavior of the cells. A combination of cells and extracellular matrix components, soluble factors delivered to the tissue from the vasculature, and the growth factors produced by the cells govern all aspects of the behavior of stem cells. For example, in the intestinal mucosa, the pericryptal myofibroblasts that surround the crypts may serve as niche cells, whereas in the hair follicles, the region just below the sebaceous glands seems to be a stem cell niche. The niches themselves control many dynamic facets of the stem cells, intrinsically regulating the internal signaling, synthesis of structural and metabolic proteins, their mitotic activities, axes, and growth pattern. These events certainly play a pivotal role in leading intrinsic and extrinsic factors that will define the physiological function of stem cells or the first step in the pathological transformation of stem cells in carcinogenesis.

General Classification of Stem Cells

Because adult somatic stem cells consist of a different population of the cells that share some common characteristics, it is difficult to rigorously divide the cells into some classi fications. A new theory has currently proposed that stem cells are generated from a single cell source. Thus, we review here adult stem cells according to the commonest classification as follows:

1. Hematopoietic stem cells (HSCs)
2. Mesenchymal stem cells (MSCs)
3. Multipotent adult progenitor cells (MAPCs) isolated by fluorescent-activated cell sorting (FACS) from the bone marrow
4. Side-population phenotype cells (SPs)
5. Tissue-specific cell progenitors (TSCPs)
6. Umbilical cord blood-derived stem cells (UCBDSs)

Bone marrow stem cells

The bone marrow has been considered to provide an adequate microenvironment for stem cells to survive forever. Stem cells in the bone marrow can migrate into blood vessels, circulate around the body, and return home when needed. A long time ago, only a few stem cells were recognized in humans and they were thought to be a restricted population with a limited potential to differentiate in a single organ system. Such reasoning was examined through the study of bone marrow, which contains a wide range of cell populations. The complex constitution of bone marrow also attracted the interest of scientists. Such investigations changed the original thought to a new one, which implies that stem cells also have the ability to give rise to the cells of other tissue types as well as to the cells of the original, referred to as the "plasticity of stem cells." Bone marrow has been described to contain at least two different types of stem cells. One type includes HSCs, which produce the entire progeny of blood cells of the body, and the other includes MSCs, which are a promising source for tissue repair. It is also believed that another population exists, called MAPCs, which could be generated from the adult bone marrow of several species, and can differentiate into multiple cell types *in vitro*.

General Characteristics of Stem Cells

Stem cells possess a wide range of different characteristics, which have made them an attractive cell source for cell biology, ontogeny, toxicological studies, and cell therapy. Several types of stem cells have been reported, and each possesses particular characteristics that determine their potential.

Hematopoietic Stem Cells (HSCs)

Characteristics

For the past three decades, HSCs have been considered important cells. In 1963, the origin of hematopoietic cells was first reported. One of the main characteristics of HSCs is the capacity to give rise to intermediate precursor or progenitor cell populations that partially differentiate and commit to various types of blood cell lineages. HSCs need to possess the hallmark properties to equilibrate cell self-renewal, whereas the cells quickly generate progenitors as a workforce as well as additional stem cells without depleting the reserves. Therefore, HSCs need to be multipotent; that is, a single HSC can produce several different lineages of mature blood cells and proliferate to yield a broad number of mature progeny. HSCs in the bone marrow of the mice are a rare population with a frequency of 1 in 10,000 to 100,000 of total blood cells, and the cells may be even less in humans. HSCs are thought to be relatively in-active in the adult hematopoietic system, with 1–3% in the progression of the cell cycle and approximately 90% in the cell cycle G0. The cells divide only a few or not at all until they are required to differentiate. Abnormal clonal expansion of HSCs may result in chronic myelogenous leukemia, polycythemia vera, and myelodysplastic syndromes. HSCs are believed to have the ability to live for a long period of time, probably a lifetime in the recipient after bone marrow transplantation. In fact, HSCs require the bone marrow microenvironment, which regulates their migration, proliferation, and differentiation, to maintain active hematopoiesis throughout their lifetime.

Isolation and phenotypic characteristics of HSCs

Recent experiments have demonstrated that HSCs in bone marrow from many different species can be purified by FACS as SP cells. In 1994, multipotent cells committed to the hematopoietic lineage in mouse according to their different array of cell-surface markers were isolated. This cells were described as KTLS c-kit$^+$ (K), Thy-1.1^{low} (a marker on stem cells) (T), Lin$^{-/low}$ (Lineage-marker) (L), and Sca-1$^+$ (Stem cell antigen-1) (S). The cells showed >80% for hematopoietic multilineage differentiation and represented only 1/2000 cells in the bone marrow. HSCs were proposed to be divided into three compartments based on both the expression of the surface markers and their self-renewal ability.

1. Long-term HSCs (LT–HSCs): LT–HSCs habitually reside in the bone marrow and have for all intents and purposes six developmental alternatives: remain quiescent, differentiate, self-renew, migrate, enter senescence, or undergo programmed cell death. The cells represent only 0.007% of cells in the bone marrow. In young adult mice, approximately 8% of LT–HSCs arbitrarily enters into cell division per day, and half of their progeny are LT–HSCs to maintain the level of steady state. LT–HSCs perform self-renewal perpetually without depleting the pool of stem cells, and the cells are in charge of producing proliferative short-term HSCs. LT–HSCs express the surface markers of Thy1.1^{low}Flk-2$^-$. The expression of Flk-2 is upregulated and the expression of Thy-1.1 is downregulated as self-renewal capacity of the cells diminishes.
2. Short-term HSCs (ST–HSCs): ST–HSCs engender the lineage-committed progenitors to produce the billions of differentiated hematopoietic cells in the peripheral blood daily. The self-renewal life span of ST–HSCs is 6–8 weeks, and afterward, the cells fade away from the bone marrow. ST–HSCs represent 0.01% of the cells in the bone marrow of young adult C57BL mice and have the phenotype of thy1.1^{low} Flk-2$^+$.
3. Multipotent progenitor cells (MPs): MPs have restricted self-renewal potential for less than 2 weeks. The expression of thy1.1$^-$Flk-2$^+$ is also identified in MPs. The offspring of HSCs have been characterized and lineage restricted oligopotent progenitor cells for *lymphoid*, common lymphoid progenitor (CLP), and *myeloid*, common myeloid progenitor (CMP), granulocyte-monocyte progenitor (GMP), and megakaryocyte-erythrocyte progenitor (MEP) lineages.

Comparable phenotypic Mmarkers of HSCs in human and mouse

CD34 was the first marker found in human hematopoietic progenitors. Most human HSCs express CD 34, which is also expressed in the committed progenitors and nonhematopoietic progenitors. The characteristic phenotype of human HSCs includes the lack of expression of lineage markers (Lin-) and expression of Thy-1, c-Kit, and Sca-1, CD45 without CD38 expression. Nonetheless, some human HSCs can be found in the fraction of CD34-negative population. CD34-negative HSCs are a precursor fraction of CD34-positive HSCs. Human HSCs also express Bcrp, known also as ABCG2 transporter, which outflows particular molecules as Hoechst-33342 staining. Detection of CD34 expression in HSC could be performed by the use of HCC-1 antibody in CD59 family members (the sca-1 antibody for mouse detects CD59 family members). Recently CD133 has been identified and could be used as another marker for human HSCs instead of CD34. It is important to remember that the CD34⁺ bone marrow population denotes 1–6% of the cells in bone marrow, whereas the HSC compartment corresponds to only 0.05%. Hence the CD34⁺ population includes HSCs and a small fraction of the non-HSC cell population. Most quiescent LT-HSCs are CD34⁺Thy⁺Lin⁻CD38.

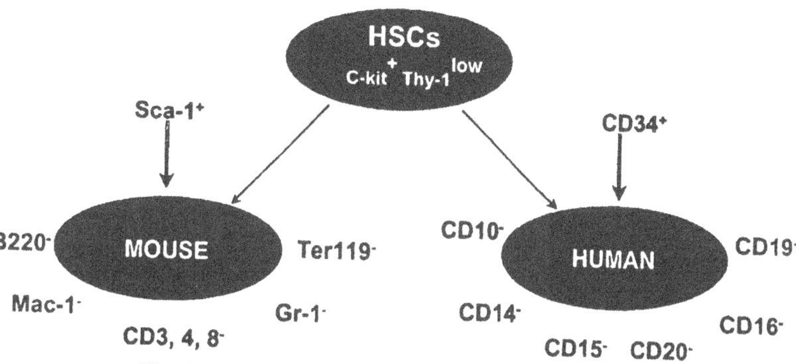

Fig. 2.1. Marker profiles of HSCs in human and mouse.

Mechanism of activation cycle of HSCs

During the late phase of embryonic development, HSCs are located in the fetal liver, where they undergo massive expansion before they enter into the bone marrow and express AA4.1 and Mac 1, which are usually absent in HSCs in a quiescent state. It has been generally believed that the microenvironment affects the fate of the cells. When HSCs are unperturbed in their quiescence niche, the cells express receptors associated with metabolism and aging (IGF1R) and show the activity of tyrosine kinase Tie1, which allows the cells to respond to multiple mitogenic signals. HSCs also express high levels of transcription factors, such as c-fos and GATA-2, which enable quick activation of the cells. HSCs are ready to act in response to changes in their environment "*state of readiness.*" Immediately encountering the stress, HSCs pause totally by remaining quiescent in their niche, while they prepare to proliferate. This phase is mediated by upregulation of TIMP and serine proteinase inhibitor A-3g and by antiproliferative genes, such as Tob1, p21, and Btg3.

Interferon-induced genes are also upregulated, indicating that HSCs are responding to pro-inflammatory signals caused by the stress. The signals induce a proliferative status, which is divided into early and late proliferation phases. In the early phase, the expression of genes involved in the regulation of replication and repair of DNA is enhanced in HSCs. In the late phase when most of HSCs are in cycle, other genes related to energy production are expressed, indicating an increase in the metabolic activity of HSCs. In this context, two proposed approaches are associated with the proliferation state, mobilization and migration. HSCs need to move out of their quiescence niches and enter into a proliferative zone.

Down-regulation of á-4 integrin is necessary for proliferation of HSCs, and downregulation of c-kit has been linked to mobilization of HSCs. At the final phase, HSCs are required to return to their niches in order to stay at the initial state of bone marrow. This step usually starts the day when the damage is ameliorated, when several cells in cycle decrease, and is related with the expression of antiproliferative genes.

Plasticity of HSCs

The hematopoietic tissues such as the bone marrow and peripheral blood have heterogeneous stem cell populations, including hematopoietic stem cells, mesenchymal stem cells, multipotent adult progenitor cells, and endothelial precursor cells. HSCs have been widely used to study the plasticity of adult stem cells. Stem cell plasticity can be defined as a unique property of tissue-specific adult stem cells. Approximately more than 80% of studies reporting plasticity of adult stem cells have been performed using the cells derived from the bone marrow or mobilized peripheral stem cells. Although a previous concept was that differentiation of HSCs was restricted only to a hematopoietic lineage, current studies have reported that HSCs derived from bone marrow can give rise to hematopoetic precursors and multiple "unexpected" cell types, such as neural cells, hepatic cells, cardiac muscle cells, and skeletal muscle cells. Many attempts have been proposed to define the mechanism for how stem cell plasticity occurs. Despite these efforts, there is still no clear evidence regarding whether stem cell plasticity really exists. Some investigators have suggested "*trans-differentiation*" as a possible cause of stem cell plasticity, and others have proposed the cell fusion effect. Even though many theories about plasticity have been proposed, nobody knows for certain whether stem cell plasticity is common or infrequent, whether it might be a vestige of the potential expression during embryonic development, or whether it has a physiologic role in the repair and homeostasis of the tissues. The plasticity of adult HSCs, even though it is rare, has suggested that the environment can reprogram the fate of the cells.

Potential implications of HSCs

Studies on bone marrow cells differentiating into nonhematopoietic lineages have proposed that the cells are a representa-tive source of cell "replacement" in the treatment of numerous diseases. To amplify and generalize this issue for clinical translation, we should accumulate the useful processes of regeneration of blood formation by HSCs, skin replacement by putative epidermal stem cells, and the benefits reported in treating patients with myocardial infarction with bone marrow cells, mobilized peripheral HSCs, or hematopoietic progenitors.

Mesenchymal Stem Cells (MSCs)

Characteristics

MSC is a wide population that exists in the niche of the bone marrow and has attracted the attention of researchers by their potential for self-renewal and differentiation into functional cell types in the intrinsic tissue where they reside. These cells have also been isolated from the fat tissues. MSCs can be expanded in culture for several passages without losing their differentiation potential and have been widely accepted as stem cells due to their usefulness in the clinical treatment of osteogenesis imperfecta, bone tissue regeneration, and hematopoietic recovery.

Self-renewal and multilineage differentiation potential of MSCs

Characterization of MSCs is subject of active investigation, because diversities of techniques to isolate the cells and different ways to analyze the self-renewal ability of the cells have been documented. Considering the lack of reliable specific markers and locating site of MSCs, further experiments are needed to address these issues. To identify MSCs, a combination of several monoclonal antibodies has been tested. As of now, markers for MSCs include SH-2, SH-3, SH-4, SB-10, CD29, CD44, CD90, and STRO-1. In addition, MSCs are negative to hematopoietic markers CD34 and CD45 and the cells are human leukocyte antigen (HLA) class I-positive and HLA class II-negative. The first experiment supporting the presence of MSCs was conducted in the early 1960s. Aspirated bone marrow cells were cultured at low density. The resultant cells formed colonies of fibroblasts, and they were responsible for osteogenesis. Murine MSCs showed self-renewal activity, and the cells differentiated into many types of cell lineages, such as osteoblasts and chondroblasts, adipocytes, neuronal progenitors, and myocytes with the stimulation of cytokines, growth factors, and chemicals *in vitro*. However, it is controversial whether such plasticity of MSCs is induced *in vivo* even after minimal injury. To address this issue, researchers have used animal models of injury. Such experiments have shown that MSCs contribute to the repair or regeneration of damaged bone, cartilage, and infracted myocardial tissues.

Isolation of MSCs

Since 1980 when the characterization of human bone marrow fibroblast colony-forming cells (CFU-Fs) was performed, which was the gold standard to identify MSCs, many researchers have attempted to develop different methods for isolation of MSCs. Now MSCs can be identified by their ability to adhere to a static surface and their proliferat-ing potential. Approximately 30% of human bone marrow-aspirated cells adhering to plastic culture dishes are considered to be MSCs. MSCs in the bone marrow are a heterogeneous population that contains not only putative cells but also tripotent (ability to differentiate into osteocyte, chondrocyte, and adipose lineage-osteo/chondro/adipo), bipotent (osteo/chondro), or unipotent cells (osteo).

Future prospectives of MSCs

Adult MSCs have shown great promise in cell therapy in humans due to their multipotentiality, capacity for extensive self-renewal, and lack of induction of immune response. MSCs may be a valuable source to introduce foreign genes and could be a useful tool for gene therapy for bone regeneration and tissue engineering. Researchers have also proposed MSCs as a useful means to protect the brain tissue from ischemic damage. MSCs ameliorate functional deficits after stroke in rats probably by releasing protective cytokines by the cells. Another potential clinical application is the use of MSCs as a drug delivery vehicle for the treatment of invasive malignant tumors. The behavior of MSCs has been exploited as a tumor-targeting gene therapy in gliomas. Many studies regarding genetically modified MSCs have revealed extraordinary antitumor effects of the cells in experimental models of gliomas. MSCs have the advantage of easy propagation *in vitro*. Moreover, implantation of autologous MSCs into patients with malignant gliomas is ethically nonproblematic.

Multipotent Adult Progenitor Cells (MAPCs)

MAPCs are bone marrow-derived stem cells with an extensive *in vitro* expansion ability, more than 80 population doublings, as well as a capacity to differentiate *in vivo* and *in vitro* into tissue cells of all three germinal layers; ectoderm, mesoderm, and endoderm. These cells have been isolated from three different species, including mouse, rat, and human.

Isolation and culture of MAPCs

MAPCs of different species require different isolation and culture procedures. Human MAPCs are isolated after seeding bone marrow mononuclear cells (BMMNCs) of $CD45^-$ $GlyA^-$ at low densities ($1\text{–}3 \times 10^3/cm^2$) onto fibronectin-coated plastic dishes, with <2% FCS (fetal calf serum), EGF (epidermal growth factor), and PDGF-BB (platelet-derived growth factor). During the culture, depletion of the mono-nuclear cells is observed. The remnant clones that emerge over time are then harvested, and approximately 20% of the total cells seeded. The cells should be plated again at a density of $0.5\text{–}1 \times 10^3$ cells/cm^2. Maintenance of the stem cell phenotype is critically dependent on such low-density inoculation. The culture conditions of mouse MAPCs are similar to those described in human MAPC culture, except for the addition of the leukemia inhibitor factor (LIF).

Phenotypic characteristics and proliferation capacity of MAPCs

Human MAPCs are characterized by the lack of hematopoietic markers such as CD34 and CD45 and the presence of the low expression of VCAM, CD44, MHC class I, and endoglin. The cells can be cultured *in vitro* for more than 50–8 0 population doublings, while preserving their normal karyotype. Mouse MAPCs are positive for CD34, CD45, CD44, c-Kit, CD3, Gr-1, Mac-1, and CD19 and negative for major histocompatibility complex (MHC) class I and class II. The cells express a lower level of Flk1 and Sca1 and a higher level of CD13 and SSEA-1. Mouse MAPCs express pluripotent markers of Oct-4, rex-1, and nanog, which were observed only in ES cells. The cells can be cultured for more than 80–150 population doublings, but the karyotype of the cells becomes unstable.

In vitro differentiation of MAPCs

The differentiation of MAPCs to several lineages is achieved when the cells are re-plated at high density (1–2 × 10^4 cells/cm^2). The cells were cultured in the absence of the serum, but with lineage-specific cytokines required for the differentiation of the desired tissues.

1. *Mesoderm*. By the use of VEFG, the differentiation of MAPCs has been demonstrated into functional mature endothelial cells expressing endothelial markers such as CD31, flk-1, and vWF. Such MAPC-derived endothelial cells are capable of contributing to neoangionesis and wound healing *in vivo*.
2. *Ectoderm*. Verfaille et al. have shown the potential characterization of MAPCs to differentiate into functional neuroectodermal cells, including astrocytes, oligodendrocytes, and neurons.
3. *Endoderm*. MAPCs can differentiate into hepatocyte-like cells by using FGF4 and HGF. Such cells expressed hepatic markers of CK19, AFP, CK18, albumin, HepPar-1, and CD26 and produced albumin, urea, and glycogen.

In vivo differentiation of MAPCs

The potential of multipotency of MAPCs has also been examined *in vivo* by intravenous transplantation of the cells into postnatal murine recipients treated either without radiation or with sublethal irradiation. The observation of chimaerism in many somatic tissues of the mice derived from blastocysts demonstrated the engraftment of MAPCs in various tissues, including hematopoietic, lung, gut, and liver. In these tissues, MAPCs have acquired phenotypic characteristics of the respective cells, indicating their multipotenty.

Future prospectives of MAPCs

MAPCs have been compared with ES cells, for their similar *in vitro* potential to give rise to tissue cells of all three germ layers. MAPCs have shown the same ability as ES cells *in vivo* experiments, although MAPCs do not develop tumors. Due to the nontumorigenecity, MAPCs can serve as a source for the production of a wide spectrum of transplantable cells with an enormous promise for the treatment of many degenerative or inherited diseases. Taking it into account that MAPCs can be recovered from the patients themselves, the clinical use of the cells would be advantageous, avoiding the need for immunosuppressive therapy. MAP Cs provide a prospectively beneficial tool to study developmental biology of the stem cells as well as drug discovery.

Side-Population Phenotype Cells (SPs)

Purification of stem cells was reported based on an efflux of fluorescent dyes, such as Rhodamine 123 and Hoechst 33342. The purified cell population, referred to as SP, has been identified as a small fraction in the bone marrow in all species examined. SP cells can yield about 0.05–0.1% from total bone marrow cells by the use of a flow cytometry cell sorting. Despite being a small population, it possesses interesting capacities, including extensive proliferation and multipotential to generate the entire adult hematopoietic cell lineages. Indeed, only a single transplantation of 200 SP cells can fully repopulate the bone marrow of lethally irradiated mice. It has been reported that a successful expression of dystrophin is achieved in a mouse model of Duchenne's muscular dystrophy after transplantation of SP cells. SP cells have contributed to regenerate the infarcted myocardium by developing cardiocytes and vascular endothelium cells. SP cells have been identified in others several tissues, such as Posterior, by identifying the expression of the ABC transporter Bcrp1/ABCG2. Because of Hoechst 33342-related toxicity, other strategies have been proposed to recover SP cells by using monoclonal antibodies. Even though SP cells seem to be a small source for basic research and possible cell therapy, the cells have shown greater potential. Since SP cells were identified in the bone marrow, the cells have held great promise due to their plasticity and replicating capacity *in vivo* without any tumorigenic transformation. *In vivo* differentiation of SP cells has succeeded in only mesoderm tissues (skeletal muscle, cardiocytes, and vascular cells). Studies have shown that hematopoietic stem cells in the bone marrow are capable of trans-differentiating and giving rise to neuronal progenitor cells, but that such trans-differentiation has not occurred in SP cells.

Tissue-specific SP phenotype cells from different compartments

For a period of time, the SP phenotype cells were identified in many other different tissues, including the brain, pituitary gland, skin, corneal and limbal epithelial ocular tissue, mammary glands, skeletal muscle, lung, heart, liver, spleen, pancreas, small intestine, kidney, testis, peripheral blood, and in umbilical cord blood.

Main characteristics of SP cells from diverse compartments

A variable number of SP cells have been distributed in the different tissues of the body. The SP cells are a heterogeneous population that possesses the ability to give rise to their lineage-specific progenitor cells. Some of these cells have been analyzed and found to be multipotent. *In vitro* cultures of SP cells have shown differences in their propagation capacities and quiescent state.

Tissue-Specific Cell Progenitors (TSCPs)

Neural cell progenitor

The cells involving the development of mature central nervous system (CNS) are precisely regulated by both temporal and local patterns of differentiation, which determine the appropriate cell function. The role of niches shows plasticity coordinated by both the intrinsic factors and the extrinsic soluble signals. Therefore, the specific neural differentiation is affected by this regional patterning. Neurogenesis involves the opposing soluble signals that determine dorsal and ventral patterning: Sonic hedgehog (Shh), bone morphogenetic protein (BMP) antagonists, chordin, and noggin are secreted from the floor plate, whereas other signals originating from the roof plate result in the creation of the gradient of signal concentrations. Precise concentration and ratio of each independent signal derive the development of the specific neuronal phenotypes at different points in accordance with these gradients. Such phenomena cause the different expression patterns of the cells and create the groups of neurons with different patterns of cell division and differentiation. At the beginning, the CNS stem cells divide symmetrically to enrich their population pool, or asymmetrically to generate more differentiated progeny, which become mature cells of neuronal and glial lineages. The spinal cord can produce both oligodendrocytes and neurons from common precursors, and the final decision of the cell fate depends on extrinsic signals and specific patterns of transcriptional activation.

General characteristics of neural progenitor cells

In rodent models, neural progenitor cells have been identified in specific regions of adult CNS. The cells isolated from different sites of CNS are not identical and thus show different growth characteristics, trophic factor requirements, and specific patterns of differentiation. Growth factor requirements can define at least two major types of neural progenitor cells isolated from CNS. One cell type requires a high dose of EGF and can be expanded as floating neurospheres, while preserving their phenotype after many passages, and eventually they come to be FGF-responsive. In contrast, another cell type isolated from CNS is exclusively FGF-dependent. Such cells can be propagated, as adherent cultures with FGF-dependent and the cells do not respond to EGF. The cells do not express EGF receptor either *in vivo* or *in vitro*. As these cells have been isolated from multiple brain areas, it is likely that both of neural precursor cells coexist. Both cells can self-renew and differentiate into the three neural cell types *in vitro*. Differentiation of the cells in tissue culture can be induced by withdrawal of growth factors or by induction of specific signals. It seems that distinct stem cell populations are programmed to differentiate into specific cell types during the CNS development based on their response to growth factors. Moreover, some of these phenotypes expressed in progenitor cells in CNS have been observed in progenitors isolated from the pancreas of adult mice, which can generate neural and pancreatic lineages.

Epidermal progenitor cells

Keratinocytic populations can be grown *in vitro*, while displaying clonal growth. Keratinocytes can generate normal epidermis when they are appropriately grafted. Furthermore, the proliferative heterogeneity of the keratinocytes reveals the presence of stem cells, that is, epidermal progenitor cells. β1 integrin seems to play a central role in the regulation of the progenitor cells. When β1 integrin binds its ligand of type IV collagen, the cells exhibit high proliferative capacity, while maintaining their undifferentiated state. Therefore, the number and patterning of progenitor cells *in vivo* are autoregulated by the stem cell niche and turnover of the cells provides regulatory feedback signals. The differentiating potential of epidermal progenitor cells has totally denied the previous speculation, implying that the cells were not multipotent.

Progenitor cells in the respiratory tract

The respiratory tract seems to have a local progenitor population, which gives rise to mature respiratory cells and preserves the native architecture along the tract. Consequently, tissue homeostasis is maintained by these cells, in which the trachea and bronchus segments, bronchiole, and alveolus are maintained by mucous secreting basal cells, by Clara cells, and by type II pneumocytes, respectively. These cells serve as structural and functional parenchyma and work for quick regeneration if any injury occurs in the respiratory tract. In addition, the recent reports have demonstrated that progenitors existing in the populations of basal cells, Clara cells, and type II pneumocytes are not only able to provide tissue function, but also possess renewal capacities. These progenitor cell populations contain both SP cells and hematopoietic markers-expressing cells and are capable of repopulating the bone marrow as HSCs do. These findings have sustained the theory that bone marrow stem cells serve as the whole postnatal stem cells and their own progenies to provide a common interchangeable cell source.

Skeletal muscle progenitor cell or satellite cells

The embryonic mesoderm generates skeletal musculature. Satellite cells are skeletal muscle progenitor cells that are responsible for postnatal growth and repair. Injury in skeletal musculature results in detriment in skeletal muscle mass, but injury itself triggers muscle regeneration of muscle tissue, which is accomplished by differentiation of native progenitor cells. The tissue-specific cell progenitors are so-called satellite cells. Despite the replenishment of the satellite cell pool during muscle growth, the number of satellite cells, which is highest in postnatal muscle, declines with aging. This unique population of the cells exists between the muscle fiber sarcolemma and its covering basement membrane. Anatomically, the satellite cells can be clearly defined. The cells are quiescent lying outside the myofibers but beneath the basement membranes.

Quiescent muscle satellite cells are characterized by the expression of surface markers such as M-cadherin, syndecan 3 and 4, and CD34. Even using a standard dissociation technique of the muscle tissue, an efficient isolation of myogenic progentior cells has not been achieved. Many growth factors are implicated in the regulation, chemotaxis, proliferation, and differentiation of satellite cells. Basic fibroblast growth factor (bFGF), platelet-derived growth factor (PDGF), transferring, and hepatocyte growth factor (HGF) have been identified as potent mitogens for satellite cells. HGF, bFGF, and IGF-1 and TGF-β can also promote chemotaxic activity of satellite cells in tissue culture [179, 182]. Based on their SP phenotype, Hoechst 33342 dye efflux-used FACS has become the easiest way to isolate skeletal muscle progenitor cells. This SP population can generate terminally differentiated skeletal muscle cells and completely repopulate the bone marrow after transplantation.

Hepatic cell progenitors

Hepatocytes possess the ability to rapidly respond to the parenchymal loss with turning on active mitosis. After massive loss of hepatocytes induced by two-thirds partial hepatectomy, the remaining hepatocytes make a cell-cycle progression at two to three times to restore preoperative cell volume. Such an enormous repopulating capacity is con-ducted by unknown potential and properties of hepatocytes. These crucial properties that defines a stem cell are capable of generating a large progeny. This phenomenon can be observed at least in some hepatocytes. Putative hepatic stem cells have been identified by the cell membrane markers, such as the lowered expression of the asialoglyco-protein receptor. Induction of a massive liver damage compromises the regeneration of hepatocytes, and then facultative hepatic progenitor cells distributed along the small branches of the intrahepatic biliary trees are activated to divide. Oval cells that express the same markers as HSCs (c-kit, flt-3, Thy-1, and CD34) transiently amplify the biliary population and then differentiate into hepatocytes. This particular phenomenon may provide information as to how the liver provides niches for facultative stem cells or offers an opportunity for cell fusion.

Progenitor cells in the gastrointestinal tract

The presence of progenitor cells in the intestinal crypts has been observed. Intestinal crypts and gastric glands are considered as specific niches that contain noncommitment and probably multipotent stem cells. The epithelial intestinal cells form the lining invaginates with numerous crypts and finger-shaped projections along the gastrointestinal tract and possess a rich population of neuroenteroendocrine cells disseminated throughout their epithelium. The plasticity of progenitor cells in the intestinal epithelium has been shown by differentiation of the cells to insulin-secreting cells using GLP-1. Intestinal crypts and gastric glands are enclosed by protective fenestrated intestinal subepithelial myofibroblasts and disperse in the lamina propria with merging blood vessels. The myofibroblasts secrete HGF, TGF-beta, and KGF to regulate the differentiation of the intestinal epithelial progenitor cells. Thus, myofibroblast cells play a central role in regulating the differentiation of the progenitor cells located in Lieberkühn crypts.

Adult pancreatic progenitor cells

The adult pancreatic tissue is composed of the exocrine and endocrine cells. During embryological development, the pancreatic tissue is generated from differentiation of the ductal epithelium. The exocrine tissue is first differentiated and then endocrine tissue is differentiated. Islets of Langerhans under physiological conditions turn over continuously, but slowly. Terminally differentiated pancreatic beta cells have a life span of approximate 50 days. The cells have a balance of apoptosis and replacement, which is conducted by replication of differentiated beta cells. The replicating capacity of the beta cells is limited.

The presence of pancreatic progenitor cells that can give rise to pancreatic and neuronal cell lineages has been demonstrated. Ductal and acinar cells have been proven to have plasticity to differentiate into insulin-secreting cells or to trans-differentiate into hepatocytes. The beta cells certainly replicate; however, the senescence of the cells still determines their potential. Otherwise, beta cells may be reprogrammed by cell fusion. *In vitro* culture human islets gradually lose their insulin expression, but they preserve the expression of PDX-1. Recent research has suggested that adult pancreatic islets contains progenitor cells. Pancreatic progenitor cells may also exist in the non-endocrine tissue. These progenitor cells are capable of generating terminally differentiated endocrine and exocrine progeny. They are identified by the positive expression of nestin, referred as to nestin-positive progenitor cells (NIPs), and are dispersed in the whole pancreatic tissue. In addition, SP phenotype cells were observed in NIPs and the cells can give rise to vascular and neuronal progenies.

Umbilical Cord Blood-Derived Stem Cells (UCBSCs)

Stem cells were isolated from umbilical cord blood (UCB) and cultured *in vitro*. Umbilical cord blood-derived stem cells (UCBSCs) had been proposed as an alternative source of regeneration of hemopoietic tissue by allogeneic transplantation. The successful hematopoietic reconstitution in a patient with Fanconi's anemia has proved the potential of UCBSCs. Usually small cell fractions are recovered from the cord blood, but the primitive hematopoietic population possesses a high proliferative capacity. UCB cells contain a larger hematopoietic population of $CD34^-$ as well as a subset of $CD34^+$ and $CD38^-$, of which population ratio is about fourfold higher than that in bone marrow cells.

Moreover, the most primitive phenotype ($CD34^+CD38^-CD45RA^{low}CD71^{low}Thy\text{-}1^+c\text{-}kit^{low}Rh^{low}$)-expressing cells present in UCB at 0.003% of the entire population of nucleated cells. Their proliferative capacity reach to a 50-fold expansion of colony forming cells. Successful *in vitro* expansion of the cells depends on the cytokines contained in the culture. Such cytokines include SCF, IL-1, IL-3, IL-6, GM-CSF, G-CSF, M-CSF, erythropoietin, and thrombopoietin. The cells also possess multipotent characteristics and outstanding plasticity. Therefore, there have been several approaches of differentiation of non-hematopoietic tissues ongoing in the clinical tissue regeneration settings and *in vitro* toxicological studies.

Heterogeneous Populations of Stem Cells in Bone Marrow

Bone marrow contains two main well-defined populations of stem cells, HSCs and MSCs. They renew by themselves and give rise to all of the terminally differentiated blood lineages. In addition, bone marrow possesses a small subset population of nonhematopoietic stem cells (NHSCs). This population of NHSCs is identified by the expression of $CXCR4^+$, $CD34^+$, $AC133^+$, lin^-, and $CD45^-$. Moreover, there is evidence that tissue damage in the body itself is capable of triggering the bone marrow stem cells to get into the circulation. Subsequently, the stem cells modify their phenotype in accordance with the tissue where they migrate. Specific activation of membrane surface receptors and subsequent activation of transcription factors determine a modulation of the phenotypes and migratory properties of the stem cells.

Chemotactic or homing signaling is involved in the regulation of the migration. The bone marrow stem cells have an exceptional ability to adapt and survive in different microenvironments. The cells can respond to several cytokines and growth factor, such as HGF, VEGF, LIF, and bFGF. The axis SDF-1-$CXCR4^+$ seems to be the most crucial regulatory factor, which is involved in honing of the stem cells. Therefore, it may be considered that bone marrow stem cells can serve as the source of all adult somatic stem cells. UCBSCs are considered as HSCs because of their strong proliferative capacity. UCBSCs certainly display higher potentials compared with adult stem cells and have been proposed as the best candidate for regenerating the damaged tissues in the clinical setting among the stem cells.

Uses and Applications of Stem Cells in Toxicology

Besides the further clinical application of stem cells, utilization of the cells in the pharmacological field is also of great interest. As mentioned, stem cells are specialized cells found within many tissues of the body, in which they have the role to maintain homeostasis and repair of the damage tissue. The advantages of unlimited proliferation and subsequent differentiation of the stem cells can be of great use for *in vitro* screening of the newly developed drugs, allowing us to predict possible adverse effects without the need to test them in animals. For example, hepatocytes derived from stem cells can be routinely screened for new drugs and chemicals to evaluate their liver toxicity.

Artificial Cells

A major limitation to the clinical application of cell therapy and drug discovery is the current inability to isolate an adequate number of functional and transplantable cells. Unfortunately, the number of human organs available for transplantation or cell isolation is severely limited. Considering the cost and difficulty in some cases of cell isolation and the need for immediate availability of consistent and functionally uniform cell preparations, human cells cannot be isolated on a scale sufficient to treat more than a fraction of the patients who need organ transplantation. The use of animal cells would result in additional concerns related to the transmission of infectious pathogens and immunologic and physiologic incompatibilities between donors and humans. Thus, other alternative cell sources, such as stem cells, have been explored. In particular, embryonic stem cells have unlimited proliferative capacity and theoretically can differentiate all kinds of cell types. In contrast, somatic stem cells have finite proliferation ability in the currently available culture system.

The cultivation of mammalian cells is an important experimental procedure that is a fundamental tool in biological studies. Establishment of methods to control differentiation and proliferation in stem cells is not yet achieved. Thus, possible tumor development will be occurred after de-differentiated or trans-differentiated stem cells. To overcome this issue, great efforts have been made to construct immortalized human cell lines with an unlimited replicative potential. However, despite the widespread use of the culture system, we have recently begun to understand the essential mechanisms that control cell growth and division. This section discusses recent advances in our understanding of the molecular mechanisms that regulate the life span of cell lineages *in vitro* and an approach to construct human cell lines with currently available genetic manipulation for cell therapy and the study of pharmacology and toxicology.

The definition of cellular immortality is infinite survival with an unlimited proliferative potential. In fact, primary human cells in tissue culture rarely undergo spontaneous immortalization process. Thus, researchers tried to immortalize human cells by using x-ray and chemical carcinogens, but it turned out to be very inefficient. Currently, human cells have been immortalized by an introduction of the transforming genes of DNA tumor viruses, such simian virus 40 large T antigen (SV40LT), papillomaviruses, and the catalytic unit of the human telomerase reverse transcriptase.

Immortalization of Human Cells

Limited proliferative life span or senescence of human cells

Senescence is a terminally arrested growth state of the cells. It differs from the nonproliferative state of terminally differentiated cells. As senescent cells remain viable, senescence can be distinguished with cell death processes such as apoptosis or necrosis. Senescent cells are arrested at the G1/S phase of the cell cycle and are thus distinct from nondividing G0-arrested quiescent cells. Human cells are defined as senescent when they fail to respond to mitogens and the population of the cells does not divide in a certain period of time, for example, 30 days. Additional characteristics of senescent cells include (1) expression of β-galactosidase, (2) increased lysossomal biogenesis, (3) decreased rates of protein synthesis and degradation that are distinct from their pre-senescent ancestors, (4) increased cell size, (5) multinucleation, (6) cytoplasmic vacuolation, and (7) decreased membrane fluidity. The rate of protein, DNA, and RNA syntheses is reduced in senescent cells. Senescent cells accumulate altered macromolecules and exhibit DNA alterations such as shortened telomeres, decreased chromatin condensation, increased karyotypic abnormalities, and decreased methylation. Senescence does not lead directly to cell death, and senescent cells can persist in culture for up to 2 years if fed regularly.

Senescent cells may accumulate in aged tissue and could compromise tissue function by both their altered pattern of gene expression and their nonproliferative state, resulting in aged phenotypes of the tissues. A link between *in vitro* senescence and *in vivo* aging is suggested by the observation that the *in vitro* life span of cells from various mammalian species correlates with their *in vivo* life span and that the cells from individuals with premature ages suffering from disorders such as Werner's syndrome, Down's syndrome, and progeria have a shorter *in vitro* life span than that of the cells from normal individuals. However, evidence that the *in vitro* life span of normal human cells correlates with the donor age remains controversial.

Immortal or extended Life span of human cells

More than 30 years, ago, it was demonstrated for the first time that SV40, a DNA tumor virus of the papova virus family isolated by Sweet and Hillman, can morphologically transform human fetal and adult skin fibroblast. The transformation of mammalian cells by SV40 is known to require expression of only the early region of the viral genomes, which encodes two proteins of large T-antigen (94 kd) and small t-antigen (17 kd). Transfer and expression of specific oncogenes, such as simian virus 40 large T antigen (SV40 LT), in primary human cells can generate cell populations that propagate for extended periods of time *in vitro*, presumably because they bypass the first senescence crisis through the inactivation of p53 and Rb, and thus extend their life span by about 20 population doubling (PD). This extended life span ends in M2 crisis stage, which typically coincides with dangerously shortened telomeres, and every mitosis is accompanied by enormous chromosomal instability in the cells. Most of the cells fail to survive crisis, and the frequency rate of the cells that overcome the crisis is very low in humans.

The *in vitro* spontaneous immortalization of human cells using SV40T is approximately 10^{6}–10^{7} and is believed to result from activation of the endogenous telomerase. Such cells are infrequently tumorogenic, and tumorigenicity occurs only after long periods of continuous culture of the cells. These phenomena have suggested that establishment of permanent cell lines in culture involves two distinct processes: (1) an initial adaptation of cells to grow in the unnatural environment of culture dish, and (2) an acquired ability of these adapted cells to proliferate indefinitely in tissue culture. The life span of cells is measured in cell divisions; thus, cells must possess a molecular "clock" that counts the number of times they have divided. In a telomere model of senescence, telomere length acts as this counting mechanism.

Nucleoprotein structures that constitute the ends of linear chromosomes became the primary candidates to fulfill this role in human cells. It was for the first time described molecularly in 1981; telomeres serve to protect the ends of chromosomes from illegitimate fusions and other damage and shield the ends of chromosomes from recognition by the cellular DNA repair machinery. Telomeric DNA is maintained at a constant length, and telomeres shorten at a constant rate with progressive cell divisions in human cells. Telomere shortening occurs for at least two reasons: (1) Telomeres shorten with successive replication because the polymerases involved in conventional DNA replication cannot fully copy telomeric DNA and (2) telomerase, an enzyme responsible for telomere maintenance, is tightly repressed in most human somatic cells. Most immortalized human cells express telomerase, and telomere length is stable.

These observations have suggested that some elements of telomere structures monitor cell proliferation and order a signal of the onset of replicative senescence. The ectopic expression of telomerase in pre-senescent cells halts telomere shortening and permits cells to avoid replicative senescence. Telomerase is a ribonucleoprotein composed of an RNA subunit, *hTERC*, that is ubiquitously expressed and a reverse transcriptase protein catalytic subunit, *hTER T*, whose expression correlates with telomerase activity in immortal cells.

hTERT is indeed undetectable in most types of normal human cells, but it is readily detectable in most immortal cell lines, cells derived from human cancers, and human tumor samples. Expression of *hTERT* in pre-senescent human cells confers telomerase activity, resulting in telomere lengthening or stabilization, and it allows the cells to bypass replicative senescence. Cells expressing *hTERT* maintain the normal karyotype and continue to respond in the same manner as pre-senescent, nonimmortalized cells. Thus, activation of telomerase by expression of *hTERT* permits the cells to bypass senescence and become immortalized in a single step. Although maintenance of telomere plays an important role in replicative senescence, it has been proved that both pRB and p53 tumor suppressor pathways also play a prominent role in regulating the onset of replicative senescence.

When cells expressing SV40LT continue to repress hTERT expression and lack a detectable telomerase activity, the telomere length of the cells gradually shortens with continued cell proliferation. Eventually such cells enter the second period of diminished growth, which referred is to as crisis or M2. Telomere shortening may be one signal that activates the pRB or p53 pathway and initiates replicative senescence. These observations have suggested that both pRB and p53 pathways in conjunction with telo-mere shortening play significant roles in governing replicative senescence.

Crisis stage

Crisis (M2) is distinguished from senescence by cell death in the presence of ongoing cell division. Although most cells that enter crisis die by apoptosis, a few cells overcome crisis and become immortal. Immortal cells that have survived crisis typically exhibit aneuploidy and extensive nonreciprocal chromosomaltranslocations, which suggests that substantial genomic rearrangements accompany the selection of these rare surviving cells. These observations indicate that crisis is precipitated by critically shortened telomeres that have lost their ability to protect chromosomes in the setting of p53 loss. Immortal cells that emerge from crisis show the stabilized telomere lengths with extended passage, which suggests that only those cells that acquire the ability to maintain stable telomere lengths survive. It is important to note that, in general, immortal cells fail to form tumors in immunodeficient animals. Experimentally, the introduction of *hTERT* in post-senescent, pre-crisis cells confers telomerase activity, stabilizes telomere length, and permits these telomerase-expressing cells to become immortal. Human cells immortalized in this manner often exhibit near-diploid karyotypes, which strongly suggests that critical telomere shortening in the absence of pRB and p53 functions initiates crisis. Two barriers limit proliferative lifespan in human cells: (1) replicative senescence and (2) crisis. Furthermore, it is obvious that telomerase, pRB, and p53 play critical roles in regulating an entry of human cells into these two states.

Immortality

Several groups have demonstrated that the introduction of pairs of cooperating oncogenes, such as myc and ras, or the adenoviral E1A protein and ras into the primary rodent cells leads to direct transformation of the cells. However, several laboratories have now shown that telomere biology differs in important ways between human and murine cells. Unlike most human cells in which telomerase is tightly repressed, most murine cells express detectable telomerase activity. In addition, telomeres are maintained at much longer lengths in cells derived from inbred mice than are observed in human cells. These observations have suggested that the replicative life span of murine cells is not limited by telomere length. With extended cell division, telomere shortening activates either replicative senescence or crisis and telomeres play in protecting chromosomal integrity, which suggests that telomeres play an important role in repressing tumor formation. In contrast, the maintenance of telomere length confers cell immortality. These observations also indicate that telomeres serve as a factor that restricts and/or promotes malignant transformation. Under most circumstances, short telomeres limit the life span of the cells, depending on the status of the pRB and p53 pathways, to greatly reduce the pool of premalignant cells.

To address cellular immortality, researchers have made great efforts to establish an immortalized human cell lines. Such cell lines provide the advantage of uniformity and sterility, grow in unlimited quantity, and are far less costly than isolating the primary cells. One approach to construct clonal cell lines is transduction of the primary cells with genes from DNA tumor viruses, such as SV40, human papillomavirus, and Epstein-Barr virus. Transformation of normal cells with early region genes of

SV40, typically by transfection with expression plasmids, remains a common immortalization technique. For example, human fetal hepatopcytes were successfully transduced with pSV3neo DNA containing both large and small T antigens of the early region of SV40 and bacterial neomycin phosphotransferase gene. After G418 treatment, one line of the surviving clones, OUMS-29, grew well in the chemically defined serum-free medium without any crisis and showed liver-specific functions. When transplanted into immunodeficient mice, OUMS-29 cells were not tumorigenic. The potential risk of malignant formation of OUMS-29 cells cannot be precluded in humans. Safeguards, including the introduction of suicide genes, should be considered in immortalized cells for human application.

In parallel, cells are recovered from surgically resected tumor specimens and cultured. Cell lines have been established for the study of different pathophysiologies. These cell lines grow indefinitely in tissue culture and have been widely used all over the world. However, genetic constitution and alterations of such cells are often observed, and several important specific functions, including several receptors and transporters, have been unfortunately deregulated.

Tightly Immortalized Human Cell Lines

Transduction of immortalized cell lines with these suicide genes would provide a way to eliminate the cells after transplantation. Cells modified to express a herpes simplex virus–thymidine kinase (HSV–TK) gene become sensitive to ganciclovir (GCV). Thus, researchers have introduced the HSV–TK gene into cell lines. For example, OUMS-29/TK cells, immortalized human fetal hepatocytes expressing HSV–TK, were more than 100 times sensitive to GCV treatment than unmodified parental OUMS-29 cells. OUMS-29/TK cells stopped proliferation in the presence of 5-μM GCV.

Conditionally Immortalized Cell Lines

An approach to create a conditionally immortalized cell line is the use of a transforming gene containing a temperature-sensitive mutation. Primary rat hepatocytes were successfully immortalized with a thermolabile mutant SV40T (encoded by the early region mutant tsA58) and functioned as well as primary hepatocytes after transplantation. However, the continued presence of SV40T in the transplanted cells may increase the risk of malignant transformation of the cells after transplantation in the recipients.

Ultra-Transform Immortalized Transgenic Cell Lines

This approach has proven to be successful because the resulting cell lines showed stability in culture and sensitivity to chemical exposure. The strategy implicates the development of a bi-transgenic hepatocyte cell line to evaluate the ability of various organic and inorganic chemicals to induce the expression of the HSP70-driven reporter gene. Development of two types of transgenic mice is necessary in advance. One is a transgenic mice (Hsp70/hGH) secreting high levels of human growth hormone (hGH), and another is transgenic model (AT/cytoMet) allowing the reproducible immortalization of untransformed hepatocytes retaining liver functions. Both strains are crossed, and the resulting transgenic strain permits a reproducible immortalization of untransformed hepatocytes. Several stable hepatic cell lines (MMH–GH) showing highly differentiated phenotypes have been generated from the double transgenic animals. This strategy is valuable in the field of toxicology and in the development of chemical and physical xenobiotics. The technology provides a simple biological system that reduces the need for animal experimentation and/or continuously isolating fresh hepatocytes.

Reversibly Immortalized Cell Lines

To generate an immortalized hepatocyte cell line more suitable for clinical use, a more tightly regulated system for cell growth should be considered. An attractive system using site-specific recombination has been documented. DNA sequences intervened by loxP recombination targets can be excised after expression of Cre recombinase. A Cre/loxP system allows the construction of reversibly immortalized cell lines. To provide more stringent control over the expression of transforming genes, human hepatocytes were transduced with a retro-viral vector SSR#69 expressing SV40T and selectable positive (hygromycin resistance gene) and negative (HSV-TK) markers that were intervened by a pair of loxP recombination targets and subsequently excised by Cre/loxP recombination. One emerging clone after SSR#69-transduction, NKNT-3, was a highly differentiated hepatocyte cell line. NKNT-3 cells were sensitive to 5-μM GCV.

Adenovirus-mediated Cre recombinase expression was efficiently performed to remove SV40T from NKNT-3 cells. Intrasplenic transplantation of such reverted NKNT-3 cells significantly improved the survival of 90% hepatectomized rats. Cre/loxP-based reversible immortalization has been achieved in several types of human cells. In our studies, SV40T-transduced normal human endothelial cells (ECs) acquired an extensive proliferation capacity to population doubling level (PDL) 65 to 80, but complete immortalization was not achieved. This was explained by the absence of spontaneous activation of endogenous telomerase, which is known as one of the essential participants in cellular immortalization processes in SV40T-transduced ECs. To achieve immortalization of normal human ECs, a retroviral vector SSR#197 expressing hTERT and GFP cDNAs flanked by a pair of loxB target sequences was constructed.

Cotransduction of human ECs with retroviral vectors SSR#69 and SSR#197 facilitated establishment of a completely immortalized cell line TMNK-1 that expresses a differentiated endothelial phenotype. Feasibility of reversible immortalization in TMNK-1 cells was demonstrated by using TAT-derived HIV-mediated Cre/loxP recombination followed by GFP-negative cell sorting and drug selection. Lately, the system has been applied to establish hepatic stellate cell lines, cholangiocyte cell lines, hepatic progenitor cell lines, bone marrow-derived human cells, and human pancreatic beta cell lines. To establish immortalized human pancreatic beta cell lines, freshly isolated human pancreatic islet cells were transduced with SSR#69, followed by hygromycin selection. Then, the resultant cells were super-infected with SSR#197 for immortalization.

At the first screening, tumorigenic assay of the resulting cell lines was performed in immunodeficient mice. Then, gene expression analysis was conducted in nontumorigenic clones. Based on these findings, NAKT-15 turned out to be highly differentiated. To obtain the reverted form of NAKT-15 cells, the cells were infected with a recombinant adevovirus virus vector (AxCANCre) expressing Cre recombinase tagged with a nuclear localization signal (NLS) expressing the recombinant adenovirus vector. After AxCANCre infection, GFP-negative cell populations were recovered by a MoFlo cell sorter and then cultured in the presence of neomycin analog G418.

Applications

Numerous genomics-based technologies are now routinely applied to drug discovery. The central role for these technologies is validating the next generation of therapeutics from novel targets identified through genomics. The aim of such technologies is to accurately identify the next generation of targets that demonstrate therapeutic efficiency and safety. Immortal human cell lines will have unique attributes that can be used for drug discovery, and if cell therapy is the goal of such cells, the addition of redundant safeguards into the cells and accumulation of experimental data will be required before clinical trials. The ultimate goal of cell transplantation is an autologous setting in which the patient's own cells are genetically modified *ex vivo* with a reversible immortalization method, and then a reverted form of the cells can be transplanted back to the patient.

Immortalized or reversibly immortalized cells offer continuous availability, uniformity, and sterility, and the cells can be functionally cryopreserved for the future use. Production of such cell lines may overcome the shortage of donors, and thus, the established human cell clones may be considered as a potential cell source for the treatment of diabetic patients or liver failure patients with transplantation.

We anticipate that the production of artificial cells will be useful not only to provide carcinogenesis models, but also to develop drug discovery and possible cell therapy in the future. Reversible immortalization of human cells has important applications in biological research, biotechnology, and medicine.

The ethical issue of transplanting immortalized cells is still controversial, but clinical approval of a protocol involving transplantation of these cells depends on the balance of risks and benefits. If patients with high risk were to receive such transplants with considerable benefits, approval would be obtained after reliable accumulation of data regarding the safety and efficacy of immortalized cells. We here represent an important step in the development of a useful strategy for resolving the organ shortage that now limits the use of normal human cells for cell therapies. Such technology can be applicable to a variety of somatic cells and would potentially be used to treat a large number of patients with clinically significant pathologic conditions.

3

AUTOMATION

Man has long strived to minimize or replace fully his involvement in a variety of tasks by devising substitute machines and instruments; the chemical laboratory, the ultimate site for chemical analyses, has obviously joined in this trend.

FUNDAMENTALS AND OBJECTIVES OF ANALYTICAL AUTOMATION

The need to automate analytical processes gradually is unarguable. The earliest serious attempts at automating chemical analyses date from the 1970s. The vast amount of literature and opinion supporting time and labour investments in the automation of the analytical laboratory, aired during the 1970s and early 1980s, is now a thing of the past.

While the path travelled in this direction so far has been highly fruitful, there is still a long way to go (in fact, ways in science have no dead ends). Therefore, the following reasons, advanced to justify automation of the analytical laboratory, remain valid if things are to be further improved:

1. *Personnel release*. Replacing a human operator in routine or hazardous tasks (e.g. those involving toxic or explosive substances) results in increased safety and avoidance of subjective errors.
2. *Improved analytical performance*, particularly with regard to precision of the results.
3. *More efficient use of the effective capacity of analytical instrumentation and more rational management of chemical reagents*. Minimizing reagent consumption decreases analytical costs and results in improved environmental safety through decreased disposal of hazardous wastes or diminished exposure of laboratory staff to toxic chemicals, such as the organic solvents typically used in closed flow systems. Increasing instrumental power enables processing of very small samples or use of multi-parameter assemblies for several determinations at once.

In addition to the above 'analytical chemical' reasons, the need for laboratory automation is justified by other arguments. Thus, there are management reasons such as the need to minimize costs, extend working days in order to process large numbers of samples (e.g. in clinical laboratories) or perform analyses at odd hours (e.g. production controls, public water supply check-ups, atmospheric pollution controls in zones of heavy traffic, etc.). There are also reasons arising from social demands for increasingly higher living standards; this entails massive, continuous controls of pollution, water potability, food and drink quality, etc., all of which involve analysing large sample batches.

Improving existing automatic processes, cutting costs, automating analytical operational sequences by suppressing manual operations linking other, automatic operations, will remain pending goals until the whole analytical process, from sampling to result interpretation, can eventually be automated. Fully automated analyses are the ultimate goal of laboratory automation. This inevitably entails performing

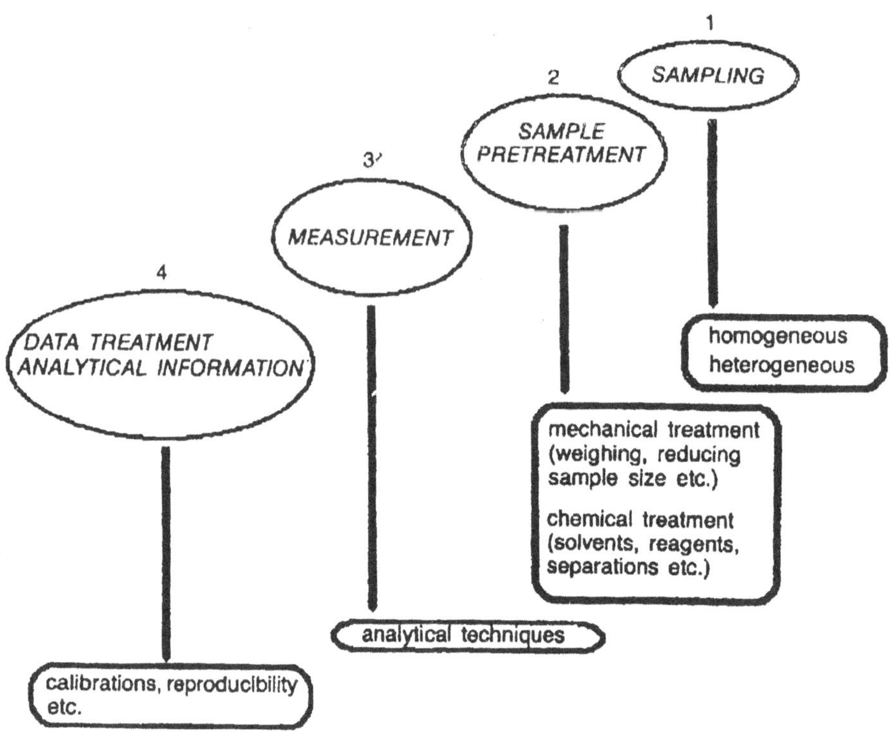

Fig. 3.1. Fundamental steps of the analytical process.

analyses 'on site', i.e. carrying out every operation, from sampling to result delivery, at the site of the sample, thereby avoiding the need to handle it for transfer to the laboratory and altering (contaminating) it during storage or transport. On-site analyses entail the use of specific monitors, mobile laboratories or even remote sensors.

The earliest available fully automatic methods were those used in mining and oil drilling; these were later followed by those employed to monitor industrial processes at some point along the productive chain. More recently, atmospheric analyses have been automated with the aid of spectrophotometric detectors installed in a mobile vehicle (a plane or van), as have determinations of control parameters in waste and drinking waters, and clinical analyses involving direct connection of the patient to the measuring instrument (there are reported instances of blood analyses where the patient's bloodstream was directly connected to the injection valve of a flow injection analysis (FIA) system). Automation of the analytical laboratory can be viewed from two different standpoints: the automation of laboratory unit operations (LUOs); and the automation of an operational sequence. It should be noted that, very often, the overall process comprises only one or two unit operations (e.g. in control analyses, determinations of melting and boiling points, pharmaceutical dissolution tests, etc.).

There are a number of commercially available devices for automating a unit operation (e.g. the dissolution of solid samples and transfer of the resulting liquid) in the sample preparation step. As regards operational sequences, the trend should be towards automating the whole analytical process, where 'whole' is meant to include every operation performed after the sample, properly stored, is received by the analyst. In this respect, it should be borne in mind that any analytical process consists of the following fundamental steps:

1. The first step involves a number of unit operations (weighing, dissolution, disaggregation, sample or particle size reduction, etc.) and management procedures (assignation of a reference number,

form filling, etc.). Disaggregation and sample or particle size reduction are the most thoroughly automated, with the aid of electronic and computer equipment.

2. The second step of the analytical process, viz. preparation of the sample for measurement, encompasses a variety of operations that can be classified into two different groups:
   (a) Initial mechanical operations.
   (b) Sample processing (usually dissolution) for 'adjusting' the measurement conditions, and any derivatization reaction needed, etc. This is usually integrated with other steps (e.g. the removal of agents which would interfere with the assay or the separation of several analytes to be determined). A chromatographic system, whether liquid or gas, performs enough operations without the operator's participation for the method to be considered an automatic method of analysis. After the operator injects the sample (if the instrument concerned lacks a sample drum and autoinjector), the eluent sweeps the sample to the detector; on the way, the sample is subjected to separations or even derivatization reactions that produce transient signals whose transduced value and meaning (in terms of concentration) are displayed by the result acquisition and delivery system (usually a straightforward microcomputer).

There are various methodologies for (partly) automating the analytical process; among them, FIA has evolved dramatically in a matter of years with the establishment of a host of efficient procedures. FIA is a flow methodology. According to the way the sample is processed, automatic methods of analysis can be classified into three broad groups:

1. Discrete or batch methods;
2. Flow methods; and
3. Robotic methods.

A fourth, heterogeneous category, comprises all those methods developed in order to automate specific unit operations.

Discrete or Batch Methods

This group comprises all those methods based on static analysis criteria (robotic methods excluded); each sample preserves its physical integrity, isolated in its own vessel from the preceding and following samples in the chain. In fact, each sample occupies a stand-alone vessel where every operation (reagent addition, heating, agitation, etc.) takes place. Occasionally, detection is also performed in the vessel itself; otherwise, the sample is transferred to the detector for measurement, which gives rise to two types of methods: with and without sample transfer.

One other possible sub-classification of this group is based on the type of path travelled by the sample to the detector: sample vessels can be links in an endless chain or make up a closed circle. The ensuing applications require using a piston pipette furnished with a valve for controlling sample or reagent loading and unloading.

Centrifugal analysers belong to the closed circuit type of automatic assembly. However, they depart from the typical operation of this type of system in that sample and reagents are placed in the same vessel but do not mix there; in fact, mixing is prevented by the non-uniform shape of the vessel, which has two different heights that allow the sample to be held in the inner bottom part—the innermost in the radial direction—and the reagents in the outer top part. After every sample has been prepared, the assembly is spun at high speed, which causes samples and reagents to mix in each vessel, from which they are transferred to the measuring 'optical cell'. This special 'cuvette' is another part of the vessel into which the sample and reagents are forced; it has an optically transparent window that permits the absorbance to be measured every time a sample passes the detector. This produces successive signals for each sample which increase with increasing reaction development until levelling off at the end. This type of assembly is designed for subjecting a specific type of sample to measurements of one or several parameters, i.e. it is a specific type of design Depending on the number of determinations which can be performed, it can be classified as single-parameter or multi-parameter.

Flow Methods

Unlike batch methods, where samples are held in individual vessels, in flow methods all samples are introduced at the same point and travel the same path. Flow assemblies consist of a variable number of lines (a manifold) through which the sample and reagents are propelled on their way to the detector. This entails establishing a liquid (or gaseous) flow called the '*carrier stream*', into which samples are inserted. The samples are propelled through the closed system as far as the detector. On its way from the insertion point to the detector, the sample is subjected to one or more reactions (or any other type of analytical operation) in order to condition it properly for the determination.

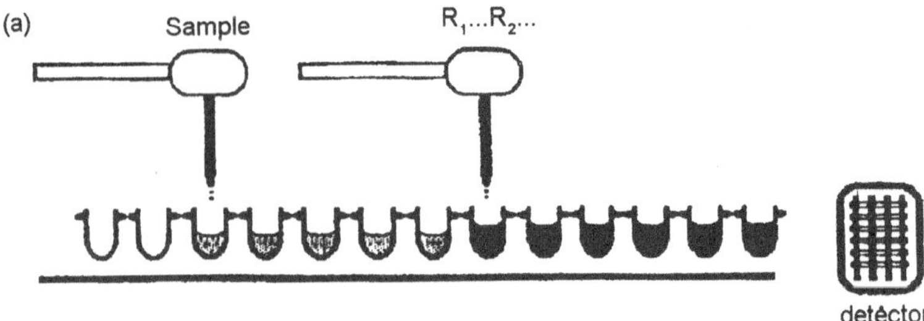

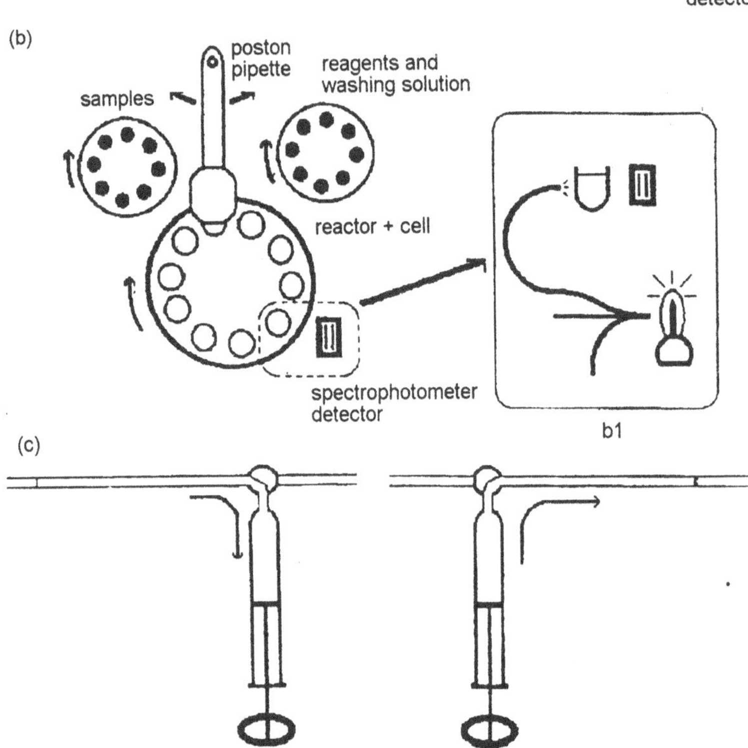

Fig. 3.2. Discrete analysers. Each sample preserves its physical integrity by being placed in a vessel, (a) Sample vessels are linked to an endless chain; (b) sample (reactor+cell) vessels make a closed circle; (b1) simultaneous determination in different cells by means of the optical fibre; (c) piston pipette for loading and unloading sample or reagent solutions.

According to the type of flow used, flow methods can be classified as:

1. Segmented-flow methods;
2. Continuous-flow methods; and
3. Stopped-flow methods.

The essential difference between the first and the second methods is that in the first, the liquid flow is periodically segmented with air bubbles. Such a difference is not merely operational, but results in two different physico-chemical methodologies.

The term '*stopped-flow methods*' is applied to kinetic methods involving mixing of the sample and reagents in the detector cell in order to perform periodic measurements for monitoring reaction development. This type of method is rarely considered to be of the automatic type. We should note that the '*continuous-flow*' concept does not exclude occasionally stopping the flow (for example, to allow the reaction to proceed without increasing sample dispersion in the carrier). Continuous-flow methods are also kinetic methods: measurements are performed during the course of the reaction without the need to wait for equilibrium to be reached. Therefore, some continuous- flow methods frequently include halting of the flow.

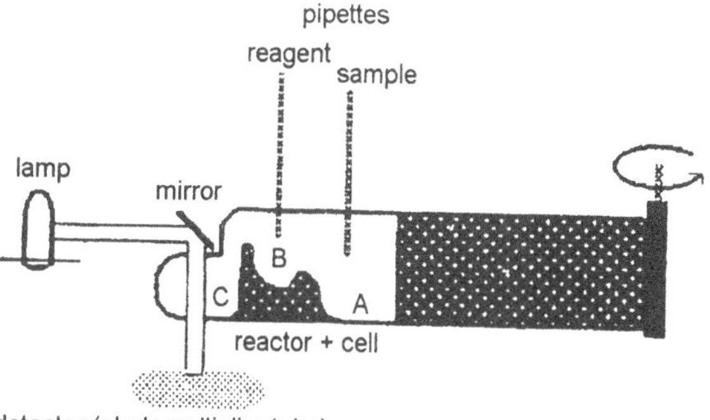

Fig. 3.3. Scheme of the reactor + cell of an automatic centrifugal analyser.

Segmented-flow Methods

As can be seen, the sample is introduced into the system by aspiration and swept to the detector by the carrier. The flowing stream is segmented by air bubbles that are primarily intended to avoid carry-over between successively processed samples. The instrumentation required has been commercially available for some time and includes the following essential elements:

1. The *propulsion unit*, which functions to produce the liquid flow. There are various types of units and pumps, the most widely used of which is the peristaltic pump (see Section 3.2.2), which allows one readily to adjust the appropriate flow-rate for each application.
2. The *sample and bubble insertion system.* Samples and bubbles are aspirated into the system by means of a moving arm. A plug of washing liquid can also be aspirated between samples. The inserted sample volume is a major variable and should therefore be highly reproducible.

   By controlling the aspiration flow-rate and time, a fixed amount of sample can be inserted into the manifold; this is the so-called 'fixed-time' procedure, the accuracy and reproducibility of which rely on dependable functioning of the peristaltic pump and timer used. Alternatively, the amount of sample that is introduced can be controlled via the *aspirated volume* by means of two strategically placed electrodes at the insertion point governing a moving pipette. This procedure is more accurate and technically more complex. Like the previous one, it entails using electronic or computer equipment to control the inserted sample volume.

   Sample insertions are alternated with volumes of a solvent or 'washing' liquid to flush any residues of the previous sample and avoid carry-over to the next. The washing liquid is usually employed at a 1:2 ratio with the sample, even though higher ratios (6:1 and 9:1) are also occasionally used. The throughput is usually in the region of 40–60 samples/h but can reach up to 150 samples/h. Inserting air bubbles between each sample and the washing liquid prevents the former from dispersing in the latter.
3. The *reactor*. The reagent solutions are merged with the sample, with which they mix as a result. The reaction zone may include heaters, dialysers, filters, columns or solid beds. Both the length and the inner diameter of the reactor, and any ancillary elements, are influential (void volumes should be minimized or completely avoided, if possible).
4. The *detector* is used to monitor continuously the solution that is passed through it; in response, it produces a signal on passage of each sample. Before it reaches the detector, the flow must be debubbled in order to avoid spurious signals arising from phase differences. This is accomplished by means of a *debubbler* located immediately before the detector. However, the debubbler can be dispensed with if the detector concerned can discriminate between the signal produced by the sample and those due to liquid-air and air-liquid phase changes.

The detectors used in segmented-flow methods are similar to those employed in other analytical methodologies with the sole exception that they must use a flow-cell. Their frequency of use by type is also similar; thus, 70 per cent of segmented-flow applications use a UV-vis spectrophotometer, followed by 10 per cent that employ a potentiometer.

The debubbler functioning is quite simple. The manifold line is split into two, of which one is aimed upwards and the other downwards. In this way, air (and some liquid) is released from the former. Debubblers are preferably integrated in the flow-cell in order to minimize carry-over between successive samples.

The signals produced by these assemblies correspond to a time after which equilibrium is reached: both chemical equilibrium (completion of the sample-reagent reaction) and physical equilibrium (attainment of a constant composition in the sample zone). Hence the analytical signal is constant throughout the sample zone. The signal obtained from empirical results is not perfectly rectangular, mainly because of mixing between adjacent segments when bubbles are removed.

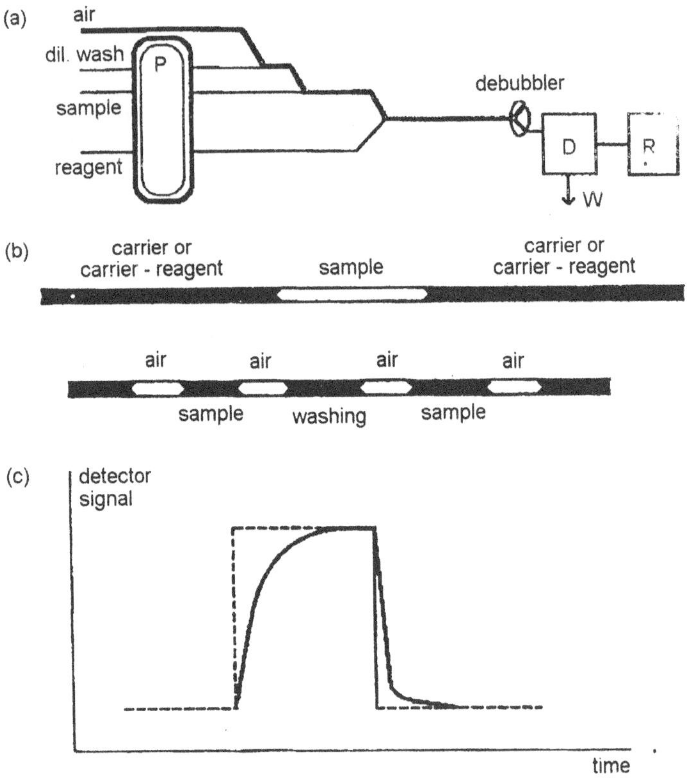

Fig. 3.4. Components of a segmented flow-analyser (SFA). (a) Scheme of a basic SFA manifold; (b) view of the segmented-flow; (c) characteristic profile of the transient signal provided by an SFA manifold.

Carry-over in this type of assembly usually arises from the tip of the moving arm that aspirates the samples (it is introduced into each sample to be processed in sequence); this entails washing the tip carefully between samples. Also, bubbles do not completely sweep sample residues adhered to tubing walls, there always remains a liquid film that prevents close contact between air and the walls, and acts as a contaminating vehicle by retaining a portion of each sample that is circulated through the tubing. Finally, in removing air bubbles from the liquid flow, two consecutive samples may mix to some extent in the absence of a physical barrier between the two; consequently, the distance from the debubbler to the detector flow-cell should be as short and the intervening path as clear as possible.

One other potential shortcoming is baseline drift, which can be quite significant after prolonged periods (physical and chemical changes can give rise to marked alterations of the signals after one hour or more of functioning). The drift is usually corrected with the aid of a computer and/or standards.

Robots in the Analytical Process

Essentially, a robot mimics the actions of a human operator. A laboratory robot usually consists of a moving arm fitted with a 'hand' that affords the movements required to transfer objects between places. For efficient operation, the objects to be handled and the instruments where they are to be placed should obviously be located near the robot. A robot's scope is limited to its close environment; this entails setting up a *workstation* where the robot and all the instruments on hand are interfaced to a computer. The computer commands the robot to perform an appropriate operation each time, and acquires and processes the data supplied by the instruments.

According to the definition of the Robot Institute of America, a robot is a reprogrammable, multipurpose manipulator, capable of moving objects and performing pre-programmed tasks. This definition encompasses the essential features of a robot that distinguish it from other automatic systems. Thus, the ability to perform tasks other than those programmed in advance endows robots with a high flexibility for adaptation that makes them more versatile analytical tools. The programming, reprogramming or even self-programming (feedback) facilities of some robots depend on the complexity of the software and hardware of the governing computer (i.e. of its 'intelligence').

The operational flexibility of a robot (or, properly, a robot station) increases with its ability to communicate with its environment. Thus, robots equipped with special sensors can not only be programmed and reprogrammed by a human operator, but also make decisions by themselves in real time. Theoretically, there are no analytical constraints to a robot's performance. Robots can take care of any type of agitation (whether mechanical, magnetic or vibrational), heating, extractions, weighing, liquid transfers, etc. Some robots can perform 'entire' analyses whereas others function as 'servers' for analytical instruments. The latter only take part in the initial analytical operations (viz. those of mechanical nature involving handling of the sample). For example, there are uncomplicated robots for weighing mineral samples: the system weighs samples, adds acids, transfers vessels to a microwave oven for digestion, dilutes the resulting solution, transfers it and, finally, flushes the vessels used in the previous steps. Other robots function to inject samples into a chromatograph or an FIA assembly, or to determine the total polyphenol content in olive oil, for example. The sample must be weighed, diluted with n- hexane and extracted twice with 60:40 methanol. The alcoholic extract is then injected into the FIA manifold. The time used in these operations is typically about 30 min and the reproducibility, as relative standard deviation (RSD), 1.6 per cent. Some robots have been used as servers for FIA systems, as in the determination of total vitamin C in foods, where the robot performs the extraction and purification involved, or in the determination of metals in lubricating oils. Both comprise the following basic elements:

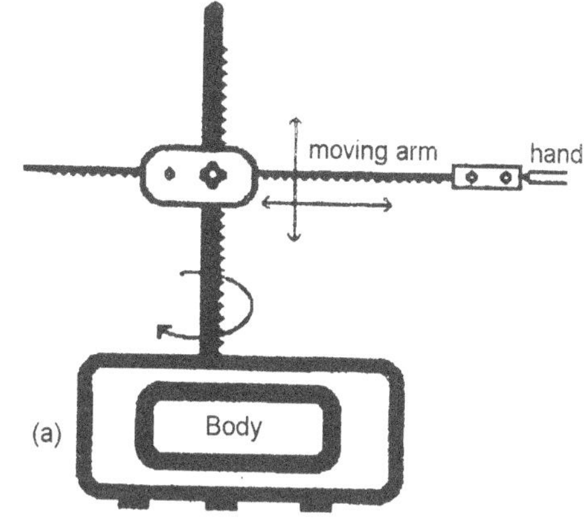

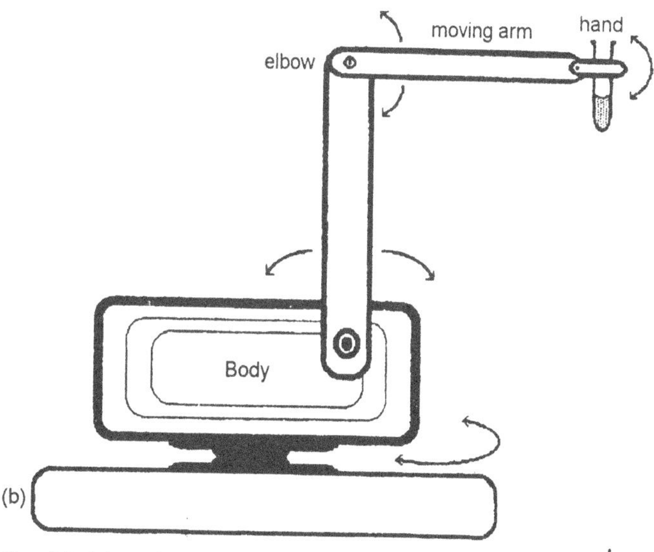

Fig. 3.5. Schematic configurations of laboratory robots, (a) Cylindrical configuration; (b) revolute configuration.

1. The *manipulator* (the part actually shown in the figure), which consists of a stand (the static portion) and an arm (the moving portion). The arm can be articulated and can include an elbow, a hand or even fingers (occasionally articulated as well).
2. The *power supply*, which should be adapted to the particular task. In analytical laboratories, the robot need not be able to carry large masses or move especially rapidly, so it requires no hydraulic or pneumatic supply; rather, it uses an electrical power supply.
3. The *controller*, which programs and commands the movements the robot is to perform. In its most simple version, this is done by point-by-point programming via a keyboard or by use of computer software at various levels (joint, coordinate and object).
4. *Sensing systems*, which can be of the stand-alone type or integrated into the '*robot body*', and are available in various types including optical, acoustic (usually an ultrasonic source), tactile, etc. The most simple optical sensor for this purpose consists of two photodetector LEDs (light-emitting diodes) at the hand that trigger the robot's movement when the light beam between them is interrupted. More recently, diode arrays have gained wide acceptance in this context. Alternatively, a conventional TV camera is equally useful.

The workstations comprise various types of connection: between the robot and the different apparatuses integrated in the station (mechanical); between the robot and the computer; and between the computer and the human operator.

Quality control applications have by far been the most receptive to the use of robots. For example, a number of pharmaceutical laboratories have installed robot workstations for content uniformity assays, dissolution testing and stability studies, among others. Between 40 and 75 per cent of the time devoted to sample manipulation in one such laboratory is used in manual, tedious operations such as weighing, sample and reagent transfer, dissolution, etc., which are a bottleneck for increased productivity and detract from quality of analytical results.

The determination of moisture by use of the Karl-Fischer method is one of the most frequently employed titrations in the pharmaceutical laboratory. The operational sequence involves the following steps: (1) addition of the solvent to the titration vessel; (2) titrating with the Karl-Fischer

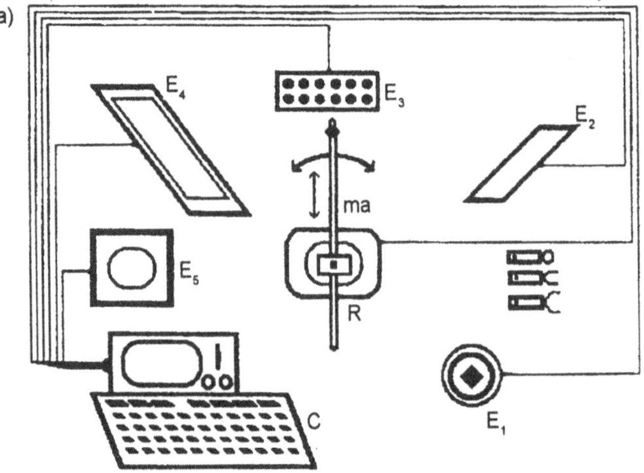

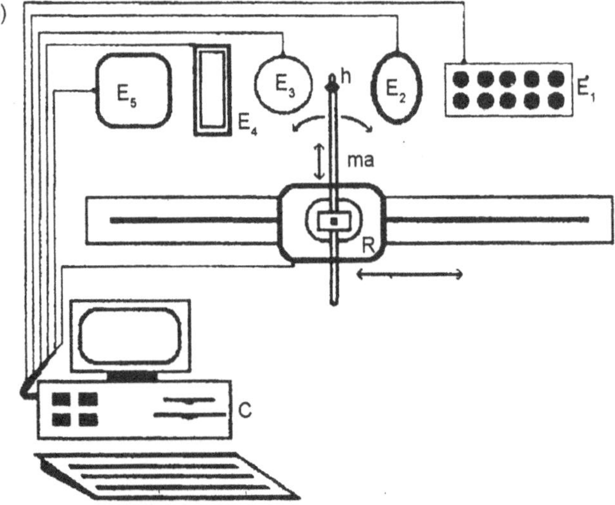

Fig. 3.6. A robot integrated in a workstation, (a) Robot operating in a circular space; (b) robot provided with displacement operating in a linear workstation.

reagent; (3) weighing the sample and placing it in the titration vessel; (4) titrating; and (5) calculating the moisture content. A dedicated workstation can simultaneously prepare and weigh several samples for subsequent titration while others are being titrated.

The operations involved in the initial manipulation of the sample are of a widely variable nature, so they escape automation unless such flexible means as robots are available. The first step in this direction is to define the laboratory unit operations (LUOs) needed and the sequence in which they are to be performed: weighing, grinding, liquid (reagent or solvent) dispensing, conditioning (heating, cooling, mixing), separation (extraction, filtration, centrifugation) and, finally, data acquisition and processing. After LUOs and their order of implementation are established, the configuration of the workstation is adapted to the specific purpose.

Analytical Uses of Robot Stations: Advantages and Disadvantages

Decreased costs aside, robot stations offer a number of assets. Thus, they are estimated to be able to perform four times as much work as a human operator in the same time—in fact, they have no coffee breaks or weekends off—and they carry out potentially hazardous operations, and ensure greater reliability in the results. In fact, replacing a human operator with a robot increases the precision of results. Humans perform differently under different conditions, whereas a robot always acts the same, whatever its 'circumstances'. Robots never make an error out of tiredness or boredom; nor do they make transcription mistakes. The limiting factor for precision in many tests is the operator's technique. By way of example, the variation (as RSD) obtained in an analysis of amino acids was decreased from 5 per cent with manual preparation of the sample to 3 per cent by use of an autosampler and, further, to 2 per cent by use of a robot.

The increasingly better precision, detection limits, accuracy and efficiency of instrumental methods is running parallel to increasingly stringent demands for results of control tests contained in the regulations issued by competent bodies worldwide. Notwithstanding the above-mentioned, well-documented advantages, robots have some shortcomings. Thus, programming a robot to perform such an ordinary task as a titration involves hundreds of steps that can easily take days or weeks to fine tune. A robot does not work like a human operator, so its actions must be optimized from a different standpoint. Some steps involve complicated processes that demand heavy programming. Also, not every robot movement can be as rapid; thus, while translational (lengthwise and vertical) movements can be fairly quick, rotation movements are invariably slow. In addition, a robot may take more time than a skilled operator to perform a routine task. All these have an impact on analysis times.

The more complicated a process is, the more error-prone it will be. For example, if a procedure comprises 100 steps and the confidence of each is 90 per cent, the likelihood of one or more mistakes being made during the process will be greater than 60 per cent. Accordingly, a robot should not always be allowed to operate unattended. Small changes in the size and shape of laboratory containers are no hindrance for a laboratory worker; on the other hand, all vessels to be handled by a robot should be highly uniform as its movements are programmed to be identical time after time. International regulations for the standardization of vessel sizes are missing in this context.

Space use in a workstation is crucial. For example, a fixed-stand robot typically operates within a radius of 60 cm horizontally and 50–60 cm vertically. A robot moving over a rectangular space or operating rectangular instruments is an oddity. The most effective way of arranging things around a robot varies with the particular task. Thus, the limited scope of the robot restricts the number and type of peripherals it can access; replacing one peripheral or the robot itself may entail reprogramming the entire process. Optimizing space accessibility entails using a mobile robot or several stationary units for transferring objects in both directions. Successful automation of a laboratory demands some conceptual changes from those that are to perform the automated analyses and those in charge of purchasing and managing the equipment needed. Operators will obviously require special training in the new operations and an open mind to the changes. State-of-the-art performance in massive routine analyses (whether clinical, pharmaceutical or environmental) rests on effective personnel training or even retraining in many instances.

Automating one or more analytical operations deprives the analyst of control over the underlying physico-chemical processes. In the long run, the detachment can lead to decreased interest in the influence of each experimental factor or parameter on the analysis as a whole. Many times, some parameters such as pH, temperature, etc., have decisive effects on quantitativeness, throughput and the accuracy of the final results, for example. It should be noted that not all samples are identical (not even those in a routine analytical batch). The above-mentioned lack of interest in turn leads to overestimating the quality of automated work and to less critical assessment of the results. One should never be blinded by the seemingly brilliant advantages of automation (increased safety and efficiency, and decreased tedious work).

The above-mentioned conceptual changes also involve management officials (to an even greater extent than operators) since automating a laboratory entails making precise decisions as regards the most suitable choice among the wide variety available today. Defining the actual needs entails determining whether certain manual operations should be automated or an automated sequence of unit operations (or even a multi-user system) be designed instead. Multi-user systems rely on full laboratory automation. They simultaneously control the work of several operators as regards manipulation of samples and standards, acquisition and delivery of results, etc. This is organized around a laboratory network. The laboratory is split into several sections, each having its own system but subject to centralized data management and decision making; the resources of every line (in each system) are accessible by all users. In addition to identifying the actual needs and choosing the best solution, there is the need to maintain not only laboratory parts and dealer supplies, but also such items as software and operators' skill (through updating and retraining courses). These pose thorny problems that demand careful planning.

Brief History of FIA Definitions

An accurate definition for a methodology or an action field of human activity is always of assistance in correctly exploiting its full potential. Faced with the dilemma of whether to develop and teach the theoretical side of a new procedure or train unskilled operators in its practice, one can reach for the highly eclectic assertion that 'nothing is as practical as a good theory'. Accordingly, many FIA workers have striven to provide apt definitions for the technique. Many definitions have become obsolete in the process. Therefore, a chronological review of FIA definitions may help one to grasp its full potential and understand its historical evolution.

The earliest definition was put forward by the parents of this technique, Ruzicka and Hansen, who in 1975 defined FIA as 'the sequential insertion of discrete sample solutions into an unsegmented continuously flowing stream with subsequent detection of the analyte'. In their later monograph on FIA (Ruzicka and Hansen, 1981), they expanded the original definition as follows: 'a method based on injection of a liquid sample into a moving unsegmented continuous stream of a suitable liquid. The injected sample forms a zone, which is then transported toward a detector that continuously records the absorbance, electrode potential, or any other physical parameter, as it continuously changes as a result of the passage of sample material through the flow cell'. This is an empirical definition that merely describes the experimental phenomenon and has no physico-chemical implications.

In 1981, Steward, another pioneer of FIA, put forward an also empirical definition that was even less concerned with the physico-chemical foundation of the technique: 'Flow injection analysis (FIA) may be defined as the sequential insertion of discrete sample solutions into an unsegmented continuously flowing stream with subsequent detection of the analyte.'

In the second monograph on FIA, published in 1984 by Valcarcel and Luque de Castro, the authors evaded an explicit definition; rather, they emphasized some key aspects', namely: FIA is an unsegmented-flow technique that involves direct injection of the sample, and its controlled, reproducible partial dispersion; also, neither physical nor chemical equilibrium is ever reached and operational timing is highly reproducible. In addition, they emphasized the straightforward, inexpensive instrumentation it requires in relation to other automatic analytical methodologies, and its high precision and accuracy.

By 1986, FIA had reached such enormous development and was so widely popular that some authors noted how early workers on this technique could hardly have envisioned what the future held. In order to avoid risking obsolescence in the near future, the following definition was proposed: 'FIA is a continuous-flow sample/reagent(s) processing approach that avoids air segmentation for dispersion control.' Actually, insertion of air bubbles after each sample plug was soon to come.

At a later stage the proponents of the first definition were more precise in stating that FIA provided 'information gathered from a concentration gradient formed from an injected, well-defined zone of a fluid, dispersed into a continuous unsegmented stream of a carrier... The absence of air segmentation, and the injection of sample solution into a continuously flowing stream, resulting in a transient output signal, appear to be the most distinctive features of FIA'. Steward (1989) also expanded his original definition by stating that 'FIA can be viewed basically as an unsegmented liquid sample handling system. Once sequential liquid samples are placed in a liquid stream, the analyte can be moved, concentrated, diluted, reacted, purified, and delivered to any detector without intervention of an operator. Such operations frequently yield assays with greater accuracy, precision, throughput, and sometimes, better sensitivity than their manual counterparts.' However comprehensive, the core of the definition is in the first sentence: 'liquid sample handling systems'. This excludes heterogeneous samples, among others. On the other hand, few authors would willingly accept that FIA is a sampling handling system, not only because they process solid or gaseous samples, but also, especially, because FIA is progressing towards the full automation of the analytical process and has been applied to non-analytical processes.

Some authors have opted for more descriptive and straightforward definitions such as the following: 'the FIA technique is based on reproducible injection of a defined sample volume into a continuous-flow liquid stream. At certain points, specific reagents are added'. This type of definition is scarcely illustrative of the potential of FIA methodology, particularly in view of the dramatic breakthroughs that followed its inception. Fang (1992) reviewed the pitfalls of the early definitions and the state of the art of FIA, which he thought should be clearly apparent from a proper definition. He therefore asserted that FIA was 'a non-chromatographic flow analysis technique for quantitative analysis, performed by reproducibly manipulating sample and reagent zones in a flow stream under thermodynamically non-equilibrated conditions'. This statement omits formerly 'non-negotiable' points as a result of Fang's critical revision of previous definitions. Thus, as regards the sample:

1. No mention is made of injection or insertion of the sample in order not to exclude reversed FIA—one might say that it is a well-defined liquid portion rather than a sample which is injected.
2. Of course, there is no injection, but rather intercalation or insertion, which is more reproducible as it does not rely on the operator's skill.
3. The sample is not always transferred to the detector; for example, in assemblies involving precipitation and retention on a filter, the sample itself need not reach the detector. This is also the case with the formation of gaseous derivatives that are separated by dialysis or volatilization (as in hydride generation procedures) and subsequently transferred to the detector and monitored in a gaseous state.

Regarding the flow, it is worth noting the phrase '*unsegmented continuous flow*'. This excludes the stopped-flow mode and the use of preconcentration (absorption or ion-exchange) columns when the sample is 'stored' for some time and then eluted. The word 'unsegmented' is also inappropriate because some applications use small air bubbles or, as stated above, the sample is converted into a gaseous derivative. Of course, Fang's definition emphasizes production of analytical information without the need for equilibrium to be reached and clearly states that the analytical information obtained is purely quantitative.

The definition admits a few additional considerations. Thus, FIA is not a chromatography, but nor is it many other things. There is no reference to the frequent use of heterogeneous (liquid-liquid, solid-liquid and gas-liquid) systems. Also, FIA assemblies used to derive non-quantitative analytical chemical information (e.g. determinations of complex stoichiometries or calculations of stability or extraction constants) are excluded, and so are FIA systems including a diode array detector, which provides qualitative information as well. Fang's definition also excludes kinetic applications of FIA. In the wait for new, more precise definitions, FIA can be described as 'a flow analysis methodology gathering analytical information, performed by reproducibly manipulating well- defined liquid zones in homogeneous or heterogeneous closed systems, under thermodynamically non-equilibrated conditions'.

The difficulty of defining FIA work arises from the fact that the methodology is not one more analytical choice; rather, it has become an unconventional working philosophy for implementation of virtually any analytical operation (gravimetry, liquid-gas separation, microwave oven digestion and column chromatography included) that was formerly addressed with conventional means. Defining FIA in a few words is thus adventurous. It is probably more illustrative and appropriate to think of it as a new approach to laboratory work, 'a comprehensive analytical methodology that is implemented in a closed system under dynamic flow conditions'. FIA is a short cut to obtaining more analytical information of a high quality with sparing use of materials, samples and reagents, in addition to reduced operational time and effort.

All in all, stating that FIA facilitates implementation of any analytical operation provides an unreal, incomplete picture of this technique. In fact, some of its applications are more physico-chemical than analytical in nature. Also, as suggested by Mottola (1986), it could be used for expeditious implementation of organic syntheses. It is therefore seemingly clear for now that defining FIA and establishing its boundaries is treading on slippery ground. The boundaries are imposed by the ingenuity of its users rather than by the present possibilities of the methodology, and will surely be expanded in the future. At this point, we might copy Reilley' s definition in his attempt at resolving the eternal dispute over what analytical chemistry was and should be: 'Analytical chemistry is what analytical chemists do.' Similarly, FIA could be said to be 'whatever its practitioners can think of'; however, no one will probably be content with such a laconic definition. That the definition is laconic does not mean that it is not true or even factual, since predicting how a methodology that can be used with virtually any analytical technique and equipment (and applied even to non-analytical problems) is going to evolve is far from easy. Putting forward a prediction is thus close to playing a game of chance.

We can state, however, that the explosion of papers on FIA has attracted widespread interest on flow techniques. On the one hand, this has resulted in a growing number of researchers adopting flow methodologies, both FIA proper and otherwise (e.g. the so-called controlled dispersion mode). On the other hand, it signals the birth of new flow methodologies that have been conceived and developed by FIA trainees and experts. This has led to improved analytical performance and increasing automation, as well as to expansion to fields formerly outside the scope of the analyst. Somewhat less adventurous and certainly not a game of chance, would be to foresee the near future from methodologies already established or at an early stage of development. I have two specific examples in mind, namely SIA (sequential injection analysis) and multicommutation techniques. In the latter, the manifold consists of several solenoid valves, one of which acts as a stand-alone commutator. The flow is established by a peristaltic pump and sample and reagents are inserted alternately as small fragments into the carrier via the solenoid valves; the result is a plug consisting of alternate sample and reagent segments. Because of the zero dispersion at contact surfaces, they tend to form a homogeneous solution as they approach the detector, the solution where the reaction of interest rapidly takes place. Even though it is still too soon to discuss and compare the features and advantages (or disadvantages) of this methodology, it is worth noting the very small sample volumes that can be used (down to 2 μl) with good reproducibility (RSD less than 3 per cent), which can result in a high throughput and, especially, low reagent consumption (about 0.7 mg per sample). The determination of creatinine in urine was carried out with sample volumes of 0.5 μl, with a sample throughput of 24 per h and an RSD of 2.9 per cent.

The distinct feature of sequential injection (SI) is that it does not rely on liquids flowing in the same direction; rather, the flow direction is continually changed in a programmed manner. The aspirated sample volume is placed in the holding coil and then supplied with an also accurately measured volume of reagent. Since the velocity on the flow axis is twice the mean velocity (that at the walls is very low), the alternate displacement in both directions leads to the central nucleus of each zone penetrating into the adjacent ones. If radial mixing is achieved by using an appropriate geometric configuration for the coil, then the final result is thorough mixing of the sample and reagent to form the reaction products. Such products can be driven to the detector or even be stopped at the flow-cell to measure their rate of formation. The technical difference between SI A and classical FIA is that the latter uses one-way flow and the former a pre-programmed swinging flow.

These two techniques signal one possible trend in the evolution of FIA to new horizons for analytical flow work. If these and further new methodologies result in improving the analytical performance of FIA and increase the automatability of the overall analytical process, they will certainly be adopted in all those areas which have long demanded flexible automation capabilities at a low cost (clinical analysis, industrial process control, etc.).

4

Electroanalytical Measurement

Electrochemical detection involves two different types of measurement: of the property of the solute (analyte) and of the electrical property of the solution. The former type relies on the transfer of charge between the analyte and the electrically active surface of the electrode. The analyte is contained in a liquid or gaseous phase and the active (conducting or semi-conducting) surface is solid or liquid (immiscible with the analyte solution in the latter case). Because a charge-transfer reaction between solute ions or molecules and the electrode is required, the detector provides isolated measurements rather than average concentrations in the flowing stream. Because of the redox reaction involved (an electron transfer between the analyte and the electrode surface), the signal obtained is proportional to the analyte concentration or activity in the vicinity of the working surface. These detectors are of the destructive type inasmuch as they are based on a redox reaction of the analyte.

In practice, however, they are non-destructive as no reaction takes place (e.g. potentiometers measure at a zero Faradaic current) or the amount of analyte that is destroyed is negligible. Potentiometry, voltammetry and coulometry belong to this group. The second group of electrochemical measurements consists of measurements of the electrical properties of the solution, including conductivity and capacitance measurements. Conductimeters are scarcely selective, non-destructive and fairly universal detectors. Their use is limited to the continuous monitoring of analytes. Their low sensitivity, high background noise and strong dependence on the working temperature are major hindrances to extensive application.

Measurements based on charge transfers are more than acceptably precise and relatively selective (the selectivity can be increased by careful choice of the experimental conditions). The very nature of the electrochemical processes involved, which take place over a small active surface, makes this type of measurement more attractive and convenient for miniature detectors than are average measurements of a given solution volume.

The most frequent problem encountered in this respect arises from interactions between the sample and the electrode surface (e.g. adsorption on the electrode surface or interference with the chemical or electrochemical reactions of the analyte at the active surface). This is frequently the result of poisoning of the electrode, which is particularly frequent with solid electrodes.

The active surface is poisoned through adsorption of foreign substances that give rise to passivation and, ultimately, decreased signals. The choice of the electrode material and measurement technique to be used is dictated by the nature of the analyte to be determined. The use of solid-state electrodes is often hindered by gradual impurification of the surface through adsorption of large molecules of surfactants or reaction products.

Continuous-flow Measurements

Flow injection analysis has been used in conjunction with a wide variety of electrochemical detectors: potentiometric, amperometric, conductimetric, voltammetric and chronopotentiometric. There is no single universal choice in this respect, and ion-selective electrodes continue to be the most frequently employed in FIA applications, followed by chemically modified electrodes (particularly enzyme electrodes).

There are two distinguishing features between flow and batch electrochemical measurements: the active surface of the sensor should be mechanically stable against the flowing stream; and except in continuous monitoring applications, the sample plug exhibits a characteristic length and profile, so the residence time in the detector is limited. Therefore, the time constants involved (from sample insertion into the carrier to acquisition of the analytical signal) should be small enough to suppress any distortions in the sample profile or signal. In addition, the small cells used in continuous-flow applications (particularly liquid chromatography) exhibit a high impedance and deviate from the general rule that the dimensions of the electrochemical cell should be much greater than the thickness of the diffusion layer. Consequently, the detection conditions should always be established from measurements made with a flow-cell rather than those provided by large cells in batch experiments.

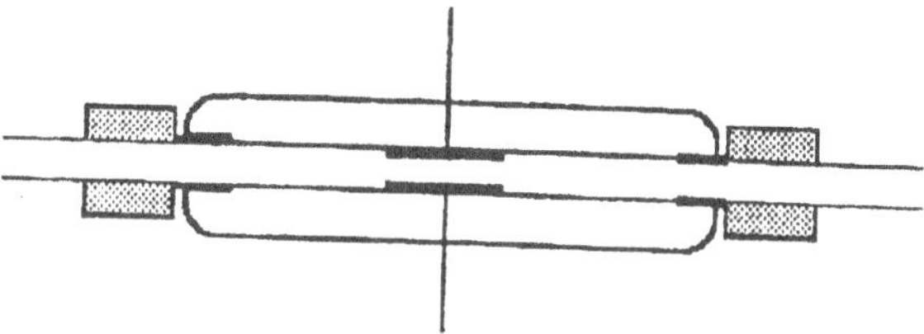

Fig. 4.1. Conductimetric flow-cell.

Flow-through electrochemical detectors can be classified according to design features such as the geometry of the indicator electrode (the location of the active surface) into annular, rod-shaped and impingement detectors. Annular detectors are rings of the same diameter as the inner diameter of the transport tubing. Rod-shaped detectors are pieces of metal wire that are placed in the middle of the flowing stream.

Finally, impingement detectors receive the flowing stream normally or tangentially to the active surface, which can be planar or otherwise (usually spherical). Electrochemical detectors used in FIA can also be classified according to the location of the reference electrode, which can be placed next to the working electrode in the same cell or in a terminal cavity by which the flowing stream is passed prior to being discarded. However, FIA electrochemical applications are usually classified according to the type of electrical parameter that is monitored and hence the detection technique used: potentiometry, amperometry, etc. In summary, electrochemical detectors feature a high sensitivity, wide linear range, selectivity against non-electroactive species, low cell dead volume and reduced costs. However, many electrodes have too short a service life or poor stability and selectivity. Improving their performance—particularly with regard to flow-through detectors—is a pressing need for dealing with complex samples or performing large batches of routine analyses such as those involving clinical and environmental samples.

Conductimetry

FIA conductimetry has been scarcely implemented in various types of conductimetric cells. Different home-made designs can be found in the analytical literature (but none have been used with pharmaceuticals). The annular type is placed at the end of the manifold; two electrodes are screwed into its walls, opposite each other, in such a way that both are brought into contact with the flowing stream. Another reported design consists of a chamber accommodating a copper sheet onto which two gold lines are deposited for electrodes; the two gold mounds run in the same direction as the flow. Another model comprises two stainless steel junctions (swagelok type) which act as electrodes and are connected by a piece of tubing through which the flowing stream is circulated.

Coulometry

Coulometric processes are those in which the analyte is electrodically oxidized or reduced over a long enough period to ensure its quantitative conversion to a new oxidation state. The amount of electricity required to effect the change allows determination of the amount of analyte originally present. Coulometric methods of analysis require no calibration against standards; the relationship between the measured quantity and the mass of analyte is derived theoretically. It should be noted that FIA assemblies are intended to operate fully automatically from sample introduction to detection; however, the calibration graph is run from standard solutions that are manually prepared from a stock solution. Therefore, FIA coulometric applications involve less manipulation than is typical of FIA analyses. Coulometric methods are implemented analytically in two primary ways depending on whether the electrogeneration is performed at a constant potential (potentiostatic technique) or a constant current intensity (amperostatic technique) in the working electrode. Flow injection coulometry relies on measurements of the integrated currenttime peak obtained by injecting a small amount of sample containing one or more electroactive species into an FIA manifold. For the electrode to operate in the coulometric mode (i.e. with 100 per cent efficiency), it should have a sufficiently large surface. The amount of charge to be passed through it in order to electrolyse the analyte is given by:

$$Q = n\mathrm{F}VC$$

where C is the analyte concentration and V the sample volume.

Most controlled-potential electrolytic cells operate amperometrically, i.e. the fraction of electroactive species that is electrolysed is usually less than 10 per cent of the overall amount, in contrast to 100 per cent in the coulometric mode. The methodology for application of the electrical signal and measurement of the response current is identical for coulometric and amperometric detectors, so, in principle, a given cell can be operated in both modes. However, designing coulometric cells poses some serious problems that have made them less popular than amperometric detectors.

Coulometric electrodes should have a large area and volume; consequently, they are largely incompatible with FIA and HPLC work. Thus, continuous-flow applications demand a large electrode surface area, but also as low a cell void volume as possible. Hence the scarcity of FIA coulometric applications. These shortcomings can be circumvented by refining cell construction procedures. One effective strategy in this respect is the use of two instead of the usual three electrodes (one of them, the reference electrode, also serves as the counterelectrode). In this way, the cell volume is reduced and the need for a potentiostat avoided (a low-voltage source is more than adequate). On the other hand, these cells require an appropriate electrolyte in order to ensure constancy in the potential of the reference/counter-electrode. Even if constant, such a potential cannot always be known since the potential of the working electrode does not coincide with the externally applied potential.

Ilcheva and Dakashev (1990) developed a coulometric cell for use in FIA systems, comprising a saturated calomel electrode and a porous Pt working electrode. Two earlier attempts at building appropriate coulometric cells for use in FIA included an ensemble of serially arranged electrodes aligned with the flow direction, and a radially arranged electrode set that was found to alter the shape of the current-potential curves and improve the selectivity of the coulometric detector.

Strohl and Curran (1979a,b) constructed a flow-through vitreous carbon electrode for amperometric or coulometric use in the determination of ferricyanide ion by reduction, and ascorbic acid, adrenaline and L-dopa by oxidation. Samples were injected into the carrier electrolyte, which was kept at a fixed potential. At low flow-rates (below 2–3 ml/min), the integral of the *i-E* curve represented the total conversion of ascorbic acid. The throughput was 20–30 samples/h. Complete conversion was unnecessary in many cases (the same assembly could be used in the coulometric and amperometric mode); also, increasing the flow-rate shortened the time needed to quantify the above-mentioned compounds. With a miniature electrode, the conversion was so rapid that the sample addition time was the determinant; at a flow-rate of 33.5 ml/min, the residence time in the valve-cell connector was 0.2s and that in the electrode 3.4s. The injection frequency was dependent on the interval between successive injections. For adrenaline, an intervening time of 14 s resulted in a throughput of 264 samples/h. The precision was not so good as that of classical controlled-potential coulometric techniques. The experimental set-up included a dampener for suppressing pulses produced by the peristaltic pump or changes in the flow-rate as the injection valve was opened or shut. Unlike most FIA modes, the cell volume here exceeded the sample volume. The other two electrodes were made of platinum and saturated calomel.

In subsequent work, the electrode was found to be too large and unsuitable for HPLC use. A new cell accommodating a reticulated vitreous carbon working electrode was thus designed, the most salient feature of which was the geometric symmetry (in the radial direction) between the working electrode and the counter-electrode. The reticulated structure of the working electrode resulted in a favourable area-to-volume ratio that permitted rapid coulometric conversion without significant band broadening in FIA or HPLC—operationally, band broadening was similar to that produced by a UV-vis flow-cell of 10 μl. The cell-electrode assembly was used to determine catecholamines and amoxycillin with detection limits (FIA) of *ca.* 0.1 ng (0.05 for hydroquinone) and a linear determination range of $4.6 \times 10^{-7} - 9.1 \times 10^{-6}$ M for amoxycillin, for example. The sample volume used was 62.8 μl in FIA and 20 μl in HPLC. In the determination of dipyrone or analgin, the sample was injected into an aqueous stream of 0.1 M HCl at a flow-rate of 0.3 ml/min. The drug was oxidized over a porous Pt electrode at a potential of 0.75 V against the saturated calomel electrode (SCE). The ensuing method was used both to determine the purity of bulk drugs and the dipyrone content in tablets and vials.

Coulometric Titrations

In a coulometric titration, the titrant is electro-catalytically produced by a current of fixed intensity. The product of the current intensity (in amperes) multiplied by the time (seconds) needed to reach the titration end-point gives the number of coulombs used, which is proportional to the analyte concentration. Therefore, some device (indicator) is needed to delimit the end of the reaction (i.e. the point where the entire analyte has been consumed). Most available end-point indication procedures (colour changes, potentiometric, conductimetric and amperometric measurements, etc.) can be used for this purpose. Only the titrant is electrogenerated in some cases (e.g. in the classical titration of halide ions by silver ions produced by oxidation of a metal silver anode). In others, the generating electrode also interacts with the analyte. In any case, the process should be 100 per cent efficient. Patriarche (1963) demonstrated in the 1960s the suitability of coulometric titrations for pharmaceutical analyses and the need to use no stable reagents or standards.

The procedure by which a coulometric titration is implemented in a flow assembly is as follows: the sample is injected into a carrier that leads it to a magnetically stirred mixing chamber of 0.7–0.95 ml capacity. There, the carrier stream is halted for a preset time in order to allow a fraction of the sample to enter the chamber. Inside it, two working electrodes (usually Pt) and a counter-electrode produce the titrant electro-catalytically. Therefore, the chamber is also the place where the analyte is titrated. The end-point of the titration can be indicated spectrophotometrically, using a fibre-optic lead to transfer a light beam to the chamber, which serves as the spectrophotometric flow-cell as well; alternatively, the end-point can be detected by potentiometric, conductimetric or amperometric means. After the end-point is reached, Faraday's law is applied to calculate the amount of analyte titrated. The determination range is a function of the time during which the flow is stopped and the amount of current produced. The system must be calibrated at a preset stop time.

The FIA-coulometric titration couple is applicable over wide analyte concentration ranges; because only a portion of sample is introduced into the titration chamber, a wide range of dilutions can be realized without the need for additional chambers or flow channels. The manifold is quite straightforward as it comprises a single channel, and the gradient chamber, generation chamber and detector flow-cell are the same thing. The system includes no membranes or filters, nor any other devices potentially altering the flow or deteriorating with use. The reagent is produced *in situ*, which avoids external preparation and storage; no standards are required.

The FIA-coulometric assemblies reported to date were all controlled via a computer that governed sample injection, halting of the flow, application of the titrant generating current, detection of the end-point, and reading and acquisition of the analytical signals. Reported continuous-flow coulometric titrations include those of acids and bases, phenothiazines, Karl-Fischer, olefins and other components of petroleum distillates (titrated with bromine electrogenerated by anodic oxidation of a bromide solution), and starch and corn syrup (titrated iodonuetrically). Not all these uses are FIA applications proper, even though they employ some typical FIA modules. Thus, in the determination of moisture by the Karl-Fischer method, an FIA injection valve was used as an auxiliary means for recirculating the active reagent (iodine) from the coulometric titrator. In this way, the sample was mixed and transferred to the titration cell. Similar comments can be made on the continuous-flow coulometric titration of various phenothiazines (chlorpromazine, promethazine, diethazine and trifluoperazine) in pharmaceutical preparations by the so-called 'triangle programmed titration technique', which is a flow technique but involves no injection of discrete volumes of sample or controlling its dispersion. The foundation of such an original titration lies in the continuous circulation of a sample stream that is merged with another of reagent which is electrogenerated with the aid of a triangular programmed current-time diagram.

One recent application of coulometric titrations in flow systems also dispenses with the injection valve. The analyte solution (sample) is prepared and made to an appropriate volume with the reagent to be electrolysed; a similar operation is performed with distilled water instead of the sample for blank runs. Two phenomena occur during the time that the required fraction of titrant is transferred from the generation cell to the detector: a chemical reaction between the analyte and titrant; and dispersion of the latter in the flowing stream. Therefore, the interaction of the titrant depends not only on the volume where it is produced, but also on those factors affecting its dispersion (flow-rate, inner diameter and length of the path to be travelled, and size of the generating and detection cells). Detection can also rely on the analyte (the electrogenerated titrant) or some reaction product.

5

Calorimetry in Pharmaceutical Research

Calorimetry is the measurement of energy changes within a material that are either manifested as exothermic (heat liberating) or endothermic (heat consuming) events. Changes in energy (not absolute energies) are conventionally determined, and quantitative measurements may be made if the mass of the sample(s) is accurately known. Recently, nanocalorimetry or calorimetry microarrays are expanding the application of calorimeters to high throughput screening (HTS), providing high throughput thermodynamic measurements at the microgram scale. Preliminary studies using these microchip calorimeters have shown interesting potential for their applications in studying biological macromolecules in solution, such as protein ligand binding and measuring heat capacities on samples as small as 10 μg. Additional applications could include the study of the thermal properties of drug molecules in HTS.

The most common applications of calorimetry in the pharmaceutical sciences are found in the "subfields" of differential scanning calorimetry (DSC) and microcalorimetry. State-of-the-art DSC instruments and microcalorimeters are extremely sensitive and are powerful analytical tools for the pharmaceutical scientist. Differential scanning calorimetry usually involves heating and/or cooling samples in a controlled manner, whereas microcalorimetry maintains a constant sample temperature. The DSC instruments are considered to be part of the "*Thermal Analysis*" armamentarium. The beginning of this article gives a brief introduction to thermodynamics. A description of DSC, which includes instrumentation, calibration, and applications, follows. A section on microcalorimetry is next, with a brief introduction into microcalorimetry, instrumentation, calibration, and applications. The article ends with a general comment on the regulatory aspects of calorimetry. A general description of the underlying physical or chemical transitions/reactions can be found in the section on DSC.

Thermodynamics

A calorimeter consists of a container that is isolated from its exterior surroundings, where the heat exchange that occurs between the system and the environment can be measured. The "environment" is defined as the calorimeter and its contents, and the "system" is either a chemical reaction or physical change of state. The system can either absorb (endothermic) or lose energy (exothermic) to or from the environment. Exothermic changes will require the temperature of the environment to increase because it is the environment that is receiving the energy lost by the system. The energy of an isolated system remains constant and the energy exchange of the system must be equal but opposite in sign to the energy of the environment (First Law of Thermodynamics, Conservation of Energy). Endothermic changes in the system will involve a decrease in temperature of the environment because the environment is providing the energy absorbed by the system.

Based on the assumption that the system is closed, which is usually the case in DSC and microcalorimetry, any reaction or change in state is independent of the path and can be subdivided into small reversible steps (Hess' Law of Summation). The First Law of Thermodynamics states that energy may neither be created nor be destroyed. It defines the internal energy, dU, as the sum of the change in heat that has been transferred to the system, dq, and the work done on the system, dw.

$$dU = dq + dw \qquad \ldots(1)$$

When operated at constant pressure, Eq. (1) can be written in terms of the enthalpy, H. The total energy exchange between the system and the environment, the enthalpy change (dH), is the sum of the change in internal energy of the system, dU, and the change in the amount of work, PV

$$dH = dU + Pdw \text{ (at constant pressure)} \qquad \ldots(2)$$

At zero net work and negligible change in volume (a close approximation for solids and liquids), the equation reduces to

$$(dU)_P = (dH)_P = (dq)_P \qquad \ldots(3)$$

Thus, the enthalpy is effectively equal to the heat added or lost from the system, and changes in enthalpy can be measured directly in a calorimeter as dq (heat flow).

A

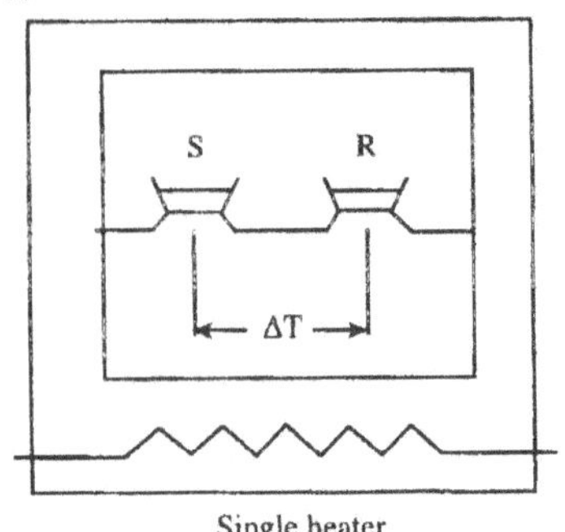

B

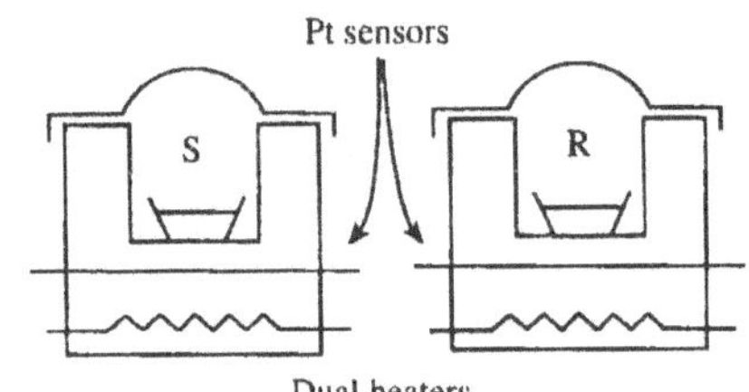

C

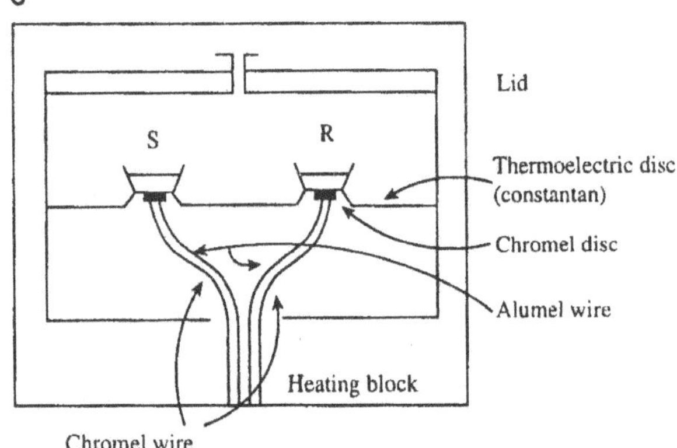

Fig. 5.1. Schematic diagrams of the (A) differential thermal analysis (DTA); (B) power-compensated DSC; and (C) heat-flux DSC cells.

The heat exchange, dq, entering or exiting the system is equal to the change in enthalpy, dH, which is related to the heat capacity, Cp

$$dq = dH = \int_{T_2}^{T_1} CpdT \qquad \ldots(4)$$

The increase in temperature of the system (from T_1 to T_2) is a function of its heat capacity. If Cp is large, then the transfer of a given amount of heat to a system results in only a small temperature increase.

Two principal DSC designs are commercially available—power compensated DSC and heat flux DSC. The two instruments provide the same information but are fundamentally different. Power-compensated DSCs heat the sample and reference material in separate furnaces while their temperatures are kept equal to one another. The difference in power required to "compensate" for equal temperature readings in both sample and reference pans are recorded as a function of sample temperature. Heat flux DSCs measure the difference in heat flow into the sample and reference, as the temperature is changed. The differential heat flow to the sample and reference is monitored by chromel/ constantan area thermocouples.

Modulated Temperature Differential Scanning Calorimetry/Dynamic Differential Scanning Calorimetry

Conventional DSC measures a sample's total heat flow. This total heat flow is comprised of a heat capacity component and a kinetic component

$$\text{total heat flow} = \text{heat capacity component} + \text{kinetic component}$$

$$dq/dt = CpdT/dt + f(T,t) \qquad \ldots(5)$$

where dq/dt = heat flow, Cp = heat capacity, dT/dt = temperature rate, $f(T,t)$ = heat flow from kinetic component as a function of temperature and time. Variations of conventional DSC have been used to extract additional information from these experiments. Two such techniques are modulated differential scanning calorimetry (MDSC) and dynamic differential scanning calorimetry (DDSC). Unlike conventional DSC, MDSC and DDSC determine the total heat flow, dq/dt, and the heat capacity component of heat flow, $CpdT/dt$. Eq. (5) then leads to the indirect determination of the kinetic component of heat flow, $f(T, t)$.

MDSC, developed by TA instruments, is based on the conventional heat flux DSC furnace design. The temperature programs differ in that a sinusoidal modulation is overlaid on the conventional linear heating or cooling rate to produce a continuously changing non-linear sample temperature. This can be viewed as running two experiments at once. The first experiment consists of heating the sample at a constant linear rate to obtain the total heat flow much like the conventional DSC. During the second experiment, the heat capacity component of the heat flow is obtained by continuously varying the temperature sinusoidally with a zero net temperature change during the course of the modulation. The experimental parameters may be optimized by modifying three variables—the average heating rate, the period of modulation, and the temperature amplitude of modulation. Fourier transformation of the modulated heat flow signal is used to calculate an average heat flow value, which is similar to the total heat flow obtained by conventional DSC. The heat capacity is determined by the ratio of the heat flow amplitude to the modulated heating rate amplitude. The heat capacity of heat flow is then obtained by multiplying the heat capacity by the average heating rate. The kinetic component heat flow is obtained by the difference between the total heat flow and the heat capacity component.

$$dq/dt = Cp(dT/dt + A_T w^* \cdot \cos wt) + f'(t; T) + A_K(\sin wt) \qquad \ldots(6)$$

where $(dT/dt + A_T w^* \cos wt)$ = measured heating rate, $f'(t,T)$ = kinetic response without temperature modulation, and A_K = amplitude of kinetic response to temperature modulation.

DDSC provides heat capacity and kinetic component information differently from MDSC. The temperature program consists of an "Iso-Scan" whereby the traditional heating rate program is combined with several isothermal holds or a "Heat-Cool" program, which consists of combined heating and cooling temperature programs. The user selects the appropriate method depending on the type of experiment being performed. From the dynamic component of the sample response, the complex heat capacity can be calculated. The complex heat capacity, Cp^*, is the vector sum of the storage, Cp', and loss heat capacity, Cp''. It is generally the same as the storage heat capacity except in the melting region where heat losses dominate. The storage heat capacity is associated with molecular motions within the sample in a manner similar to the storage modulus in dynamic mechanical measurements.

The out-of-phase component, the loss heat capacity, Cp'' is associated with the dissipative properties of the material. The loss heat capacity is out-of-phase with the temperature change because heat flow has resulted in molecular structural changes in the material. The loss tangent is the ratio of the loss heat capacity to the storage capacity and is a measure of the relative importance of each component.

$$Cp^* = Cp' + Cp'' \quad \ldots(7)$$

where Cp^* = complex heat capacity, Cp' = storage heat capacity, and Cp'' = loss heat capacity.

High Speed DSC

High speed DSC or HyperDSC is a proprietary technology developed by Perkin Elmer to be used with their power-compensated DSCs. It enables the use of very fast heating and cooling rates (100–500 K/min) that provides increased sensitivity with the compromise of reduced resolution. In the pharmaceutical industry, HyperDSC has been used for the detection of very small signals arising from weak transitions or small sample sizes (μg range). For example, some researchers have used HyperDSC to detect 1.5% amorphous content in amorphous/crystalline lactose blends. Using a fast heating/cooling rate also enables the measurement of samples while minimizing the potential for recrystallization or reorganization. The thermal properties of two polymorphs of the drug carbamazepine, Forms I and III, were studied using HyperDSC. Previously, accurate determination of the heat enthalpy of fusion of Form III had not been possible using conventional heating rates owing to concurrent exothermic recrystallization to the higher-melting Form I. The use of HyperDSC enabled the measurement of the heat of fusion by altering the kinetics of melting, where it was inhibited. Owing to its speed of analysis, it has also been proposed that HyperDSC can be used as a HTS tool for the analysis of well-understood samples.

Sample Preparation and Calibration

DSC samples are generally analyzed in small metal pans that consist of inert or treated metals (aluminum, platinum, silver, stainless steel, etc.). Several pan configurations exist such as open, pinhole, covered, or sealed. Reference pans should be made of the same material as the sample pan and in identical configurations. Typical DSC sample sizes are 3–5 mg for pharmaceutical materials. The material should completely cover the bottom of the pan to ensure good thermal contact. The pan should not be overfilled to prevent thermal lag from the bulk of the material to the sensor. Physically stable compounds that consist of large granular particles should be ground to reduce unwanted thermal effects. Accurate weights are imperative if quantitative data of the sample's energetic parameters are desired.

A scanning technique that is usually used for relative rather than absolute measurements is DSC. The meaningfulness of the results depends on the care taken in calibrating the instrument as close to the transition temperatures of interest as possible. The accuracy of any thermoanalytical instrument is strongly dependent on the use of high purity calibration standards. Well-defined standards are especially important when analyses are carried out using different instruments and at different times. In general, metal calibration standards such as indium, tin, bismuth, and lead are utilized owing to ready availability and ease of use. Low melting metals such as mercury and gallium, are used to a lesser extent because of toxicity and handling problems. Organic compounds have been recommended as standards when studying organic material to minimize differences in thermal conductivity, heat capacity, and heat of fusion. It is likely that metals will continue to be popular temperature and enthalpy standards because of availability and ease of use, and organic standards may be used predominantly at temperatures below 300 K.

The results of the DSC are dependent on the calibration of the instrument, sample preparation, and sample configuration. Some researchers argue that power compensated DSCs need to be properly calibrated upon both heating and cooling at the same rates to maintain a high level of accuracy. Standard procedures can be obtained from the American Society for Testing of Materials (ASTM). In addition, all results obtained by DSC are a function of the scanning rate used and should be reported with the scanning rate. The shape, the area of the transition or change of baseline, and particularly the temperature of the transition will be dependent on the scanning rate; it will move to higher temperatures with increasing heating rate. Increasing the scanning rate increases sensitivity, while decreasing the scanning rate increases resolution. To obtain thermal event temperatures close to the true thermodynamic value, slow scanning rates should be used (e.g., 1-5 K/min).

Definitions and Applications of DSC

The purpose of this section is to define the various parameters that are measured by DSC. The following sections will describe some of the more fundamental thermal events. Examples from the pharmaceutical field will be given to illustrate the techniques. The examples will be based on either single components such as drug substance and bulk excipients or on a mixture of components such as physical blends of drugs and excipients, solid dispersions, formulated drugs after granulation, and/or compression.

Melting

Melting is a first order endothermic process by which the compound takes in a net quantity of heat (molar heat of fusion). Through DSC, melting can be seen as an endothermic peak. The broadness of the peak defines the purity of the crystalline compound undergoing melting, with the less pure and less perfect smaller crystals melting first followed by melting of the purer larger crystals. The melting temperature is the temperature at which the three-dimensionally ordered crystalline state changes to the disordered liquid state. It is defined either as an extrapolated melting temperature onset, T_e, obtained at the intersection of the extrapolated baseline prior to the transition with the extrapolated leading edge, or as the peak melting temperature, T_m. Other temperatures that describe the melting process are the onset of melting, T_o, and the extrapolated end of the transition.

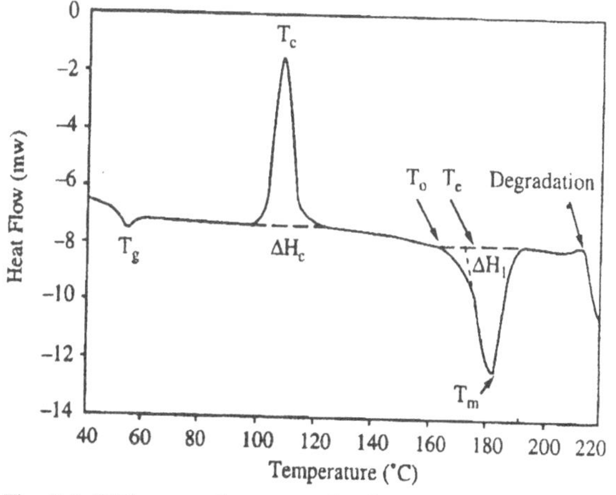

Fig. 5.2. DSC scan of sucrose showing the glass transition temperature, (T_g), recrystallization exotherm temperature (T_c) and enthalpy (ΔH_c), onset of melting (T_o), extrapolated melting onset (T_e), peak melting temperature (T_m) enthalpy of fusion (ΔH_f), and onset of degradation at 10 K/min.

The enthalpy of fusion, ΔH_f, is obtained from the area of the endothermic transition. The area of the transition is affected by the selection of the baseline. The baseline is generally obtained by connecting the point at which the transition deviates from the baseline of the scan to where it rejoins the baseline after melting is completed. For some materials that undergo a significant change in heat capacity change on melting, other baseline approximations (such as a sigmoidal baseline) are used.

Purity

The purity of crystalline compounds can be calculated using the van't Hoff equation from the enthalpy of fusion and melting temperature obtained by DSC.

$$T_{s(i)} = T_e - RT_e^2 X/(\Delta H_f F_i) \quad \ldots(8)$$

where $T_{s(i)}$ is the sample temperature at equilibrium corrected for thermal lag effects (K), T_e is the melting temperature of the pure compound (K), R is the gas constant (8.314J/mol/K), X is the molar

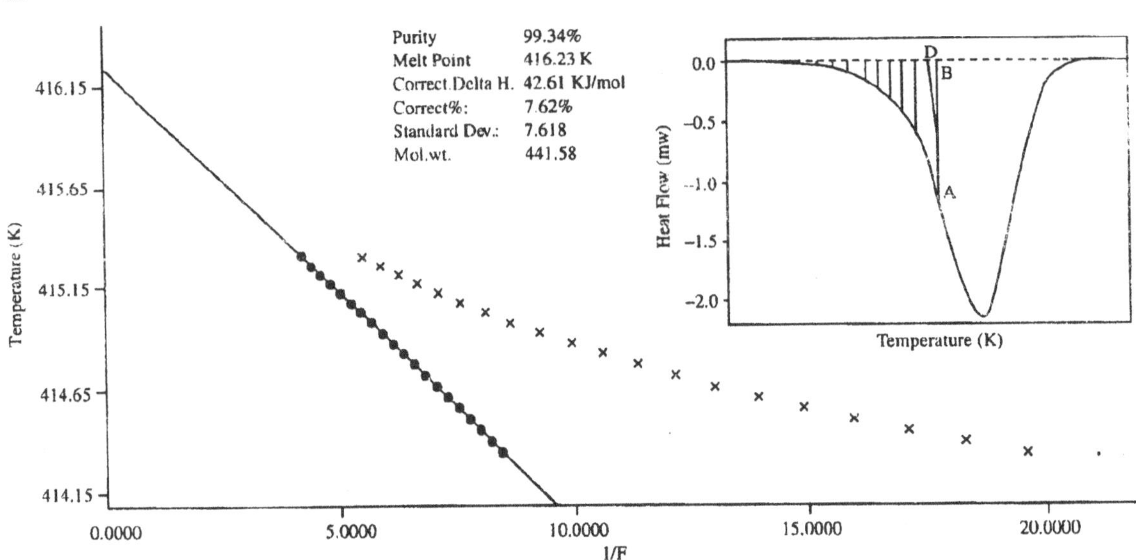

Fig. 5.3. DSC scan of drug substance divided into segments, A_i, for purity calculations of a compound of total enthalpy or area, A_T.

fraction of impurity, ΔH_f is the enthalpy of fusion of the pure compound (J/mol), and F is the fraction of the sample that is molten at $T_{s(i)}$. The melted fraction is equal to the area of the section melted (A_i) divided by the total area of the melting endotherm (A_T). The melting depression, (T_e - $T_{s(i)}$) is equal to the slope, $(RT_e^2/\Delta H_f)\ X$, of the straight line obtained when $T_{s(i)}$ is plotted as a function of $1/F_i$. The theoretical melting temperature is obtained on extrapolation to $1/F_i = 0$. A straight line may not be obtained owing to thermal lag, sensitivity, lack of a eutectic point detection, and formation of solid solutions. In addition, a significant amount of material may have melted before a measurable heat flow is observed by using DSC.

As a result, a correction constant K_{corr} is added to the measured areas (each fraction) to correct the curvature of the plot of $T_{s(i)}$ as a function of $1/F_i$. The melting depression (T_e - $T_{s(i)}$) is then obtained when $F_i = 1$.

$$1/F_i = (A_T + K_{corr})/(A_i + K_{corr}) \qquad ...(9)$$

It is necessary that the melting curve is obtained with a calibrated DSC using small samples (1-3 mg) and slow scanning speeds (<5 K/min, preferably 2 K/min). The purity of a compound should be determined at several scanning speeds to ensure that the compound does not undergo any solid-solid transitions, such as polymorphic conversion or degradation. The three advantages of obtaining purity by DSC are: (1) its speed of measurement; (2) the type of impurity does not have to be known; and (3) a minimal amount of sample is required. However, in the case of salts, excess base or acid is counted as an impurity.

Calculations of drug purity using DSC were used to assess the quality of progesterone and lipoic acid, and to define specifications for the drugs. The enantiomeric purity of (-)ephedrinum 2-naphthalenesulfonate has also been determined using DSC.

Crystallization

Crystallization can occur on cooling from the melt and/or heating above the glass transition temperature of amorphous materials. The temperature at which this occurs is the crystallization temperature, T_c. Through DSC, crystallization is observed as an exothermic transition with an enthalpy of crystallization, ΔH_c. The energy released when the molecules, atoms, or ions organize into a 3-D solid state is related to the crystal lattice energy. Some compounds can crystallize into different molecular arrangements called polymorphs, discussed later.

Quantification of Crystallinity

The crystallinity of drugs and excipients before and after formulation processing can be determined using calorimetry. In some cases, crystalline compounds can be converted during pharmaceutical processing to the amorphous form, which is a thermodynamically less stable form. Amorphous compounds consist of non-ordered molecules. This can have important implications for the chemical and physical stability of the formulations. The effect of grinding on the crystallinity of different crystal forms of indomethacin was evaluated using DSC and other techniques.

An exothermic transition can sometimes be observed by DSC on crystallization of the amorphous form. This can be used to quantify the amorphous content of crystalline drugs. A calibration curve that consists of a plot of the enthalpy of crystallization as a function of crystalline content was used to determine if the lyophilized MK-0591 drug substance was completely amorphous or contained some crystalline compound.

Polymorphism

Polymorphs are crystalline compounds of the same molecular structure that have a different arrangement of molecules in the unit cell. Polymorphs have the same chemical composition but have unique cell parameters. Therefore, polymorphs can have very different melting temperatures, densities, solubilities, chemical and physical stabilities, dissolution rates, and bioavailabilities.

Polymorphs are either enantiotropic or monotropic. Enantiotropic polymorphs have a thermodynamic conversion temperature where one form is more stable above this temperature while the other is more stable below this temperature. Processing the least stable form, dissolution/recrystallization, and certain storage conditions might cause enantiotropic polymorphs to later convert. If there is no conversion temperature below the melting temperatures of the polymorphic pair, then the different crystal forms are monotropic. That is, there is only one crystal form that is thermodynamically stable at all temperatures and pressures. Calorimetry can be used to determine which polymorph is the more stable form. The DSC can provide accurate unambiguous melting temperatures and enthalpies of fusion. Based on the melting temperature and the enthalpy of fusion, the relative thermodynamic stability of the polymorphic pair can be determined.

DSC and complimentary thermal techniques such as temperature X-ray powder diffraction were used to determine the thermodynamic relationship of the six anhydrous polymorphs of tetracaine hydrochloride. The phase diagram of the polymorphic conversion of diflunisal in polyethylene glycol 4000 solid dispersions was obtained as a function of polymer content.

Heat Capacity

Accurate heat capacity, *C*p, measurements may be obtained by DSC under strict experimental conditions, which include the use of calibration standards of known heat capacity, such as sapphire, slow accurate heating rates (0.5–2.0 K/min), and similar sample and reference pan weights. MDSC or DDSC also have been used to determine the heat capacity of several pharmaceutical materials.

Glass Transition

By the use of various pharmaceutical manufacturing processes, (e.g., lyophilization or comminution techniques), drugs or excipients may be made amorphous. Amorphous compounds are defined by their lack of long-range molecular order and structural periodicity. Their high-energy state is of great interest to the pharmaceutical industry as it can lead to fast dissolution rates and increased bioavailabilities. However, amorphous compounds are thermodynamically unstable, although depending on their glass

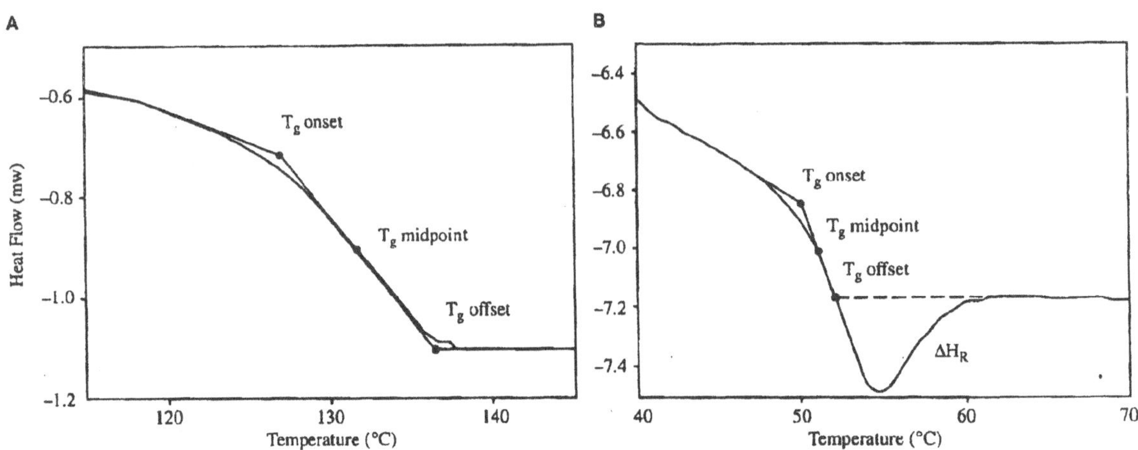

Fig. 5.4. A-DSC scan of the glass transition temperature of a miscible blend of a MK-0591 with 10% PVP, showing the onset, midpoint, and offset glass transition temperatures. B-DSC scan of the glass transition of sucrose with the enthalpic relaxation endotherm and enthalpy (ΔH_R)

transition temperature, they may be kinetically stable for extended times. Amorphous compounds are characterized by a glass transition, which by DSC is seen as an increase in heat capacity change.

$$\Delta Cp = Cp_{liq} - Cp_{glass} \qquad ...(10)$$

where Cp_{liq} is the heat capacity of the liquid, and Cp_{glass} is the heat capacity of the glassy phase. The glass transition temperature is measured either at its onset or at its midpoint. Structural relaxation can occur owing to the restricted but finite mobility of the molecules below the glass transition. This gradual volume or enthalpy change is observed by DSC as an endothermic peak superimposed on the glass transition, and this may lead to difficulties in interpretation of the transition. Modulated temperature DSC can sometimes be used to separate the enthalpic overshoot from the glass transition temperature.

Defining the glass transition temperature is important to the development of stable amorphous pharmaceutical materials. A leukotriene biosynthesis inhibitor, MK-0591, has been shown to be kinetically stable in the amorphous phase at normal storage temperatures if protected from moisture, because of its elevated glass transition temperature of 125°C. In lyophilized systems, a high T_g', defined as the apparent glass transition temperature and observed as the change of the heat capacity of the lyophilized formulations, is important to define the stability of such formulations. MDSC has been used to select optimal freeze-drying conditions to avoid cake collapse. The glass transition temperature of amorphous multicomponent mixtures can be used to determine the miscibility of the components. If the mixture is miscible, then a single glass transition temperature is usually obtained. Various equations can be used to predict the glass transition temperature of miscible mixtures. Examples include the Gordon–Taylor equation [Eq. (11)] or the Fox-Flory equation [Eq. (12)].

$$T_{g\ mix} = [w_1 T_{g1} + K w_2 T_{g2}]/(w_1 + K w_2);$$
$$K = \rho_1 T_{g1}/\rho_2 T_{g2} \qquad ...(11)$$
$$1/T_{g\ mix} = 1/T_{g1} + 1/T_{g2}$$

where ρ_1 and ρ_2 are the densities of the two components and T_{g1} and T_{g2} are their respective glass transition temperatures.

Temperature Dependence of Molecular Motions in Amorphous Materials

A critical attribute that dictates the stability and performance of any amorphous material is the manner in which its rate of molecular motions (τ) varies with changing temperature (T) (i.e., $d\tau/dT$).

At temperatures that are approximately 0–100 K above the calorimetric glass transition temperature (T_g), this property is known as the fragility of the material. Several workers have suggested that $d\tau/dT$ below T_g (in the non-equilibrium glassy state) is the most appropriate descriptor of amorphous pharmaceutical materials as this is the normal state for the storage and processing of such systems. A simple graphical plot of τ vs. T can be constructed at temperatures below T_g from the results of enthalpy relaxation experiments. These measurements can be performed using either a conventional DSC or a microcalorimeter. Alternate calorimetric methods of estimating $d\tau/dT$ at T_g have been described in the literature, but the applicability of these methods to pharmaceutical materials has not yet been clearly demonstrated.

Degradation, Decomposition, Stability Determinations, and Drug-Excipient Compatibility

The degradation, decomposition, and stability of drugs, or formulations can be determined by DSC or microcalorimetry. The advantages of the techniques are their speed of measurement and the small amounts of sample required. At times, interpretation of the results can be difficult, particularly when simultaneous reactions occur. Decomposition kinetics is generally determined using the Arrhenius equation. The samples are stored at elevated temperatures for known periods of time and analyzed by DSC. Alternatively, they can be held isothermally in the DSC at different temperatures, followed by scanning at heating rates sufficiently fast to avoid additional decomposition. A rate constant is calculated for each storage condition by plotting the logarithms of the areas of the transitions (e.g., the decomposition endotherm, etc.) as a function of time. The natural logarithm of the reaction rates, k, are then plotted as a function of $1/T$ as per the Arrhenius equation.

$$k = Ze^{-(Ea/RT)}; \ \ln k = \ln Z - E_a/RT \qquad \ldots(13)$$

where Z is the Arrhenius frequency or preexponential factor, E_a is the Arrhenius activation energy (J/mol) for the reaction, and R is the gas constant. The activation energy and preexponential factor are assumed to be constant and independent of temperature.

Alternatively, the reaction peak maxima may be determined at different heating rates (φ) and used to calculate the activation energy, assuming first order kinetics.

$$E_a = -2.19T \frac{d \log \varphi}{d(1/T)} \qquad \ldots(14)$$

The energy of activation is obtained from the slope of the log of the heating rate (φ) as a function of 1/T. It is assumed that only one reaction occurs during the transition and that the peak maximum represents a point of constant conversion for each heating rate. The method cannot be used with compounds that decompose on melting or undergo isomerizations at the reaction temperature or any other simultaneous reaction. Some modification of DSC may be needed to determine the degradation kinetics of compounds under different environmental conditions. DSC is often used for the rapid screening of excipients for drug-excipient compatibility studies. Certain assumptions have to be made, which include that the thermal properties of these mixtures are the sum of the individual components when there are no interactions between the components. The method does not take into consideration: (1) effects owing to thermal conductivity (thermal lag effects); (2) mixing effects that can lower the purity of each component resulting in slightly broader, lower melting temperatures; or (3) sample geometry effects that result in variations in peak shapes and peak temperatures. In addition, reduction in enthalpies of fusion can occur as a result of the solubilization of the drug in molten excipients. This latter phenomenon can be used in part to determine the solubility in different molten excipients.

Interactions with Water/Solvents, Hydrates

Water can have a significant impact on the physical and chemical stability of drugs. Water may be present as part of the crystalline lattice (hydrate), or it may be on the surface ("free") or more tightly incorporated ("bound"). The evaluation of the type of water present in a pharmaceutical material has been determined using subambient DSC (thermoporosimetry), such as in the case of magnesium stearate hydrates, as well as thermogravimetric techniques. Free or surface water can crystallize and the melting enthalpy of this free water can be used to calculate the surface water content of compounds from the melting enthalpy of pure water. The state of water in hydroxypropyl methylcellulose gels with and without drugs such as propranolol hydrochloride or diclofenac was determined in this way by DSC.

MICROCALORIMETRY

Microcalorimetry is used to monitor thermal changes associated with physical and/or chemical events that do not require heating or cooling for their initiation. Such events include dissolution, precipitation, reaction, and crystallization. In a typical microcalorimetry experiment, these events are "triggered" in a controlled manner by mixing two preequilibrated and separate phases (e.g., water vapor and amorphous drug, solvent and crystalline drug, or protein and carbohydrate solutions). Solid-state processes may also be measured such as in the case of drug degradation or during drug-excipient screening studies. Microcalorimetry techniques are sometimes referred to by the processes that are monitored (e.g., immersion calorimetry, solution calorimetry, titration calorimetry, etc.). Differential scanning calorimeters may be operated in isothermal mode; however, for highly accurate and reliable isothermal measurements, specially designed microcalorimeters are required.

Thermodynamics

Microcalorimeters have the ability of directly measuring the order of the reaction (n), the rate constant (k), the reaction enthalpy ($\Delta_R H$), and the equilibrium constant (K_{eq}). For example, solution microcalorimetry may be used to determine the free energy of dissolution of a solid compound, which is particularly important in pharmaceutical research for dissolution studies and in the determination of the relative thermodynamic stability of polymorphs. The change in the Gibbs-Helmholtz free energy, ΔG_{sol}, on dissolution is

$$\Delta G_{sol} = -RT \ln K_{eq} \qquad \ldots(15)$$

where T is the temperature (Kelvin, K), R is the gas constant (8.314 J/mol/K), and K_{eq} is the equilibrium constant for the change of the compound from the solid state to the dissolved liquid state. The equilibrium constant can be determined, at low concentrations, from the ratio of the concentration of the compound in the solution, or its solubility, to that in the solid state (where by definition, $[C]_{solid} = 1$).

$$K_{eq} = [C]_{soln}/[C]_{solid} = [C]_{soln} \qquad \ldots(16)$$

The ΔH_{sol} is the enthalpy change that occurs on dissolution of one mole of compound in a solvent. The solution microcalorimeter may be used to obtain the enthalpy of solution directly. The change of free energy can be calculated from the concentration using the enthalpy obtained. The change in the entropy of solution ΔS_{soln} can then be determined from the Gibbs-Helmholtz equation.

Alternatively, the change in free energy of solution ΔG_{soln} can be calculated from the van't Hoff equation

$$\delta(\Delta G_{soln}/T)/\delta T = -\Delta H/T^2 \qquad \ldots(17)$$

Additionally, in cases where the reaction of interest is monitored at atleast three different temperatures, the activation energy (E_a) of that reaction may be determined. Microcalorimeters can offer scientists a large range of important information provided that their systems are sufficiently well understood. Signals arising from more than one process may compromise quantitative results if they are not sufficiently separated. There are cases where concomitant processes, if occurring at sufficiently different reaction rates (at least 2X), may be quantitatively analyzed using an iterative procedure that is described in more detail by Skaria et al.

Instrumentation

The simplest type of non-scanning calorimeter is the isoperibol instrument. In this type of calorimeter, a constant environment is maintained inside an insulated reaction vessel. Typically, a silvered dewar is used, and the interacting components (e.g., solvent and solute) are held in subcontainers. Liquid phases are usually stirred and the temperature is accurately recorded using a thermometer or thermocouple. At the start of the experiment, the reaction vessel is allowed to reach a steady state, and a baseline temperature or temperature drift is recorded. The interaction of interest is then initiated by permitting the two components to mix, and the resulting temperature increase from baseline is recorded. The system is calibrated by monitoring a standard reaction (e.g., neutralization of hydrochloric acid) or by applying a controlled amount of electrical energy via a heating coil. From this, the heat capacity of the system is determined, and the enthalpy change for any monitored process can be calculated from the observed temperature change. Isoperibol calorimeters can be easily constructed from their individual components, and several different instruments are commercially available at a modest cost.

Owing to the high degree of accuracy and sensitivity that is required for pharmaceutical analysis, more sophisticated microcalorimeters are frequently used for studying pharmaceutical systems. An example of such an instrument is the TAM manufactured by Thermometrics. In this instrument, twin sample cells are used to achieve greater signal stability and to minimize the effects of spurious thermal fluctuations. Comparably, a similar instrument is available from Setaram known as a microDSC. The cells are housed in a constant temperature environment maintained via a sophisticated heater and water jacket system.

Minor changes in sample heat flow are detected with relative ease using this arrangement. The TAM and microDSC are calibrated electrically, and the commercially available sample configurations allow the mixing of solids, liquids, and gases in various proportions. Controlled gas and liquid flow rates, and changing sample environments (e.g., relative humidities) can also be achieved with appropriate accessories. A major practical advantage of this type of calorimeter when compared with less sophisticated instruments is the small sample size requirement of only a few tens or hundreds of milligrams per determination. This type of microcalorimeter has been used for detection and monitoring of crystallization events, sorption and desorption of organic and inorganic vapors, chemical reactions (drug degradation and drug interactions with excipients), molecular motions in amorphous pharmaceutical materials, ligand binding phenomena, microbiological growth, and the determination of solid heat capacities.

Sample Preparation and Calibration

Microcalorimeters are usually operated in a similar way irrespective of the source of the energy change that is being monitored. Specimens are preequilibrated at the desired measuring temperature for several hours and then introduced into the calorimeter chamber. After a short delay, the external stimulus is applied to trigger the event of interest, and then the energy that is liberated or consumed is measured. The reaction is isolated from the environment by a jacket, which serves as a thermal shield to minimize the absorption and emission of radiant heat.

Calibration of microcalorimeters is usually achieved by direct heating using an electric heating element. Extreme care is required to achieve consistent sample preparation and to maintain constant experimental procedures because the interpretation of results can be confused easily by experimental artifacts. Simultaneous thermal events of opposite sign (exothermic and endothermic) are quite common and may often confound the interpretation of data. In all experiments, an appropriate thermal reference is required as the energy changes that are measured are simply energy changes relative to the reference specimen. Common references include an empty sample container, or a sample container filled with an inert material, which has a similar heat capacity and mass to the sample.

Definitions and Applications of Microcalorimetry

Microcalorimeters have found widespread use in the pharmaceutical sciences in recent years for applications as diverse as determining the degradation rate of drugs, estimating the strength of binding between proteins and receptor sites, and monitoring metabolic processes in microorganisms.

Interactions between water vapor and amorphous pharmaceutical solids were evaluated using isothermal microcalorimetry. The desorption of water from theophylline monohydrate has been investigated using microcalorimetric approaches. The properties of surfactants and surface-active drugs in solution were studied by Attwood et al. using calorimetry, while titration microcalorimetry has been utilized to elucidate the nature of specific interactions in several pharmaceutical polymer-surfactants systems. Drug decomposition was evaluated as a function of different excipient blends in compressed tablets using isothermal heat conduction microcalorimetry. A more unusual pharmaceutical use of microcalorimetry is to study energetic changes that occur during tablet compaction. The compression calorimeter used is a custom-made research instrument that appears to have many potential applications for the pharmaceutical scientist.

Microcalorimetry has proven to be a particularly useful tool to detect different levels of disorder in pharmaceutical materials. Gao and Rytting demonstrated the validity of solution microcalorimetry to measure changes in the crystallinity during processing of both the drug compound and the excipients. Other workers have used elevated vapor pressures to trigger crystallization of disordered materials in the calorimeter and have been able to use the measured energy output to directly quantify the levels of disorder crystallinity in their samples.

Stability studies using microcalorimetry are widely reported in the literature. Some authors have monitored exothermic degradation reactions over several days or weeks and have projected the degradation extent and rate over the shelf life of the drug or drug product. The sensitivity of modern instruments is capable of measuring reaction rates of 1×10^{-11} sec^{-1} directly at 25°C, corresponding to 0.03% degradation per year. Some researchers have also described qualitative screens for drug-excipient compatibility studies. Other authors have used microcalorimetry to monitor relaxation of amorphous pharmaceutical materials and have then calculated relaxation time constants from these data for use in shelf life predictions. The use of microcalorimetry for preformulation stability screening of a drug with potentially reactive excipients has also been described.

Regulatory Considerations

Calorimetric methods are infrequently used for routine quality control purposes because of their non-specific nature and relatively slow speed. However, data from calorimetry experiments are commonly presented in applications for new product licenses and in support of patent applications. To ensure the integrity of all calorimetry data, normal procedures for good laboratory practices, standard operating procedures, appropriate calibration methods, and regular instrument servicing are necessary. The use of DSC for the measurement of transition temperatures and sample purity is described in the United States Pharmacopoeia, and standard procedures for DSC analyses are also suggested by the ASTM.

6

CHEMILUMINESCENCE

Chemiluminescence (CL) is a phenomenon involving the emission of light (usually in the visible or infrared region) as a result of a chemical reaction. Some reaction product is obtained in an excited state and emits light on returning to its ground state. Essentially, the process by which luminescence is produced is identical to that for photoluminescence (fluorimetry or phosphorimetry) except that no excitation light source is needed. A CL process can be schematized in two steps involving excitation:

$$A + B \rightarrow C^* + D$$

and return of the excited species to its ground state:

$$C^* \rightarrow C + h\nu.$$

Chemiluminescence is produced in very few reactions since, most often, the energy released on vibrational excitation of ground states is in the form of heat. For a chemical reaction to be suitable for CL detection, it should meet three essential requirements:

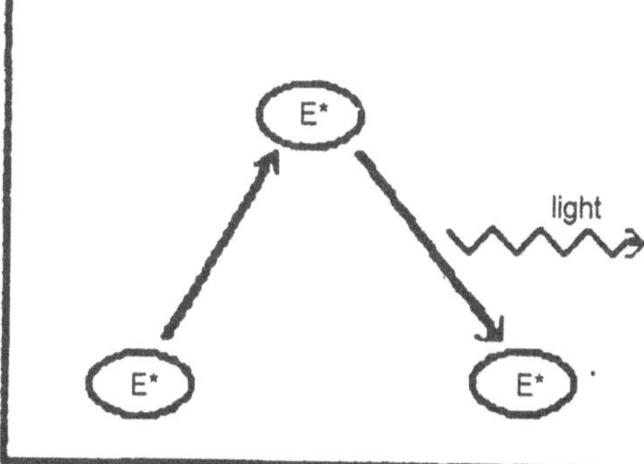

Fig. 6.1. Emission of light by a chemiluminescent molecule. 1, excitation; 2, relaxation.

1. It should release an adequate amount of energy for an electronically excited state to be obtained;
2. The pathway via which it proceeds should favour the formation of such an excited state; and
3. The excited state should be luminescent or be able to transfer its energy to another, luminescent molecule.

Photon energy in the visible region ranges from 44 to 71 kcal/mol; accordingly, for a reaction to be chemiluminescent, it must release at least 44 kcal/mol. This amount of energy is actually produced by a number of oxidation reactions (particularly those involving oxygen, peroxides and miscellaneous strong oxidants). The rates of CL reactions vary over wide ranges (from less than a second to over one day). The quantum yield, of which the light intensity produced is obviously a function, also varies widely. Thus, the yield of bioluminescent (BL) systems is typically very high (e.g. 0.88 for luciferin, which results in a detection limit of *ca.* 10^{-21} mol in the most favourable of cases). The highest quantum yields for non-biological systems (*ca.* 0.50) are provided by peroxyoxalates. Other commonplace systems such as lucigenin and luminol provide yields of *ca.* 0.01 or even lower.

The CL behaviour of a chemical system can be predicted on the basis of several empirical rules. Thus, if a given compound is fluorescent, the compound itself or its oxidation product is a good CL candidate. This rule has a number of exceptions that preclude predicting whether or not CL will be produced in many instances. It should also be noted that many CL reactions in solution involve oxidation of aromatic compounds. Notwithstanding the large number of CL applications reported in the past decade, there are few basic light-producing systems of practical use.

The chemiluminescence produced by living organisms is known specifically as *bioluminescence*, which can be *electro generated* (i.e. produced by an electrochemical reaction). In this context, it is worth mentioning *organized media* and their still incipient application to luminescence analysis. The CL phenomenon can also take place in the gas state (even inside a flame) and a solid phase.

The analytical interest of CL arises from the ability to produce fluorescent molecules with no prior irradiation, thereby avoiding various problems derived from light scatter, unselective excitation or light source instability.

Basic Chemiluminescence Systems

Non-biological Media

This group of CL systems includes non-bioluminescent substances such as luminol, lucigenin, lophine and peroxyoxalates.

Acylhydrazines

The earliest reported CL system involved interaction between luminol and various oxidants (H_2O_2, oxygen, hypochlorite, permanganate, perborate) to produce light via the following mechanism:

luminol $\xrightarrow{\text{oxidant}}$ α-aminophthalate $+ N_2 +$ light (425 nm)

The reaction is catalysed by various metal ions, of which Cu(II), Co(II), Mn(II) and Fe(II) are the most efficient. With some such catalysts (e.g. Cr(II), Cu(II), Fe(II) and Ni(II)) the CL intensity produced is increased by the presence of halides; for example, with Cr(III), such an intensity increases in the following order: $Br^- > Cl^- > F^-$. Hexacyanoferrate(III) can act as both the catalyst and the co-oxidant in the luminol reaction, which is also catalysed by haem-containing enzymes such as peroxidase. The CL intensity for the luminol oxidation with hydrogen peroxide is increased by a factor of up to 25000 in the presence of some organic compounds such as diazonium salts. The above reaction can be expanded to the following general mechanism:

reduced luminiscent reagent + oxidant + other reagents ⟶ oxidized luminiscent reagent + other products + LIGHT

This scheme clearly demonstrates the great analytical potential of the reaction. Thus, the analyte can be the oxidant, the catalyst or even a species that can be converted into an oxidant or luminescent compound (or labelled with a luminescent reagent). Determinations can also be extended, to those substances having an indirect effect such as catalyst-chelating substances (inhibitors) or sensitizers.

Imidazoles

The oxidation of lophine (2,4,5-triphenylimidazole) by H_2O_2, NaClO, H_2O_2-Fc $Fe(CN)_6^{3-}$ or oxygen in an alkaline medium is chemiluminescent. The mechanism proposed for the oxidation in dimethyl sulphoxide is as follows:

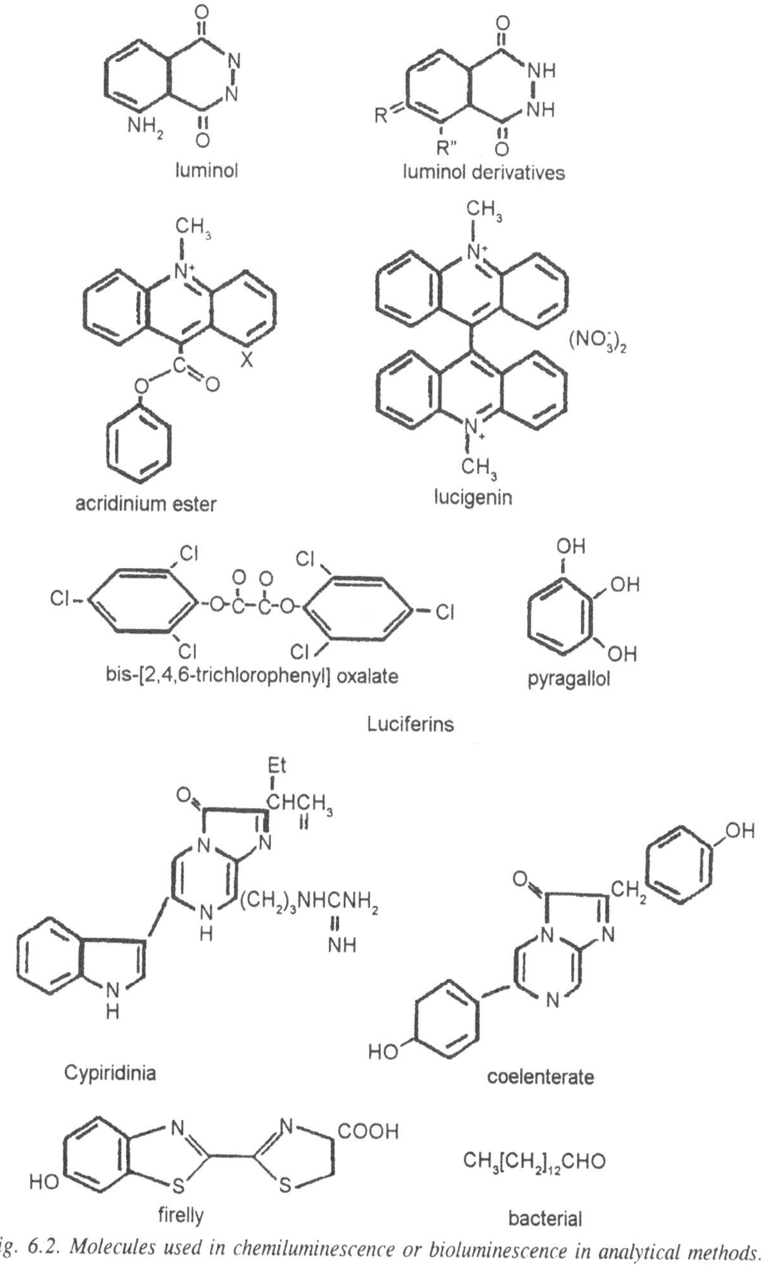

luminol

luminol derivatives

acridinium ester

lucigenin

bis-[2,4,6-trichlorophenyl] oxalate

pyragallol

Luciferins

Cypiridinia

coelenterate

firelly

$CH_3[CH_2]_{12}CHO$

bacterial

Fig. 6.2. Molecules used in chemiluminescence or bioluminescence in analytical methods.

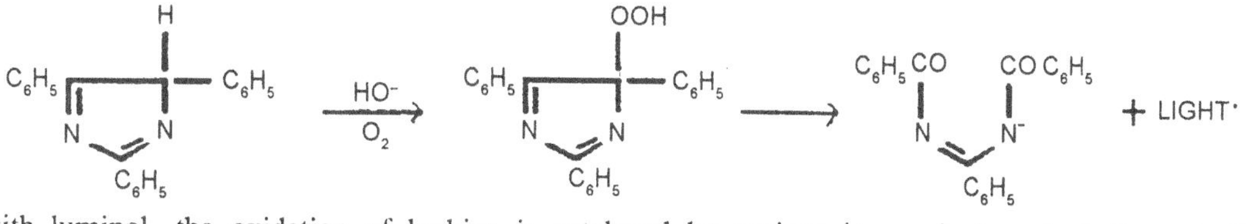

As with luminol, the oxidation of lophine is catalysed by various inorganic ions including, $AuCl_4^-$, MnO_4, and Cr(III).

Acridinium salts

The best known and most widely used CL acridinium salt is lucigenin (*bis-N*-methylacridinium nitrate), which is also oxidized by alkaline hydrogen peroxide to produce light that is emitted for a few minutes.

lucigenin $\xrightarrow{H_2O_2,\ OH^-}$ peroxide aduct → *N*-methylacridone* → *N*-methylacridone + hν

$2NO_3^-$ + lucigenin ⟶ *N*-methylacridone + light

The reaction product is water-insoluble. In order to prevent it from sticking to the manifold conduits or adhering to the cell walls, a surfactant (sodium dodecyl sulphate) is normally used. The reaction is also catalysed by metal ions, some of which (e.g. Bi(III)) have no effect on the luminol reaction.

Oxalate esters

The CL oxidation of some oxalates exhibits rather a high quantum yield (up to 0.27 according to some authors and as high as 0.50 according to others). This type of CL reaction is one of the most efficient known to date and entails the presence of a fluorophore. By way of example, the mechanism for the reaction of peroxide ion in the presence of rubrene is as follows:

bis(2,4,6-trichlorophenyl) oxalate $\xrightarrow{H_2O_2}$ 2,4,6-trichlorophenol + 1,2-dioxetanedione

1,2-dioxetanedione ⟶ FLR* + $2CO_2$ ⟶ light

The CL intensity and half-life are altered by the presence of weak bases such as triethylamine. Emission is quenched by readily oxidized species such as bromide, iodide, sulphite, nitrite, organic sulphides and substituted anilines. One major shortcoming of these compounds is their low water solubility, which entails using dioxane-water, *tert*-butanol-water or ethyl acetate-methanol-water mixtures. Attempts at preparing water-soluble esters have met with a low selectivity from the resulting compounds. The use of micellar media, reversed micelles and bilayer membrane aggregates as reaction media increases the stability of such oxalate esters in an aqueous medium.

Miscellaneous

Other, less frequently used CL-producing systems include those involving singlet-state oxygen (e.g. H_2O_2-ClO^-, triphenyl phosphite-O_3, H_2O_2-pyrogallol-HCHO, etc.).

Low CL emissions have been detected in autoxidation reactions and in the oxidation of various carbenes and Grignard reagents by oxygen, and nitrite by ferric peroxide, among others.

Bioluminescence

Bioluminescence is a naturally occurring phenomenon arising from a variety of organisms including bacteria, fungi, animals and plants, but is particularly significant in some marine species. Analytically, the two most significant natural bioluminescent systems are those in *Photinus pyralis* fireflies (quantum yield 0.88) and *Vibrio harveyi* and *Photobacterium fischeri* bacteria. Bioluminescent reactions are luciferase-catalysed oxidations of luciferins. Luciferin and luciferase are two generic names coined in 1880 and widely used at present—and the source of occasional confusion for this reason. Luciferases are enzymes that catalyse the substrate (luciferin) oxidation, which produces light. The mechanism for a basic bacterial luminescence reaction is as follows:

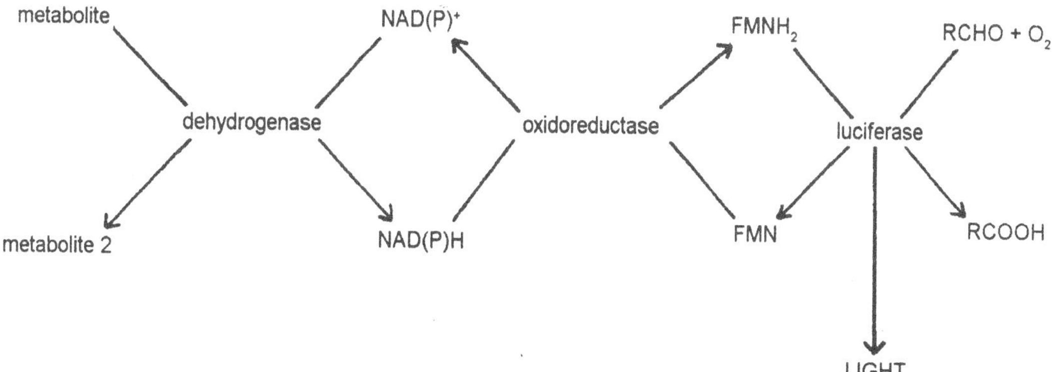

NAD^- is nicotinamide adenine dinucleotide; NADH is reduced NAD^-; mononucleotide; $FMNH_2$ is reduced FMN; RCHO is decanal.

Adenosine triphosphate (ATP) quantification typically relies on the most thoroughly studied of all bioluminescent reactions. The ATP-luciferin reaction is catalysed by luciferase, forming initially a luciferase-luciferyl adenylate (AMP-LH_2), which reacts with oxygen, producing the emitter oxyluciferin (and light), carbon dioxide and AMP (adenosine monophosphate). The pH influences the emitted light; red (560 nm) at 86 and yellow-green (615 nm) under acidic conditions (pH7.0). The reaction mechanism can be expressed as:

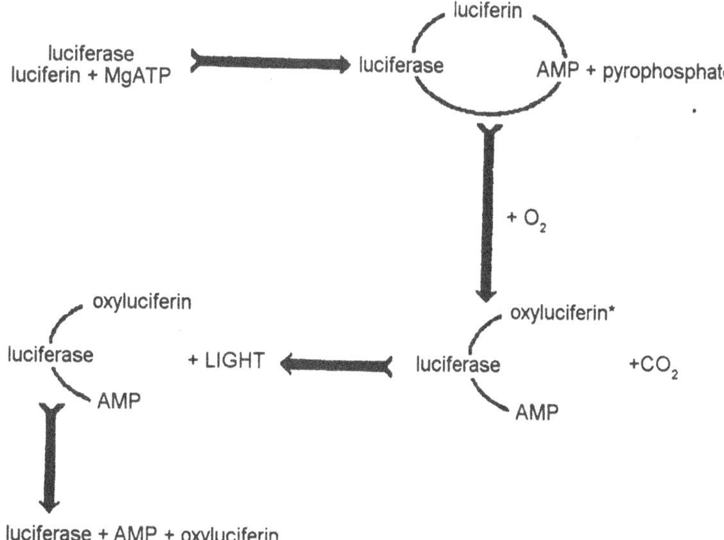

The presence of Mg(II) ions is mandatory in order to trigger luciferase activity. The amount of light emitted is proportional to the ATP concentration, so any substance involved in the production or depletion or ATP can equally be quantified. A similar effect is produced by divalent metals such as Zn(II).

Non-chemical (or Bio)-induced Chemiluminescence

Electrochemiluminescence phenomena

Electrochemiluminescence (ECL) phenomena, which arise from an electrochemically generated reagent, have been studied to a comparatively lesser extent than have Chemiluminescence processes. Electroluminescent reagents can be generated over accurately controlled periods at precisely controlled sites. The CL emission is confined at the surface electrode and the reaction can be started and stopped simply by changing the electrode potential.

This detection technique has been used to some extent in HPLC and—even less often—in FIA. It shares some of the advantages of Chemiluminescence techniques including the absence of stray light from the source and the need for no sophisticated instrumentation (a straightforward potentiostat is sufficient to excite the analyte). Finally, as frequently claimed by the advocates of this technique, chemical production of CL entails including one or more reagents in HPLC eluents, which results in more time-consuming procedures relative to ECL. On the other hand, the greatest pitfall of the ECL technique lies in the fact that electrochemiluminescence is quenched by water present in the eluent.

By *in situ* electro-oxidation in the presence of oxygen or hydrogen peroxide, luminol produces luminescence. The ECL intensity due to peroxide injections overlaps with the background emission of oxygen. Such background noise, however, does not detract from the detection limit for peroxide *(ca.* 1 μM*).* The net ECL (after subtraction of background noise) peaks at pH 10. The optimal electrode material for this purpose is gold, even though glassy carbon also surpasses platinum and results in maximum intensity at a positive potential of 0.4–0.6V. The stability of the ECL signal can be improved by using alternate potentials: luminol is first oxidized at a positive potential and then reduced at the electrode surface at -0.2V.

The additional work required to remove moisture completely fostered research into the mechanisms and analytical accessibility in aqueous systems. There are several available selective methods for the determination of metal traces based on the electrogeneration of luminol at a Pt electrode. Alternatively, luminol can be generated by using an oxide-coated aluminium electrode for multi-determinations of trace inorganic ions, fluorescent organic compounds and micelle-encapsulated polynuclear aromatic hydrocarbons (PAHs). Haapakka *el al.* (1990) developed a straightforward detector based on one such electrode for implementation in a continuous-flow system.

Irradiation sources

The photoinitiation of peroxyoxalate chemiluminescence was first reported in 1990. The classic chemical procedure based on peroxyoxalate chemiluminescence is:

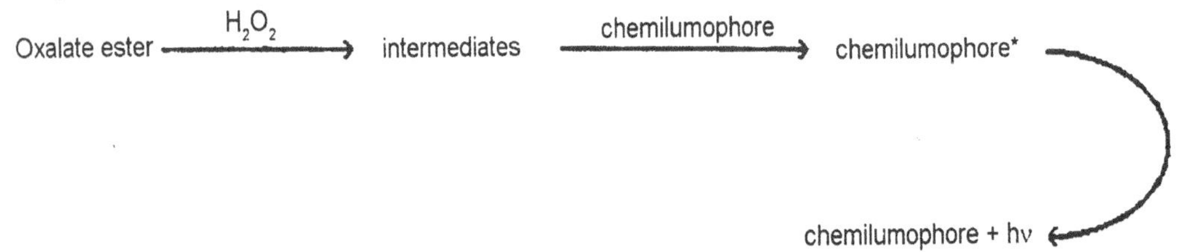

which presents side reactions and is very sensitive to experimental parameters such as solvent composition, pH and temperature. The photoinitiation leads to a simplified procedure by elimination of hydrogen peroxide. The procedure is also enhanced by use of the imidazole as a base catalyst. The mechanism proposed begins with hydrogen abstraction by the triplet-excited state (oxalate ester) followed by addition of oxygen. Chemiluminescence is observed only when hydrogen-atom-donating species were present. Hydrogen donors include alcohols, ether, aldehydes and ketones. The chemiluminometric procedure may be initiated by a low-pressure mercury lamp.

Analytical Procedures

Traditional analytical applications of chemiluminescence involve highly sensitive reactions with lifetimes of several minutes, which therefore allow for monitoring with fairly simple analytical instrumentation and procedures. The sample is held in a cuvette that is placed inside the chamber, and a few drops of the chemiluminescent or bioluminescent reagent are added with the aid of a syringe, after which the emitted light intensity is measured by means of a photomultiplier tube. Because only a single substance in the reaction medium emits light, no wavelength discrimination is needed. Recent advances in analytical instrumentation have facilitated mechanization or automation of reactant addition, data acquisition and processing, the use of multiple cuvette holders, etc., with no substantial modification of the basic process.

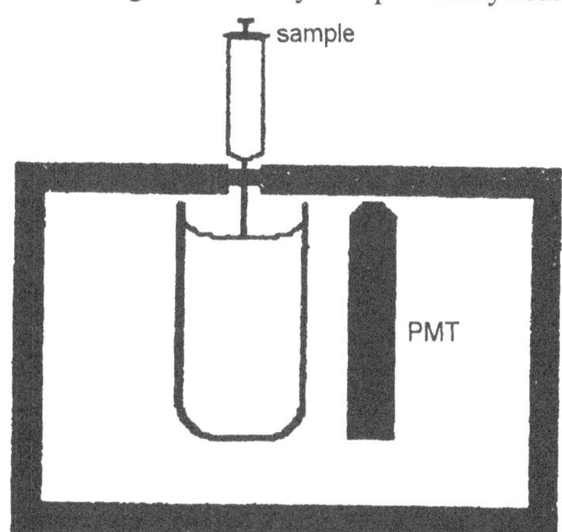

Fig. 6.3. Batch chemiluminescence arrangement. The sample is injected into the cell placed close to the photomultiplier tube (PMT).

Continuous-flow Procedures

The essential elements for a continuous-flow CL photometric determination are a flow-cell, a reactant mixing chamber, a photodetector and an electronic device for acquiring and processing data. Some instruments designed for other purposes include all these elements for CL or BL measurements. As a result, customized, unsophisticated systems are commonplace in FIA work. The sample is inserted into a carrier at an appropriate pH. The reagent, which is circulated along a different line, is merged with the sample-carrier stream as close to the mixing chamber as possible; once in the chamber, the reaction mixture is monitored by means of the phototube. Experimental set-ups for CL determinations are usually optimized with regard to both the type of connectors used at channel merging points and the cell size and configuration.

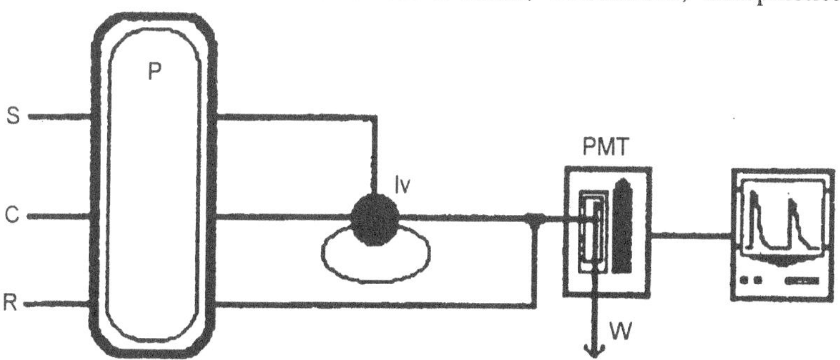

Fig. 6.4. FIA-chemiluminescence assembly. S, sample; C, carrier; R, reagent; P, pump; Iv, injection valve; PMT, photomultiplier tube; W, waste.

Sample-Reagent Reaction

A CL reaction in an FIA system takes place as usual, i.e. on merging two streams containing the sample and reagent, respectively. Mixing should be done near the cell for obvious hydrodynamic reasons. CL measurements can be made within a few seconds after mixing, which is particularly useful for monitoring rapid kinetics. Most often, the FIA manifold consists of one or two channels that converge at the cell. Based on purely empirical results, many authors claim that a T-shaped connector is the most effective choice for mixing the two streams, whereas others feel that Y- shaped connectors are equally efficient.

Heterogeneous systems involving solid-phase reactors have a promising future in continuous-flow CL applications. The CL intensity depends on the kinetics of the chemiluminescence reaction involved and the way in which the sample is brought into contact with the reagent. The stopped-flow mode offers valuable technical assets in association with FIA and other techniques. After the sample and reagent are efficiently mixed, the reaction mixture is halted at the flow-cell in order to perform kinetic measurements based on intensity-time recordings. The kinetic information provided by the whole signal (the rise and decay rate) can be related to the analyte concentration with a higher precision and selectivity than the peak height or area of the light intensity-emission time curve.

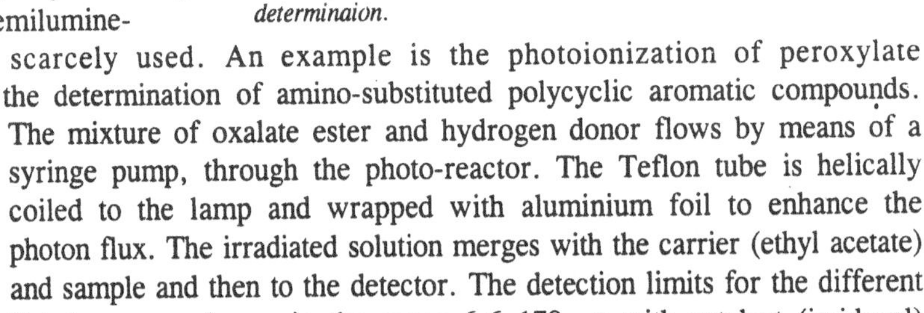

Fig. 6.5. Flow injection manifold with photoreactor and chemiluminescence determinaion.

FIA manifolds combining a photochemical reactor with the chemiluminescence detection have been scarcely used. An example is the photoionization of peroxylate chemiluminescence applied to the determination of amino-substituted polycyclic aromatic compounds. The mixture of oxalate ester and hydrogen donor flows by means of a syringe pump, through the photo-reactor. The Teflon tube is helically coiled to the lamp and wrapped with aluminium foil to enhance the photon flux. The irradiated solution merges with the carrier (ethyl acetate) and sample and then to the detector. The detection limits for the different listed compounds are in the range 6.6–170 μg with catalyst (imidazol) or 59-500 pg without catalyst.

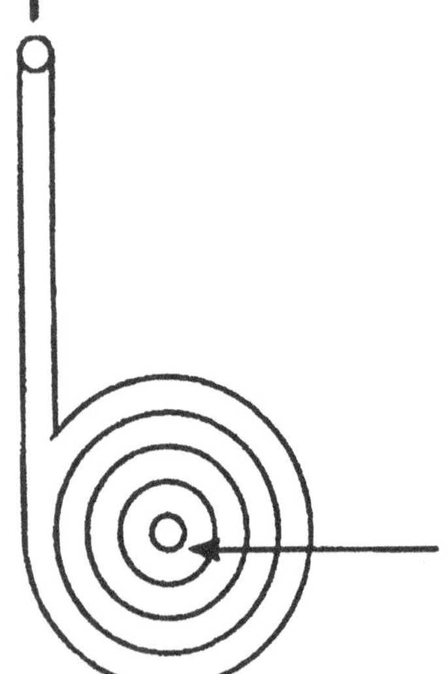

Fig. 6.6. The most usual design for the flow-cell in an FIA monitoring chemiluminescence manifold.

Monitoring Cells

Cell design is one other variable of interest. In fact, the cell location and distance to the detector must be highly reproducible. Dispersion and reflection phenomena pose no problem here as they affect samples and standards identically. Seitz (1981) studied various cells for continuous-flow CL measurements and determined which were the best suited to each technical mode. The cell design most frequently used in FIA is a spiral geometry that is placed as close to the photomultiplier tube (PMT) as possible.

Unlike flow-cells used in other spectrophotometric (absorption and emission) methods, CL cells have fairly large volumes, partly because of the need to collect a greater amount of emitted light, and partly because the background signal is normally ascribed to the '*chemical blank*' (i.e. the presence of contaminants in the reaction mixture, which precludes use of miniature cells). Anomalously high noise occasionally arises from side reactions, for example, adenylate kinase converts ADP to ATP in the determination of creatinine kinase activity based on firefly luciferase, thereby increasing background noise. Also, CL emitted in the peroxyoxalate reaction is very weak in the absence of a sensitizer and the required signal amplification produces a high background noise and results in a very low signal-to-noise ratio. It should be noted that background noise can arise from some experimental variables and the chemical system, but never the detector.

The essential requisite as regards cell design is that the maximum light intensity should be emitted while the analyte-reagent mixture is in front of the detector. This entails rapid mixing (particularly with fast reactions) and a cell of an appropriate volume for the emission peak to be measured. The analytical signal increases with increasing spiral length; the minimum acceptable length is dictated by the reaction rate. Using an unnecessarily long tube results in no extra gains. In order to minimize sample dispersion, the injection valve and the cell should be located as close to one another as possible—unless the carrier also functions as the reagent, in which case the reaction pathway must be optimized in order to make the best possible compromise between dispersion and reaction.

New types of chemiluminometric cells have been developed, with the aim of exposing to the photomultiplier tube a large surface reaction with the smallest possible cell volume. A cell similar to those used for thin-layer electrochemical cells has been formed by sandwiching a thin spacer (which determines the volume of the cell) between a Plexiglas front- and a Teflon back-piece. The area exposed to the detector was 0.5×1.5 cm and the cell volume was 40 μl. More recently, Lan and Mottola (1994) described a flow-through detection cell comprising a rotating disc to facilitate reaction with concomitant enhancement of the signal. The disc and the cell body were constructed of PTFE; the upper part of the cell accommodated two inlets and one outlet for solution passage. The surface of the disc was smoothly polished to reduce light scatter and to increase light reflection.

Detectors

While ordinary spectrophotometric and fluorimetric cells allow recording of chemiluminescence and bioluminescence spectra, the spectra thus obtained are distorted as a result of the light intensity changing with time by effect of reactant consumption. This shortcoming can be circumvented by performing a rapid scan (i.e. one taking a much shorter time than the reaction to complete) or using a flow-through cell. In the latter case, the decrease in the reactant concentration as the reaction develops is offset by the supply of fresh reagent. In this way, the light intensity is kept constant. Detectors based on PMTs, where impinging photons cause electrons to be emitted and the emitted electrons are amplified to electron cascades, are suitable for a variety of CL applications. While PMTs are much less efficient than liquid scintillation counters (LSCs), for example, they remain the most popular choice for this purpose. Because the spectral response is not uniform, the PMT used must provide an appropriate response at the wavelength or in the wavelength region where the CL is emitted. With low CL intensities, the measuring precision depends on the PMT used. In this respect, the PMT of choice will be that resulting in the maximal signal-to-noise ratio. Thus, with strong CL emission, the detector signal can be measured analogically, whereas, with weak CL emission, LSCs provide better signal-to-noise ratios. Scintillation counters are essentially two-channel photon counters provided with a variable discriminator. The sample is placed between the two detectors to ensure a high optical efficiency. The discriminator is set for transmission of photon impacts and rejection of small background pulses. This type of detector performs quite well with low CL intensities, but results in counting errors through saturation and dead- time losses, and provides non-linear relations between the CL intensity and the overall number of counts. This latter shortcoming can be circumvented by appropriate dilution of the sample and reagents, by decreasing the reaction rate or by reducing the fraction of light that is transmitted.

Applications to Pharmaceutical Analysis

Direct Oxidation of the Drug

A number of pharmaceuticals have been determined by the CL produced during their direct oxidation by a strong oxidant (usually an inorganic, commonplace reagent). Thus, acid potassium permanganate has been used for the determination of morphine, buprenorphine hydrochloride and the benzodiazepine loprazolam. In the three applications, the sample containing the drug was injected into a phosphoric acid stream that was subsequently merged with the oxidant stream. The experimental procedure is extremely simple, economic and effective. The determination of morphine was subsequently improved by placing a mirror beneath the spiral cell.

Permanganate ion in tetraphosphoric acid oxidizes morphine to its dimer pseudomorphine. The sample is inserted into the acid carrier channel (pH1.2), which then converges with the oxidant solution (6×10^{-4} M potassium permanganate). Both the acid and the oxidant concentration are highly influential on the emitted light intensity. Out of 35 potentially interfering analgesics studied, six (normorphine, dihydromorphine, 6-monoacetylmorphine, N-oxide morphine, nalorphine and buprenorphine) produced CL of roughly the same intensity as morphine, and a seventh (naloxone) emitted approximately half that CL intensity. These substances are structurally very similar to morphine. All other pharmaceuticals assayed, however, produced virtually negligible CL by reaction with the permanganate. The reaction mechanism for mornhine oxidation is as follows

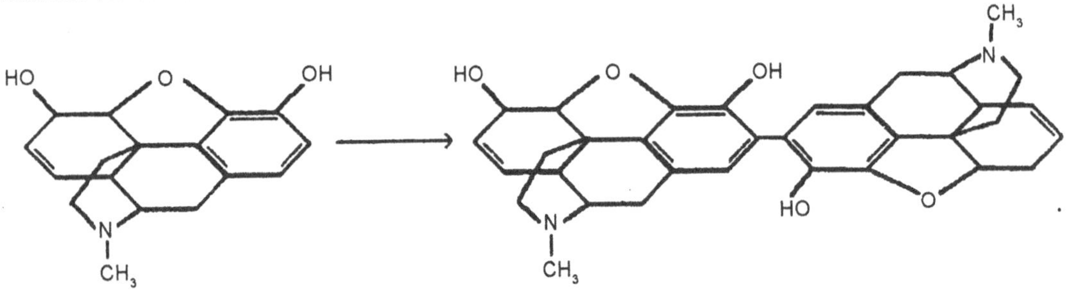

Some of the arguments used to account for CL production in this reaction (or the fact that pseudomorphine is highly fluorescent) stress the fact that the presence of the phenol group at C_3 activates the C_2 position towards quinone-like tautomerization and hence to dimerization. This assertion is supported by the following: the seven above- mentioned pharmaceuticals producing a high CL intensity bear a phenol group at C_3; and those compounds whose C_2 position is blocked by an alkyl (codeine) or acyl group (heroin) exhibit no chemiluminescence or fluorescence. One other structural argument for CL production is the presence of the furan oxygen bridge; in fact, those compounds that possess it exhibit much less intense CL. The only pharmaceutical assayed that gave a similar response to morphine was the narcotic analgesic buprenorphine (also in phosphoric acid).

Later studies revealed the CL spectra of morphine, oripavine and pseudomorphine to be identical, with a maximum at 608–611 nm. The differences lay only in the emitted intensity. The coincidence of the three spectra and other kinetic similarities observed suggested that the emitting species was very similar or even identical for the three drugs. On the other hand, acid permanganate solutions produce similar reddish- orange CL with morphine and with such compounds as ascorbic acid, hydroquinone and p-phenylenediamine. Townshend (1990) found Mn(II) to increase considerably the emitted light intensity.

Tsaplev *et al.* (1991) suggested that the CL produced by permanganate arises from the following reduction:

$$Mn(III) \rightarrow Mn(II)^* \rightarrow Mn(II) + h\nu$$

which is quite sensible because Mn(III) is fairly stable in an acid medium and is produced from both MnO_4^- and Mn(II). These authors studied the structural similarity between various compounds yielding analytically useful CL (i.e. those bearing a phenol group at C_2 and a furan bridge between C_4 and C_5), and put forward the following explanation: Mn(II) may be complexed by the phenyl and furan oxygen atoms and the complexes formed be oxidized to Mn(III) in the presence of acid potassium permanganate. If the Mn(III)-alkaloid complex is then reduced via a tertiary amine (between C_9 and C_{16}) to an electronically excited Mn(II) complex, then the resulting complex will be that emitting the CL. This mechanism is analogous to that described above for CL generation by reduction of Ru(III) chelates. Accordingly, the differences observed between the alkaloids reflect the relative ease with which they form the Mn(III) complex.

Benzodiazepines are the most commonly prescribed psychotropic drugs, which has led to widespread abuse and addiction. The great chemical similarity between these pharmaceuticals led Andrews and Townshend (1989) to investigate light emission in the reactions of seven diazepines with eight different inorganic oxidants and seven (also inorganic) reductants. Only loprazolam was found to produce analytically useful emission on reaction with potassium permanganate in 0.94M formic acid, with no structural reason for its disparate behaviour relative to the other benzodiazepines studied. Of various metal ions tested (Ca, Mn, Mg, Cu, Co, Zn, Ni, Cr, Al, Fe and Ag), only Mn(II) and Fe(II) were found substantially to alter (decrease) the emission intensity (by 40.6 per cent and 12.1 per cent relative to their absence). Neither of the sensitizers tested (rhodamine B and fluorescein) exhibited any activity in the process. Loprazolam was determined in tablets by dissolution and direct injection with no prior sample filtration.

Different chemiluminescence procedures have been proposed for the determination of catecholamines, most being based on the oxidation of these drugs. No emission is detected after mixing aqueous solutions of the drug with inorganic strong oxidants such as ferricyanide, dichromate or bromate. However, the light emission is high when the drug solution is treated with potassium permanganate in acidic medium. The CL is enhanced by some common sensitizers; the CL is increased up to about ten times when formaldehyde is present. This sensitizer was selected for the determination of adrenaline, noradrenaline, dopamine and L-dopa by oxidation with potassium permanganate in acidic medium. The sample is injected into an acidic stream which merges with the aid of a Y-shaped connector with the oxidant solution stream.

The reaction with tris-2,2'-bipyridine-Ru(III) has been exploited for the determination of erythromycin and amino acids, peptides and proteins. The detection limits achieved for the 21 amino acids assayed varied widely. The lowest (viz. those for histidine, tyrosine and tryptophan) cannot be ascribed to the substituents as they are at least one order of magnitude higher than those for the isolated structural units (imidazole, phenol and indole, respectively). The presence of hydroxyl groups was found to result in poorer responses that were ascribed to a quenching effect.

The reaction mechanism proposed for aliphatic amines involves oxidation of the starting compound by the $Ru(bpy)_3^{3+}$ complex:

$$R{-}\overset{R'}{\underset{}{N}}{-}CH_2R'' + Ru(bpy)_3^{3+} \longrightarrow Ru[bpy]_3^{2+} + R{-}\overset{R'}{\underset{}{N}}{-}CH_2R''$$

The cationic radical obtained can react with the water to yield the corresponding secondary amine and aldehyde:

$$R{-}\overset{R'}{\underset{+}{N}}{-}CH_2R'' + H_2O + Ru(bpy)_3^{2+} \longrightarrow 2H^+ + R{-}\overset{R'}{N}{-}H + \overset{O}{\overset{\|}{C}}HR'' + Ru(bpy)_3^{+}$$

Finally, the reaction between the initial ruthenium complex, $Ru(bpy)_3^{3+}$, and that formed at a later stage, viz. $Ru(bpy)_3^{+}$, gives rise to the intermediate species $[Ru(bpy)_3^{2+}]^*$, which releases light on returning to its ground state:

$$Ru[bpy]_3^{+} + Ru[bpy]_3^{3+} \rightarrow Ru[bpy]_3^{2+} + Ru[bpy]_3^{2+} * Ru[bpy]_3^{2+} * \rightarrow Ru[bpy]_3^{2+} + Light$$

Bromine is used for CL production from tetracycline hydrochloride. The determination is carried out in a carbonate-buffered aqueous medium at pH 10.4 by using 9.3×10^{-3} M bromine. Tetracycline had previously been determined by oxidation with potassium persulphate and 1,3-dibromo-5,5-dimethylhydantoine, which produced 6–7 times less light than the bromine-based system. Alternative oxidants such as sodium hypochlorite at pH 10.0 and permanganate in polyphosphoric acid proved to be much less efficient than bromide. Neither potassium periodate nor hydrogen peroxide had any effect on the drug—the latter not even in the presence of the enzyme peroxidase. Because the structure of tetracycline contains a number of potential anchoring points for chelation by metal ions, one such ion might be used to alter emitted light. The experimental results showed ferric iron to increase the CL intensity by a factor of 1.44 and all other metal ions tested to decrease it to levels as low as 11 per cent of the reference value in the case of aluminium.

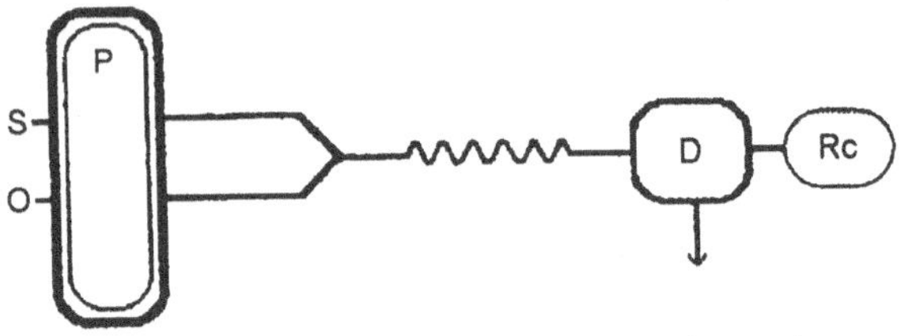

Fig. 6.7. Schmeatic diagram of a continuous-flow analyser.

In some chemiluminescence determinations of pharmaceuticals by direct oxidation, the sample is continuously aspirated into the system and merged with the reagent, the reaction mixture then being driven to the detector cell. Technically speaking, these are not true FIA systems because the sample is not inserted into a carrier. However, the instrumental similarity with an FIA system is very high, so some examples warrant inclusion here as they can be readily translated to an FIA assembly. Such examples include: the determination of thiamine with hexacyanoferrate(III) in 2 M $Fe(OH)_3$; that of paracetamol with Ce(IV) in 4 M $HClO_4$; that of tetracyclines by oxidation with hexacyanoferrate(III) in an acid medium or by degradation in an alkaline medium following reaction with lucigenin; that of isoniazid with *N*-bromosuccinimide; amiloride and streptomycin by oxidation with *N*-bromosuccinimide; and that of dihydralazine, rifampicin and rifamycin in tablets and capsules by oxidation with alkaline *N*-bromosuccinimide.

Indirect Methods

A typical example of the catalytic action of ferrous ion is the determination of ascorbic acid in juices and different pharmaceutical formulations (tablets, syrups and capsules). The method used for this purpose is based on the reduction of ferric ion and subsequent measurement of the light intensity emitted by luminol in the presence of hydrogen peroxide. A 30-μl sample aliquot is injected into a 1% solution of Fe(II) in metaphosphoric acid. The mixture is merged with a stream of 3×10^{-3} M H_2O_2 prior to entering the detector cell. The last merging point is provided by a T-shaped connector and the analytical signal is influenced by the Fe(III) concentration, pH and flow-rates. The most severe interferences are by oxalate, sulphite and sulphate ion, which affect the reduction of Fe(III) by ascorbic acid.

The oxidation of adrenaline by injection of the drug solution into a stream of Fenton's reagent was carried out for determination of the catecholamine. After injection the carrier-reagent stream merges with a mixture of hydrogen peroxide in alkaline media and acetonitrite. The detection limit was 0.3 nM.

Decreasing the concentration of hydrogen peroxide results in decreased chemiluminescence of the system luminol-H_2O_2-hematin (as catalyst). The photoreduction of riboflavin and riboflavin-S'-phosphate by ethylenediamin-etetraacetic acid (EDTA) for an FIA indirect determination is easily performed.

The photolysis cell (thermostatically controlled temperature 25 ± 0.2°C and under nitrogen atmosphere) contained phosphate buffer (pH 6.0) EDTA, iron(III) ammonium sulphate, hydrogen peroxide and the corresponding volume of standard or sample solution. The mixture was irradiated for exactly

60s; the photolysed solution was then drawn into the FIA manifold with the aid of the peristaltic pump. A phosphate buffer solution acted as a carrier, transporting the injected sample aliquot to merge with the luminol and hematin solution, and then to the detector.

Use of Sensitizers

Not all excited states of CL reaction products are effective '*emitters*'; in any case, the excited state in question can be transferred to an 'effective' fluorophore added to the system in order to increase the CL intensity substantially. The most salient asset of chemical excitation is the low background noise involved, which results in very low detection limits (frequently in the sub-femtomol region).

Twenty-eight amines were determined using two different FIA systems and post-column HPLC derivatization (the analytes included amino acids and other compounds of pharmacological interest). The procedure was based on the oxidation of an aryl oxalate by hydrogen peroxide in the presence of a base (the amines assayed, among others) and a fluorescent substance used as sensitizer. The species to be detected was the amine concerned rather than the hydrogen peroxide. The aryl oxalate used was bis[4-nitro-2(3,6,9-trioxadecyloxycarbonyl)phenyl] oxalate (TDPO) and the sensitizer was sulphorhodamine 101 in acetonitrile. The sample was injected into a stream containing 2×10^{-2} M H_2O_2 in 9:1 v/v acetonitrile/water. The mixture was subsequently merged with a stream of 5.0×10^{-4} M TDPO and 1.10×10^{-7}M sulphorhodamine in acetonitrile.

Some chemiluminescent redox reactions between inorganic compounds can be used to exploit the action of sensitizers for analytical purposes. Typical sensitizers include riboflavin for the reaction between permanganate and 3-cyclohexylaminopropanesulphonic acid (CAPS). CAPS-structurally related compounds can also act as sensitizers. Their effect is ascribed to the presence of the cyclohexyl group, yet no irrefutable evidence has to date been provided in this respect. Because cortisone and hydrocortisone contain a cyclohexyl group, the CL released in the reaction between Ce(IV) and sulphite should be increased in their presence. However, the light emitted in the oxidation of sulphite ion is ascribed to the formation of excited SO_2 molecules. The process was exploited for the determination of five corticosteroids in an air-segmented continuous-flow system (not an FIA system). Subsequent experiments involving the reaction between sulphite and bromate revealed no appreciable advantages over the previous reaction.

Nagakama *et al.* (1989) performed a long series of screening tests in order to develop CL systems for the determination of polyphenols and indoles. Of the 48 compounds assayed, four (dopamine, noradrenaline, L-dopa and normetanephrine) were of pharmacological interest. Experiments were carried out in an FIA assembly where the oxidant and reaction medium were merged prior to converging with the carrier stream (a solution containing the inorganic ion) immediately before the cell, opposite the photomultiplier tube. Seven different redox systems were tested: MnO4 - in two different acid media and the presence of Ce(IV) or Cu(II), or an alkaline medium and the presence of Cu(II); H_2O_2 in three different alkaline media and the presence of ClO^-, Fe(II) or Co(II), respectively; and alkaline persulphate in the presence of Ag(I). The results obtained revealed the influence of the oxidant chosen for each compound on the emitted light intensity, as well as the lack of specificity of acid permanganate and the high selectivity or even specificity of the H_2O_2 and persulphate systems in alkaline media.

The reaction between Ce(IV) and sulphite ion produces little CL; this is, however, markedly increased by the presence of 3-cyclohexylaminopropanesul-phonic acid (sodium cyclamate, a sweetener). This last is not a fluorophore, so it cannot take part in an energy-transfer process; its sensitizing action on the chemiluminescence is not fully understood. The CL intensity of the system Ce(IV)-sulphite is sensitized by other compounds with similar molecular structure, such as 2-cyclohexylaminopropane-sulphonic acid. The enhancement is maximal from compounds containing groups such as cyclopentyl and cyclohexyl. Light emission is strongly dependent on the organic solvent (miscible with water) used; acetone does not allow the determination of numerous steroids due to its considerable quenching effect. Acetonitrile-water solutions have been successfully used for measurement of steroids in FIA and post-column LC.

A simple FIA manifold in which the sulphite ion solution acts as a carrier of the sample and then merges with the Ce(IV) solution has been proposed for determination of several steroids in commercial formulations; cortisone, hydrocortisone and dexamethasone were determined in aqueous solutions; and prednisolone, methylprednisolone, progesterone, corticosterone and testosterone were determined in acetonitrile solutions.

The same system. Ce(IV)-SO_3^{2-}, is sensitized by well-known fluorophores which are excited by the energy transfer from the redox reaction. Quinine and quinidine are among the fluorophores excited by this redox system and their determination has been carried out by means of a segmented-flow (no FIA) analyser.

Mechanisms Based on Chemiluminescence Quenching

The conversion of luminol to 3-aminophthalate is catalysed by two different types of species: metal ions such as Co(II), Cu(II) and Fe(III), and compounds containing them; and enzymes such as peroxidase, microperoxidase and myeloperoxidase. The catalytic action of metal ions (without quenching) has also been applied to pharmaceutical analysis; vitamin B_{12} (or cyanocobalamin) may be determined by merging the carrier-sample stream with the mixture containing luminol and hydrogen peroxide.

Analytical exploitation of the quenching effect of metal ions involves using a chelating agent for the catalyst. The decrease in the free catalyst concentration through masking by the chelating agent results in a decrease in the CL produced by luminol in the presence of such a catalyst.

This process was exploited for the FIA determination of amino acids based on the Co(II)-luminol-H_2O_2 system. An FIA manifold was used to monitor the CL released by the system in an alkaline medium. On injection of the amino acid into the Co(II) solution, the metal ion was partly complexed and the emitted light intensity decreased as a result, thereby giving rise to a negative signal proportional to the amino acid concentration. The procedure allows amino acid concentrations between 0.004 and 2 nmol to be determined with a precision of 1–4 per cent as relative standard deviation. This procedure was also used for monitoring amino acids by HPLC with post-column derivatization.

The quenching effect of Cu(II) on the previous reaction was used to determine the amino acid cysteine and several other pharmaceuticals containing a thiol group. A solution containing the compound in question was injected into a 5×10^{-3} M luminol stream at pH 10.4 and the mixture was subsequently merged with a Cu(II) stream, and then with a 10^{-2} M H_2O_2 stream. In this way, a negative signal was also obtained. The emission intensity and copper concentration were found to be linearly related over the Cu(II) concentration range 5×10^{-6} to 1×10^{-4} M (i.e. 0.3–6.3 ppm Cu(II)).

Sixteen a-amino acids were determined by their CL quenching effect (masking of the catalytic activity of Cu(II)) on the luminol-H_2O_2 system. The detection limit obtained for L-aspartic acid, for example, was 2.7 ng.

Promethazine was also determined using a similar procedure. The CL produced by the luminol-H_2O_2-Cr(III) system in 0.1 M carbonate buffer was quenched by the presence of the drug. Such ions as Fe(II), Cu(II) and Cr(III) gave rise to different emission intensities in the presence and absence of promethazine (the difference between the peak height for the three ions was 0.64, 16.3 and 29.7 mV, respectively). The quenching mechanism was postulated on the basis of the reported CL of luminol:

$$\text{luminol} + [\text{oxygen}] \rightarrow \text{peroxide adduct} \rightarrow \text{aminophthalate}^* \rightarrow \text{aminophthalate} + h\nu.$$

According to some authors, oxygen solutions contain two forms that may play a prominent role in the luminol reaction, viz. singlet oxygen and superoxide ion (O_2^-). The former species is unstable in alkaline solutions, so only superoxide ion can be involved in luminol oxidation. The half-life of O_2^- is only a few milliseconds (even in an alkaline medium). Addition of promethazine to the luminol-H_2O_2-Cr(III) system shortens the period over which the CL is emitted. This is probably not the result of the formation of a peroxide adduct between promethazine and superoxide ion, which accelerates the decomposition of O_2^-. If the luminescence species were the aminophthalate (in the presence or absence of promethazine), the promethazine-peroxide adduct could react with luminol in a superoxide-exchange reaction. In short, if promethazine were the rate-determining factor, then the decrease in the CL intensity would be proportional to its concentration. The inhibiting effect of kanamycin on the reaction of lucigenin-hydrogen peroxide-cobalt(II) is the basis of an FIA-CL method for determination of the drug. Cobalt(II) is the catalyst of the lucigeninH_2O_2 system. The reaction mechanism can be expressed similarly to that above, with lucigenin instead of luminol:

$$\text{lucigenin} + [OH_2] + H_2O_2 \rightarrow \text{peroxide adduct} \rightarrow N\text{-methylacridone}^* \rightarrow N\text{-methylacridone} + h\nu.$$

According to the above-reported two forms of oxygen which may play a relevant role in the oxidation of lucigenin and the life-span of the superoxide anion, the addition of kanamycin to the lucigenin-H_2O_2-Co(H) system shortens the duration of CL. This inhibition probably indicates the formation of a peroxide adduct (by combination of the drug with the superoxide anion) which accelerates the decomposition of the superoxide. The kanamycin-peroxide adduct may react with lucigenin to exchange superoxide anions.

Enzyme catalysis has also been used for the determination of amino acids. Yung- Xiang *et al.* (1992) employed metalloporphyrins instead of peroxidase for this purpose. The catalytic activity of metalloporphyrins in the CL reaction between luminol and hydrogen peroxide is inhibited by some amino acids, which is ascribed to the formation of a mixed complex between the amino acid and the metalloporphyrin. The two axial positions of the metalloporphyrin in the complex formed (the catalytic activity sites) are occupied by the amino acid, so that the activity of the former is suppressed. Of over 20 amino acids tested, only L-cysteine, L-tyrosine, L-tryptophan and L-cystine proved to be effective quenchers for the emitted CL.

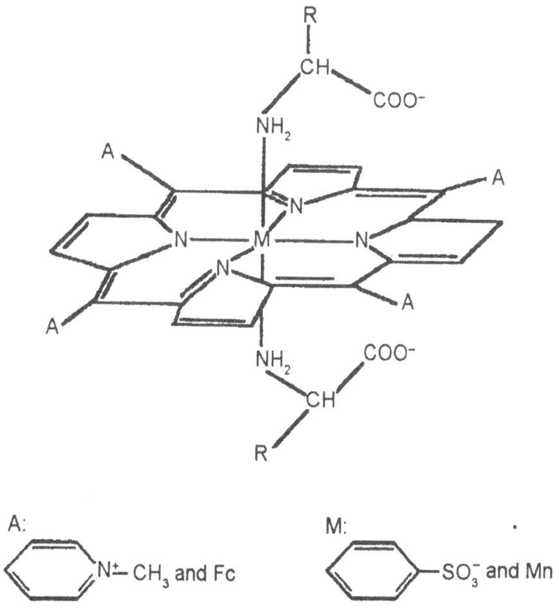

Fig. 6.8. Structure of the mixed ligand complex amino acid-metalloporphyrins.

One other method that can be considered to be based on an inhibition phenomenon was developed for the determination of cysteine and drugs containing a thiol group, using two redox reactions. The sample (via its sulphide ion or thiol group) reduced sodium hypochlorite on injection, and residual hypochlorite subsequently oxidized luminol on merging with a stream of the CL reagent in carbonate buffer at pH 11.2. The FIA assembly used for this purpose included a dispersion (gradient) tube for implementation of the method as an FIA titration. The calibration curve was linear from 10^{-4} to 10^{-1} M cysteine, N-acetylcysteine, N-penicillamine, 2-mercaptoprionylglycine and 2-thiouracil.

Analytical Reactions in Organized Media

Reversed micellar systems favour reactions between substrates that are water-soluble and others that are not. Reversed micelles (or microemulsions) are aggregates formed in non-polar solvents containing water. One of the distinct features of these micelles is their ability to accommodate large amounts of water in their core. As a result, they provide advantageous media for development of reactions between water-soluble and water-insoluble compounds.

Among other applications, these beneficial effects of *micellar media* have been used for the determination of amino acids by formation of a strongly chemiluminescent Schiff base with a suitable aldehyde (e.g. phenylacetaldehyde) in an appropriate medium (e.g. bis(2-ethylhexyl)sulphosuccinate). The Schiff base is oxidized by Fenton's reagent (31% ferrous ammonium sulphate plus H_2O_2, made fresh daily). The sample is injected into a methanol carrier following conversion into the Schiff base, and then merged with the Fe(II) and H_2O_2 solutions at the same point. After a tentative mechanism for the CL produced was put forward, the effect of micelles on the formation of the Schiff base was investigated. The results showed the formation rate of the Schiff base to increase considerably with decreasing micelle size and to be also affected by the amino acid hydrophobicity. A new FIA manifold was proposed for the determination of amino acids at lower concentrations (1–130 pmol).

Finally, the 0.15 mM 3,5-dibromosalicylfluorone-0.2M H_2O_2(0.1M NaOH)-Co(II) system allows the determination of 0.5–200 ng/ml Co(II) in cyanocobalamin and vitamin B_{12} samples.

Electrochemiluminescence

FIA electrochemiluminescence applications to substances of pharmacological interest involve, among others, the electrochemical reduction of oxygen to hydrogen peroxide in the presence of acridine esters, which produces intense light. The procedure can be applied with the ester in free form or as an analyte label. Lysine (the analyte) is complexed by the ester in the presence of N-hydroxysuccinimide and determined with a detection limit of 10 fmol. The *in-situ* generation of ruthenium(III) bipyridil was tested by a flow-injection manifold and applied to detection of amino acids after being separated in a chromatographic column. The sample (amino acid solution) is injected into the carrier solution formed by $Ru(bpy)_3(ClO)_2$ in boric acid-sodium borate buffer of pH 10; a vitreous carbon electrode at 1.2 V vs. saturated calomel electrode is the generating electrode. Detection limits, over the range 0.1–22 pmol, were affected by dissolved oxygen.

Other applications of interest related to pharmacological analysis include the determination of oxalate in urine and that of oligopeptides and albumin in bovine serum by use of a modified electrolytic cell in which the electrode is located opposite the quartz window. In this application, luminol generated at a Pt working electrode exhibits strong ECL. Non-luminescent compounds can be detected by previous labelling with luminol.

Liquid-Liquid Extraction

The liquid-liquid extraction/CL binomial has been used for the determination of steroid sulphates and steroid glucuronides, among other analytes, with lucigenin as chemiluminescent reagent and extractant. The CL is produced as the steroid sulphate-lucigenin ion-pair is extracted from the organic phase through a separation membrane. Addition of alkaline hydrogen peroxide starts the chemiluminescence. The polarity of the solvent used affects both the extraction efficiency and the emission intensity; thus, non-polar solvents such as n-hexane, carbon tetrachloride or 1,2-dichloroethane virtually suppress the emission altogether. The same procedure can be used to determine steroid glucuronides, using sodium periodate as oxidant. A similar procedure, also using alkaline hydrogen peroxide, has been developed for determining steroid sulphates.

Reagent Immobilization

One alternative way of exploiting the analytical potential of continuous-flow techniques is by using *solid-phase reactors* or immobilized reagents. These offer some advantages, including increased sensitivity and sample throughput, over solution methods.

Luminol has been immobilized in various ways for this purpose (e.g. covalent binding to controlled pore glass or quartz and adsorption on an Ambersorb or ion-exchange resin). For covalent binding, the glass surface is silylated and then glutaraldehyde is used to bind the amino groups of luminol to those of the aminoalkylsilane formed.

Reactors packed with luminol immobilized on various supports have been used in different FIA configurations with regard to the reactor, which can be both inserted in the manifold and accommodated inside the cell. In the latter case, the cell used is a cavity (1.5 × 3.5 × 0.5 cm) rather than the usual planar spiral. The amount of luminol retained by adsorption on Ambersorb, covalent binding and ion exchange is 29, 82 and 875)μmol/g support, respectively, the detection limits afforded being 0.15, 1–2 and 5–10 μM peroxide, respectively. Immobilized luminol is inert to non-alkaline flowing streams; on the other hand, alkaline solutions release an amount of luminol (by hydrolysis of luminol-glutaraldehyde bonds) dependent on the pH and injected solution volume. By releasing the luminol immediately prior to the CL reaction, the quantum yield is substantially increased and contact with the other reactants is facilitated. Columns can be repacked *in situ* and provide as good responses as newly packed columns.

The neutral pH used to immobilize substrates on ion-exchange resins is compatible with enzyme catalysis and allows the determination of glucose, as well as that of ATP with luciferin and luciferase in a reversed FIA system.

A^{9}-tetrahydrocannabinol is the main pharmacologically active principle of cannabis (*Cannabis sativa*); it is rapidly metabolized and scarcely excreted in urine. Its main metabolite, 11-hydroxy-A^{9}-tetrahydrocannabinol, is excreted in urine for several days following administration of cannabis. Radiochemical methods are highly sensitive and specific compared to conventional methods for this determination; however, chemiluminescent compounds can be used as effective immunoassay labels as alternatives to radiochemical methods. Inclusion of some enhancer molecules in the horseradish peroxidase-luminol-H_2O_2 system increases and stabilizes the signal obtained. By using a specific antiserum for tetrahydrocannabinol and its metabolite, a donkey anti-sheep antiserum and a horseradish peroxidase-labelled antigen conjugate, the immobilized enzyme was detected via its catalytic activity on the reaction between luminol and hydrogen peroxide in the presence of *p*-iodophenol as enhancer. The *p*-iodophenol enhances CL signals to a greater extent than do other 6-hydroxybenzothiazole derivatives and decreases blank signals, thereby improving the characteristics of the assay.

The amino acids L-leucine, L-isoleucine and L-valine were determined together in an FIA manifold in which the sample was inserted into an air stream that drove the sample to a point of merging with NAD and buffer at pH9.0, after which it was passed through a reactor containing immobilized leucine dehydrogenase (LD), where the amino acids were oxidatively deaminated according to the following reaction:

$$\text{amino acid} + NAD^{+} + H_2O \xrightarrow{LD} 2\text{-oxoacid} + NADH + NH_4^{+}$$

The flow emerging from the column was then merged with the bioluminescent sueam and a new solid-phase bed containing several enzymes (luciferase included) was used to catalyse the reaction in the cell vicinity, thereby generating the luminescence. This type of bed allows over 900 samples to be processed (its lifetime exceeds two months) and features a linear response over the range 20–2000 pmol in the biological matrix.

As follows from the two examples above, the most immediate applications of solid- phase enzyme reactors pertain to the clinical, biochemical and biotechnological fields. A few examples are now given to illustrate the potential of this type of reactor in the pharmaceutical field—though not necessarily involving pharmaceutical determinations, even though some of the analytes are included in many pharmacopoeias. Thus, the reaction of luminol in the presence of 4-iodophenol as enhancer and immobilized horseradish peroxidase was used to determine ethanol at the pmol level and methanol in the presence of ethanol (the former alcohol was previously converted into formaldehyde and H_2O_2 by alcohol oxidase-catalysed oxidation). Also, the degradation of glucose catalysed by glucose oxidase was used as the basis for the determination of micromolar amounts of sucrose, maltose, lactose and fructose by measuring the HO produced following enzymatic conversion into glucose. Other, more common applications use a bioluminescent reaction (in the presence of luciferase) to determine ATP or NADH, or 3a-hydroxyacids in serum.

A Pyrex tube (2.5 cm × 5 mm) was filled with an ion exchange resin. Manganese(III)-4, 4′,4″, 4″ porphyrintetraethyltetrabenzenesulphonic acid was chelated to the resin and was used as an indicator phase for chemiluminescence sensing of adrenaline in pharmaceutical formulations. Regeneration of the column to avoid deterioration of the response was carried out by passage of 1 M NaOH aqueous solution. The detection limit was 3×10^{-3} M and the coefficient of variation (10 replicates) was 3.5 percent.

7

ENZYMATIC ANALYSIS

Analytically, enzymes play two major roles. First, they function as reagents (catalysts) by converting an undetectable species into a detectable form via a kinetically controlled reaction—the unknown in this case is the concentration of the substrate rather than that of the enzyme. Second, they act as analytes (e.g. in culture broths or physiological fluids) when their concentration in the sample is to be determined, which is a frequent occurrence in clinical analysis due to the high diagnostic value of enzymes. The enzyme content in a sample is usually expressed in terms of *activity*, viz. the amount of substrate that can be converted per unit time.

There are a few hundred commercially available enzymes of high purity, some of which, however, are very expensive and unstable. As a result, enzyme analytical processes can be costly and demand sparing use of these biocatalysts or immobilization on a suitable support for reuse. Enzymes are protein materials of a high molecular weight (10000–200000 dalton), consisting of amino acid chains linked by peptide bonds. As biological catalysts acting in complex living systems, they possess two analytical features of great significance: a high selectivity (or even specificity); and self-renewal via a catalytic cycle. The latter property is of special relevance to continuous flow work as it allows recycling and hence repeated use of the reagent. Not surprisingly, the earliest enzyme application in continuous-flow systems was also the first using a closed-loop configuration.

The selectivity of enzymes can be of various types. Some act on a specific function and thus exhibit '*group selectivity*'. Others operate on a given type of chemical bond and thus show '*linkage selectivity*'. Still others affect the reactions of an individual steric or chiral isomer, thereby exhibiting '*stereochemical specificity*'. Enzymes are frequently categorized according to the type of reaction they catalyse: hydration, dehydration, electron transfer, radical transfer, C-C bond formation or cleavage.

ENZYMES IN CONTINUOUS-FLOW SYSTEMS

Enzymes can be used in two primary forms in continuous-flow systems:

1. *Dissolved,* with or without recirculation (closed systems); and
2. Immobilized in a solid-phase reactor.

Personal preferences aside, the choice is dictated by the enzyme cost and stability in each instance. For example, glucose oxidase and uricase represent two extreme situations. The former is relatively stable in solution and fairly inexpensive relative to other enzymes; the latter is rather unstable in dissolved form and about 700 times as expensive—depending on the manufacturer—as glucose oxidase. Comparative studies of the performance of these two enzymes have led to the conclusion that, provided an enzyme is reasonably affordable and stable (i.e. if its room-temperature activity for the substrate of interest remains at a fairly constant level for a relatively long time), then it can be used for repeated determinations in a closed (recycling) system. According to Mottola *et al.* (1983), dissolved enzymes result in comparatively much higher sample throughput and similar reproducibility, enzyme expenditure and number of determinations as immobilized enzymes. Immobilized enzymes are, however, consumed more sparingly, but this is of little consequence with such an inexpensive enzyme as glucose oxidase, for example. Furthermore, immobilized enzymes result in increased reproducibility relative to dissolved enzymes.

Consumption of dissolved enzymes in an open flow system (i.e. one where the enzyme solution is wasted after detection) can be minimized by using either the merging-zones mode or a miniature FIA system. Open systems provide more desirable features than does the forced flow occasionally required by solid-phase reactors. Furthermore, immobilization is the better choice for expensive and/or unstable enzymes judging by available literature on the topic. The two primary analytical purposes of enzymes are catalytic determination of substrates and reaction products.

Catalytic determination of substrates (e.g. glucose, galactose, blood alcohol, uric acid) is particularly significant in clinical analysis, but also important in environmental chemistry (e.g. in the determination of phenol) and industrial (especially pharmaceutical) analyses such as those for penicillins in pharmaceutical preparations or fermentation broths (biotechnology) by the following reaction:

$$\text{Penicillin} + H_2O \rightarrow \text{Penicilloic acid.}$$

The *products of enzyme reactions* used in continuous-flow systems mostly include NADH or H_2O_2, which are typically detected by UV-vis, fluorescence or chemiluminescence spectroscopy, amperometrically or potentiometrically. Enzyme thermistors are based on the enthalpy changes involved in an enzyme reaction. Electrochemical detectors have gained wide acceptance recently due to the wide linear determination ranges they provide; also, they can be adapted for discrimination of electroactive compounds that are oxidized or reduced at a given potential.

Dissolved Enzyme Systems

In the simplest case, the enzyme can be dissolved in the carrier stream and its use minimized by making the residence time as short as possible. Further savings can be accomplished by using the merging-zones mode, which entails insertion of discrete sample and reagent plugs into one of various possible flow configurations. The most frequently used variant in this respect is that of '*multi-injection*', which entails using two injection valves inserted in as many channels to introduce two sample and reagent plugs that are merged immediately afterwards. Alternatively, the sample can be inserted into an inert carrier and be driven to a point of merging with another stream that dispenses the enzyme,

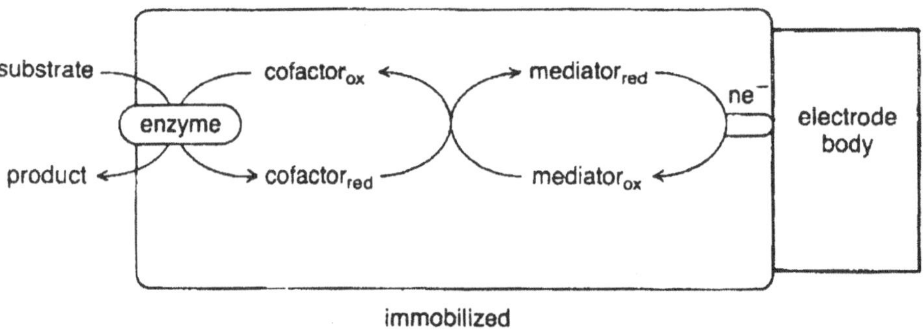

Fig. 7.1. The multi-injection technique.

but intermittently (at preset intervals), in such a way that the sample zone is supplied with enough enzyme. The sample and reagent can also be introduced sequentially into the same channel. The two aliquots are driven by the carrier to the manifold—the geometry of which determines dispersion and hence overlap—in the so-called 'chasing zones' mode. This also allows implementation of concentration gradients, thereby facilitating optimization of the working conditions.

The stopped-flow technique in its many variants can be used for measuring reaction rates as the basis for obtaining analytical results. For this purpose, the flow is halted as a sample portion reaches the detector's observation field in order to monitor signal changes over time. In this way, the residence time is lengthened without increasing dispersion—except for the negligible contribution of molecular diffusion—since the coefficient of dispersion *(D)* is time-independent. Reaction rate measurements, particularly in large numbers, result not only in increased reproducibility, but also in great reliability. While primarily used for the determination of substrates, the stopped- flow technique is equally effective for measuring enzyme activity.

Immobilized Enzyme Systems

According to the European Federation of Biotechnology, an immobilized enzyme system is one in which the enzyme is in 'any state that permits its reuse'. This is normally achieved by confining the enzyme in a water-insoluble matrix. There are two main types of analytical applications of immobilized enzymes in flow systems: chemically modified electrodes (CMEs) and immobilized enzyme reactors (IMERs).

IMERs are frequently used in flow systems including liquid chromatography (in a pre- or post-column arrangement). This type of enzyme reactor is similar to the solid-phase reactors in operational terms (e.g. location in the manifold, analytical purpose, type of support used). IMERs can be used both in isolation and in serial or parallel combinations. A single IMER can be placed at many different positions in the manifold including the sampling loop of the injection valve and the flow-cell itself. Most frequently, however, the IMER is placed between the injection valve and detector. An IMER can accommodate several enzymes immobilized on a single support, thereby ensuring that the zones where the analyte is to be subjected to various transformations lie close enough.

Immobilized enzymes combine the high selectivity of enzymatic reactions with the economy and stability ensuing from immobilization. In addition, they endow FIA applications with repeatability and a constant reactivity. Provided that a large amount of enzyme can be immobilized in a small enough volume, the resulting high selectivity ensures efficient, fast conversion of the substrate with minimal sample dispersion, which leads to an improved detection limit.

Enzyme Immobilization Techniques

For an immobilization procedure to be acceptable, it should preserve the enzyme activity while allowing a large amount of it to be loaded onto the support. There is no general rule as to what is the best immobilization procedure or support; the choice is dictated by the properties of the enzyme concerned in each instance. The immobilization procedure should never affect the configuration of the free enzyme if steric hindrance of the analytical reaction is to be avoided.

The reactors used to accommodate immobilized enzymes should be as small as possible in order to minimize sample dispersion. Therefore, efforts in this context are being aimed at obtaining high-purity enzymes, new polymeric agents (supports), optimal reactor configurations and, with multi-enzyme reactors, the optimal enzyme load proportions.

Progress of the analytical reaction in an IMER is obviously dependent on the amount of bonded enzyme. Unlike enzyme electrodes, where the small amount of enzyme present entails making fixed-time kinetic measurements, IMERs provide elevated conversions (occasionally as high as 100 per cent).

The critical reactor size depends on the kinetics of the reaction concerned and mass transfer required for the reaction to complete. If the reaction proceeds maximally, the IMER response will not be affected by the small activity losses it is bound to experience with time, nor by small changes in chemical and/or FIA variables such as pH, flow-rates, ionic strength or temperature. If a small amount of immobilized enzyme is used, however, even small changes in some experimental variables can lead to considerably decreased reproducibility. Also, the reactor lifetime increases with increasing amount of retained enzyme.

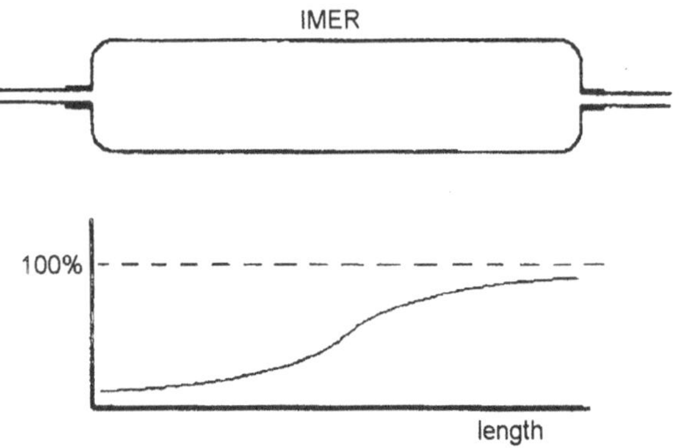

Fig. 7.2. Degree of substrate conversion vs. IMER length.

The fraction of substrate that is converted by an IMER via a first-order reaction is given by

$$X = 1 - 10^{-(aDV/Q)}$$

where a is the enzyme loading factor, D the coefficient of dispersion, V the reactor volume, and Q the flow-rate.

If the enzyme-substrate reaction is slow, the flow can be stopped in order to make reaction rate measurements, and run conversion vs. time plots. By using changes in the analytical signal rather than absolute values, several substrates can be quantified in a single sample injection, thereby also minimizing the effect of potential interferents.

Enzymes can be immobilized or anchored to an insoluble, inert support by physical or chemical means, as well as by confining them in a small volume with the aid of a semi-permeable membrane. This last procedure has been used for preparing various electrodes. Physical enzyme adsorption has rarely been used in analytical chemistry relative to covalent bonding attachment. The earliest reported instance of enzyme immobilization involved adsorbing invertase on timber coal; to the developers' surprise, the enzyme preserved most of the activity it exhibited in dissolved form. Immobilized enzymes did not gain wide popularity until the early 1950s, when carboxypeptidase and amylase were bonded to diazotized poly(*p*-aminostyrene).

Enzyme immobilization procedures, whether physical or chemical, have changed very little over the years. There are four basic types of such procedure:

1. Chemical cross-linking of the enzyme with itself or other protein molecules;
2. Trapping of the enzyme within the pores of a support;
3. Adsorption on a stiff matrix; and
4. Attachment by covalent bonding to a surface.

An additional procedure known as '*encapsulation*' has had little analytical application owing to the difficulty involved in having the substrate diffuse into the enzyme '*globule*'.

There are two chief *types of support:* porous and non-porous. Non-porous enzyme supports pose little resistance to diffusional mass transfer but offer a relatively small active surface area and hence a low loading capacity. Porous supports have much larger active surfaces and hence higher loading capacities, in addition to protection from the outer environment. However, because most of their surface area (and loaded material) lies within pores, mass diffusion is somewhat hindered. Also, porous supports, particularly those of controlled pore size, are more expensive than non-porous supports. As noted, a suitable support should feature a large surface area; high permeability; hydrophilicity; insolubility; chemical, mechanical and thermal stability; and stiffness, as well as appropriate particle size and shape, and resistance to microbial attack. Enzymes can be immobilized on a variety of surfaces including those of fibres, membranes, glass beads, polyacrylamide gel, the inner walls of nylon or glass tubes, TiO_2 beads, ion-exchange resins, carbon, etc.

Physical Immobilization Procedures

One of the simplest ways of immobilizing an enzyme is by adsorbing it on an inert support. Many metal oxides and glass are suitable adsorbents for this purpose; the attachment is established via hydrogen bonding between the oxygen-containing functions at the support surface and peripheral polar groups in the enzyme protein. Ion-exchange resins can be bonded to enzymes by ion association with charged groups at the protein surface. Adsorption attachment procedures are operationally very simple and preserve the enzyme integrity; however, the attachment may be overcome by an increased ionic strength and the enzyme is usually vulnerable to microbial and proteolytic attack.

One alternative to adsorption procedures is provided by *entrapment* between pores of a gel mesh. The gel is prepared from a solution containing the enzyme, where it is trapped as the gel sets. The high molecular weight of enzymes (frequently exceeding 15000 dalton) facilitates preparation of gels with a small enough pore size to prevent release of the trapped enzyme. A variant of this gel capturing procedure, *microencapsulation*, involves confining the enzyme in small capsules (5–300 μm in diameter) of semi-permeable membranes. The membrane thickness and permeability depend on the composition of the organic solvent, concentration and nature of the chemicals, and formation time used. Both the entrapment and the microencapsulation procedure are only applicable to those enzyme reactions involving substrates of a low molecular weight—macromolecules are obviously excluded. Substrate and product transfer are also affected by diffusional phenomena. Neither immobilization procedure causes any changes in the enzyme and both protect it from microbial and proteolytic attack.

Enzyme attachment to *semi-permeable* membranes is subject to some kinetic constraints. The effectiveness of this type of membrane relies on tight retention of the enzyme while allowing free movement of the substrate and product(s). While physical immobilization procedures do not alter enzyme active sites, the resulting preparations are less stable and have shorter service-lives than those provided by chemical procedures.

Chemical Immobilization Procedures

Enzymes can be incorporated into the propagating chain of a growing polymer by *covalent cross-linking*. The enzyme is thus attached by cross-linking between polymer molecules via a bifunctional reagent such as hexamethylenedithiocyanate, succinyl disalicylate, maleimidobenzoyl-N-hydrosuccinimide ester, etc. The low molecular weight of the cross-linking reagent allows it to reach the enzyme active sites and activate them. In order to avoid any activity losses, the enzyme is first adsorbed and then cross-linked.

By *covalent binding*, an enzyme can be attached to the surface of a pre-modified (activated) support via a peripheral group (e.g. an amino acid function that is not involved in the catalytic action of the enzyme). The process involves three steps: activation, enzyme bonding and cleavage of non-covalent enzyme bonds. Such inert matrices as glass and nylon provide the best covalent binding supports for use in continuous-flow systems. A support can be functionalized in many ways. The choice is usually dictated by the nature of the support and the enzyme stability at the immobilization pH. The bonding stability at the preparation pH and the pH at which it is to be subsequently used, which will depend on those of the sample and carrier, should also be considered. The most suitable enzyme supporting material for use in FIA applications is glass, which is functionalized by silanization, followed by cross-linking with (usually) glutaraldehyde and covalent binding of the enzyme concerned. This glutaraldehyde-based glass immobilization procedure is quite appealing on account of its simplicity and the mild chemical

$$\text{Si–OH} + (C_2H_5O)_3\text{Si–}(CH_2)_3\text{–}NH_2$$

$$\text{Si–OH} + (C_2H_5O)_3\text{Si–}(CH_2)_3\text{–}NH_2 \longrightarrow$$

controlled pore glass + aminosilane

$$\longrightarrow \text{Si–O–Si–}(CH_2)_3\text{–}NH_2 \;/\; \text{Si–O–Si–}(CH_2)_3\text{–}NH_2 + OHC\text{–}(CH_2)_3\text{–}CHO \longrightarrow$$

glutaraldehyde

$$\text{-----Si–}(CH_2)_3\text{=N–CH–}(CH_2)_3\text{–CHO} \;/\; \text{-----Si–}(CH_2)_3\text{=N–CH–}(CH_2)_3\text{–CHO} + H_2N\text{–Enz.} \longrightarrow$$

$$\text{-----Si–}(CH_2)_3\text{=N–CH–}(CH_2)_3\text{–CH=N–Enz.}$$

Fig. 7.3. Enzyme immobilization on silanized glass via glutaraldehyde.

conditions it requires—which allow application to a wide variety of enzymes—as well as the fairly high mechanical and chemical stability of glass. Glutaraldehyde is occasionally replaced with hydrazine, carbodiimide, sodium nitrate or cyanobromide as the mediator. This chemical immobilization procedure is also applicable to a different type of support in order to construct unconventional '*membrane reactors*'. There are commercially available epoxy and amino-derivatized membranes for use as enzyme supports. Some can be purchased pre-activated with glutaraldehyde; however, their efficiency can be further boosted by reactivation prior to immobilizing the enzyme.

One universal feature of chemical bonding attachment—there are few exceptions— is irreversibility: the enzyme cannot be removed from the matrix for reuse in solution. Because immobilized enzymes are heterogeneous catalysts, their properties (optimal pH, stability, Michaelis-Menten constant) differ from those in solution—for example, the activity of an immobilized enzyme usually increases with time. The analytical use of enzyme reactors in continuous-flow systems includes the determination of both substrates and, to a much lesser extent, enzyme activators and inhibitors.

Other Immobilization Procedures

All of the above-described procedures involve an aqueous medium. The fact that enzymes can act as catalysts in organic solvents allows their use in determining water- insoluble compounds and hence expands their scope in environmental, pharmaceutical and process control applications. Because enzymes are usually insoluble in non- aqueous media, they are easier to immobilize relative to aqueous solutions. In the future, enzymes may even be used in gaseous and supercritical fluid environments.

In principle, using non-aqueous solvents may expand application of enzyme catalysis to molecules of a low or zero water-solubility, and diminish microbial contamination and interferences from side reactions. In addition, the stability and service life of an IMER can be improved by attaching the enzyme to an inert support in an aqueous solution—most proteins are insoluble in organic solvents—and then using an organic solvent (carrier stream) in order to avoid sweeping the immobilized enzyme from the support. Proteins are conformationally stiffer in these solvents, so they should exhibit a higher thermal and general stability relative to a buffered aqueous solution, which can also extend the reactor lifetime. In the FIA determination of cholesterol, the analyte, dissolved in toluene, is oxidized by molecular oxygen in the presence of cholesterol oxidase; the hydrogen peroxide released is then converted to water by horseradish peroxidase, simultaneously with the oxidation of p-anisidine to a coloured product that is detected absorptiometrically. A recent procedure involved use of the immobilized enzyme-support suite in suspended form. Kojima *et al.* (1988) immobilized lactate dehydrogenase, malate dehydrogenase and horseradish peroxidase on small latex particles. The sample was injected into a carrier consisting of the latex suspension. The system was used to determine three analytes (lactate, malate and hydrogen peroxide) fluorimetrically.

Types of Reactor: Which is Best?

There are three basic types of enzyme reactor with regard to internal configuration: packed bed; open tubular; and single bead string reactors (SBSR). The most commonly used are packed bed reactors, particularly those prepared by cross-linking to a controlled-pore glass matrix via glutaraldehyde. Thermodynamic experiments with these reactors have shown the rates of the reactions they house to be more markedly dependent on some reactor properties (e.g. diffusion inside glass pores or mass transfer to the carrier surface) than on the kinetics of the catalysed reaction.

In open tubular reactors, the enzyme is normally anchored to the tube walls. Thus, enzymes can be bonded to a polycarboxylic gel applied to the inner walls of a narrow-bore nylon or glass tube. The usable enzyme anchoring surface and hence the reactor load can be increased by previously etching the inner walls of a glass tube, viz. by growing whiskers inside; some caution should be exercised, however, as continuous passage of the solvent through the tube may strip some whiskers, and the surface-expanding procedure can hardly be reproducible. One other way of augmenting enzyme loading is by anchoring the catalyst to glass particles of uneven shape (with sharp edges and vertices) that are previously inserted in the inner walls of a plastic reactor.

Tests aimed at determining which type of internal reactor configuration is the best revealed open tubular reactors to be the worst choice, and also provided some clues with regard to packed (packed-bed and SBSR) detectors, particularly in terms of size (particle diameter to tube inner diameter) ratios.

The performance of various linear, spiral, beaded and packed reactors was assessed in terms of reaction rate, sensitivity, throughput and sample dispersion by using two different enzymes: glucose oxidase and L-(+)-lactate oxidase. The enzymes were covalently bonded to the inner walls of 5-cm-long×1.12 mm internal diameter nylon tubes. The reactors filled with the larger beads exhibited 2–4 times higher activity, double sensitivity and a higher throughput than the open reactor; they also contributed minimally to physical and chemical dispersion of the sample. Packed-bed reactors were found to be superior in the determination of lactate and beaded reactors were superior in the determination of glucose. Reactors filled with beads of 1.0 mm average diameter allowed glucose to be determined over the range 10–800 μM with a coefficient of conversion of 0.056 mol of product per mol of substrate (the determination range and coefficient of conversion for lactate were 8–64 μM and 0.13, respectively). Based on other comparative studies on packing particle size, the optimal particle diameter appears to be 70 per cent of the inner diameter of the tube.

Packed-bed reactors are the best and only choice for many. Even though solid evidence is still unavailable, membrane reactors seemingly excel 'classical' (SBSR and packed-bed) reactors. A single reactor of this type can accommodate several membranes and hence different immobilized enzymes. The membranes (typically 5–8 mm in diameter) are placed in a groove carved in a plastic block. The flow impinges normally to the membrane surface it is to cross. The performance of membrane reactors is reportedly comparable to that of packed-bed reactors, with the added advantages that membranes are easier to handle and cause no flow overpressure (and hence no flow-rate oscillations), which results in typically longer service lives.

Use of Immobilized Enzyme Reactors for Determining Substrates of Pharmaceutical Interest

Immobilized enzymes have been used for a wide variety of purposes since their inception in analytical chemistry. They are compatible with virtually any type of detector intended to monitor the concentration of a substrate, reaction product, co-substrate or co-enzyme. Their potential can be further expanded by using several reactors in a serial or parallel arrangement, or by immobilizing several enzymes at once. The detection techniques commonly used with IMERs include UV-vis, fluorescence and chemiluminescence spectroscopy, amperometry, conductimetry, potentiometry (by means of ion-selective and gas sensors) and enthalpimetry.

Most FIA methods involving immobilized enzymes are concerned with biomedical and, to a much lesser extent, biotechnological analyses (viz. control and monitoring of fermentation broths). There are a large number of references to the determination of glucose and other biochemicals. However, many such compounds are also of pharmaceutical interest; for example, glucose, fructose, galactose, ethyl alcohol, ascorbic acid, penicillins, etc., which are included in many commercially available formulations. Some of the examples described below (FIA methods using one or more IMERs, irrespective of the detector type employed) do not strictly belong to pharmaceutical analysis as they involve biological matrices.

Penicillin G and V have been determined in pharmaceutical formulations (tablets and injectables) and fermentation broths, respectively, by using the enzyme penicillinase immobilized on glass via cross-linking with glutaraldehyde, upon treatment of the glass with (aminophenyl) trimethoxysilane in 95% ethanol. The enzyme exhibited maximum stability over the pH range 6–8, which was compatible with the optimal pH for glutaraldehyde binding, at 35°C. The enzyme was immobilized on glass beads that were placed in an SBSR in order to improve the results previously obtained with a packed-bed reactor. The manifold consisted of a single channel where the sample was injected into a phosphate buffer solution of pH 6.4 and ionic strength 0.10M, and pH changes were monitored potentiometrically by means of a planar electrode. The calibration graph was linear up to a 5×10^{-3} M concentration of penicillin.

Similarly, penicillin was determined using penicillinase immobilized on silica gel, with potentiometric monitoring of the penicilloic acid form via pH changes. The reactor lifetime was 600 h and a theoretical model for correlating pH (as the hydrogen ion concentration) with the analyte concentration in the sample was developed. Based on the results, the correlation between these two parameters was better than that between peak height and concentration. Prior to these experiments, penicillins were determined in continuous-flow systems by using penicillinase immobilized on silanized glass in a packed-bed reactor, or on Sepharose (via an antigenantibody reaction), with monitoring of the heat released in the catalytic reaction.

Penicillinase on a glass surface exerts its catalytic action on cephalosporin by cleaving its β-lactam ring, which results in a sharp decrease in the absorbance at 254 nm. By using a manifold consisting of two channels including the enzyme reactor and an inert reactor, respectively, two different signals are recorded, from which the analytical signal is obtained by difference. The linear determination range for cephalosporin thus achieved is 10–800 ppm, with a relative standard deviation of 0.7 per cent and a throughput of 30 samples/h.

Glutamic acid in a pharmaceutical formulation, was determined by use of an SBSR consisting of a tube of 0.8mm internal diameter filled with glass beads. The carrier (phosphate buffer at pH 7.8) drove the injected sample to a point of merging with a solution containing Trinder' s reagent in the same buffer. Detection was performed at 510nm using a spectrophotometer furnished with fibre optics for transmitting light to the flow-cell. The linear calibration range was from 10 to 500 mM, and the relative standard deviation 1.8 per cent.

Ortega *et al.* (1990) determined formate ion in pharmaceutical formulations by immobilizing formate dehydrogenase on controlled-pore glass beads previously silanized with 3-aminopropylethoxy silane, using glutaraldehyde as cross-linker. They used a packed-bed reactor and a phosphate buffer of pH 7 containing 2 mM NAD. The NADH formed was detected spectrophotometrically at 340 nm and 30°C. A linear range of 5–80 or 50–200—depending on the reactor length—and a relative standard deviation of 1.5 per cent were achieved. The method was applied to commercially available parenteral solutions.

Salicylic acid was determined in four different formulations with amperometric detection and derivatization of the analyte in an IMER containing salicylate hydroxylase (viz. salicylate 1-monooxygenase, a flavoprotein). The reactor was packed with glass beads, the surface of which was modified with aminosilane and activated with p-tetrachloroquinone. The enzyme solution, in phosphate buffer, was shaken with the activated beads for 5 h, after which the beads were stored in a refrigerator at 4°C. The enzyme was found to preserve its activity for at least one year. The process taking place in the reactor was the irreversible catalysed hydroxylation of salicylic acid to catechol. The concentration of salicylic acid in this reaction can be monitored via the disappearance of NADH or oxygen, or the formation of carbon dioxide or catechol. The latter was adopted as it provided the most accurate results. Amperometric measurements were made with the aid of a commercially available wall-jet flow-cell furnished with a glassy carbon working electrode, a Pt wire auxiliary electrode and an Ag/AgCl reference electrode. The linear determination

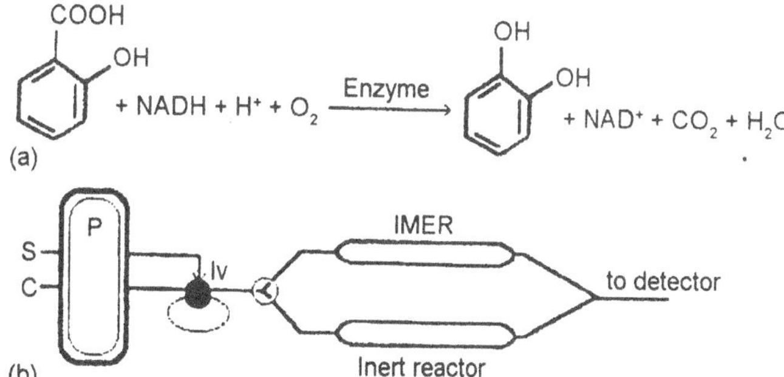

Fig. 7.4. (a) Hydroxylation of salicyclic acid to catechol; (b) schematic FIA manifold such as that proposed for salicylic acid determination in pharmaceutical formulations and ascorbic acid in brain tissue samples.

range thus achieved was 5–150 μg/ml—the optimal range for avoiding electrode fouling was 5–50 μg/ml—and the relative standard deviation 0.5–2.0 per cent.

The determination of glutamic acid in different types of sample (foods and pharmaceutical formulations) was carried out with the aid of a reactor containing immobilized L-glutamate dehydrogenase from beef liver. The enzyme was immobilized on controlled-pore glass beads modified by isothiocyanate according to the following chemical process, which includes the thioamide bonds between the free amino groups of the enzyme protein and the modified support (controlled-pore glass beads) surface:

$$R - NH_2 \xrightarrow{\text{thiophosgene}} R - NCS \xrightarrow{\text{enzyme}} R - NHCSNH\text{ - enzyme}$$

The procedure for determination of the amino acid involved injection of the sample into a carrier stream and passing it through the IMER. The NADH was produced according to the reaction:

$$\text{L - glutamic acid} + NAD^+ \xrightarrow{\text{L-glutamic dehydrogenase}} \alpha\text{ - ketoglutaric acid} + NH_4^+ + NADH.$$

The resulting NADH was fluorimetrically monitored. The flow manifold was optimized by means of the Simplex method. Although L-glutamate dehydrogenase acts on a number of amino acids, only glutamine, leucine and valine were acting as interferents.

Cholesterol is a major metabolite for a number of substrates of clinical, nutritional and cosmetic interest, as well as an emulsifier used in various pharmaceutical formulations. Massom and Townshend (1985c) determined it in blood serum, wax- wool alcohol and butter extract by injecting the sample into a phosphate buffer carrier at pH7.0. Hydrogen peroxide was released in the packed-bed reactor used, which contained cholesterol oxidase immobilized on controlled-pore glass beads via glutaraldehyde; the linear range was 0–80 mg/1, with relative standard deviation of 1.0–3.0 per cent.

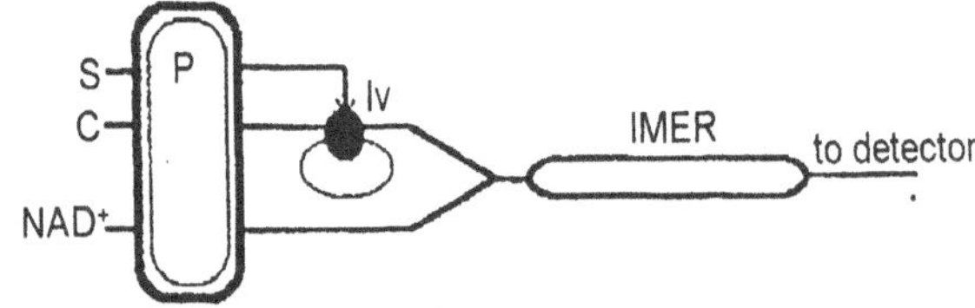

Fig. 7.5. FIA assembly proposed for determination of glutamates in pharmaceutical formulations

The essential amino acid L-lysine can be determined with L-lysine-a-oxidase from *Trichoderma viride* and horseradish peroxidase, co-immobilized in the same reactor. The peroxide produced in the reaction catalysed by the former enzyme yields a quinoneimine dye with phenol and 4-amino-antipyrine in the presence of the latter enzyme. The first step in the process is oxidation of the amino acid with L-lysine oxidase as catalyst:

$$\text{L-lysine} + O_2 + H_2O \rightarrow \alpha\text{-ketone-aminocaproate} + NH_3 + H_2O_2$$

which can be monitored via the oxygen or hydrogen peroxide. On reaction with phenol and 4-aminoantipyrine in the presence of horseradish peroxidase, the H_2O_2 gives a red quinoneimine:

$$2H_2O_2 + \text{phenol} + \text{4-aminoantipyrine quinoneimine} + 4H_2O$$

which can be monitored spectrophotometrically at 500 nm.

The immobilization procedure involves mixing the matrix (100 mg VA-Epoxy Biosynth) with lysine oxidase in phosphate buffer at pH7.4. The enzyme is covalently bonded by interaction between epoxy groups and the amino groups of the protein. The solid (resin) is isolated by filtration, dried and stored at 4°C. The same protocol is used to co-immobilize L-lysine oxidase and horseradish peroxidase, and the resins obtained are used to pack the reactor tubes. The test can be performed at a rate of 30 samples/h over the L-lysine range 1–16 mM, with a relative standard deviation of 0.5 per cent. L-lysine can also be determined in culture broths using L-lysine-2- monooxygenase immobilized on silica gel and measuring oxygen by means of a Clark membrane electrode.

One other, non-essential amino acid, L-alanine, was determined in a single-channel manifold including a reactor between the injection valve and a fluorimetric detector that was operated at λ_{ex}=340 nm and λ_{em}=465 nm. The enzyme, alanine dehydrogenase, was immobilized on pre-aminated poly (vinyl alcohol) beads. The reactor was stable for about 6 months and was used to analyse serum and beverage samples over the amino acid concentration range 0.5–500 mM, with a relative standard deviation of 0.83–0.85 per cent at a rate of 40 samples/h.

Ascorbic acid was determined in brain tissue samples using an FIA system with a split carrier channel. One of the split lines included an inert bed and the other a catalytic bed containing ascorbic acid oxidase. As the sample containing the ascorbic acid was passed through the inert bed, an amperometric signal corresponding to all electro-oxidizable matter in the sample (ascorbic acid, catecholamines and various metabolites) was obtained. The sample reaching the detector via the catalytic bed provided a smaller signal (ascorbic acid was removed by the bed) that was subtracted from the previous one in order to calculate the ascorbic acid concentration.

The determination of methanol in the presence of ethanol is one example of the use of several co-immobilized enzymes with enhanced selectivity. The system includes three enzymes: alcohol oxidase, catalase and formaldehyde dehydrogenase. The first catalyses the oxidation of methanol to formaldehyde and hydrogen peroxide; the latter is subsequently decomposed by catalase. The formaldehyde yielded in the first reaction is later oxidized to NADH, which is in turn oxidized by 1-methoxy-5-methyl-phenazinium methylsulphate. Finally, the resulting reduction product is spontaneously oxidized to an amount of hydrogen peroxide that is proportional to the initial methanol concentration. The H_2O_2 released is monitored via the chemiluminescence produced by reaction with luminol.

One other example of the use of several enzymes in a single reactor is the determination of the activity of LDH in serum samples. For this purpose, a lactate oxidase-catalase pre-column is used to remove lactate in the serum prior to reaction with lactose dehydrogenase. The chemiluminescence of ammonia is measured by means of a glutamate dehydrogenase-glutamate oxidase reactor. Finally, co-immobilized creatininase, creatinase and sarcosine oxidase in a single reactor are used to determine serum creatinine.

There are a number of methods for glucose determination based on its oxidation by oxygen in the presence of glucose oxidase, which yields gluconic acid and hydrogen peroxide. The interest in the determination of glucose is justified by its high clinical significance. Glucose oxidase was the first enzyme used in immobilized form in a continuous-flow system and has since been employed on a wide variety of supports included in a host of configurations. The hydrogen peroxide released can be detected amperometrically using two Pt electrodes at a potential difference of 0.6 V.

An IMER for glucose can be used in combination with another reactor in order to determine various sugars. Thus, an IMER placed behind a bed containing invertase and mutarotase can be used to quantify sucrose (by conversion into D-fructose and α-D-glucose, and monitoring of the latter via the H_2O_2 released in a prior IMER for glucose). Alternatively, the hydrogen peroxide can be monitored by the chemiluminescence produced on reaction with luminol. By using an appropriate IMER for each sugar, as well as a glucose IMER, various sugars including sucrose, maltose, lactose and fructose can readily be determined. Glucose is converted using two enzymes, glucose oxidase and mutarotase, in the same IMER; because the former is specific to β-D-glucose, the equilibrium concentration of which is 64 per cent, mutarotase is employed to ensure that all α-D-glucose is converted into β-D-glucose. Glucose has also been determined with the aid of a membrane reactor; the hydrogen peroxide released is monitored spectrophotometrically with the aid of a solution containing peroxidase and 2,2'-azinobis(3-ethylbenzthiazoline sulphonic acid) at room temperature. The sample volume used is 20 μl and the throughput achieved is 20 samples/h.

In other instances, several reactors, rather than a single one containing several enzymes, are used in FIA. The fluorimetric determination of fructose by use of a reactor containing mannitol dehydrogenase immobilized on poly(vinyl alcohol) beads involves a straightforward manifold into which the buffered carrier including the sample is injected and led to the detector via the IMER.

The bacterial detection of ATP is one example of the use of enzymes in their natural environment as an affordable, practical alternative to IMERs and dissolved enzymes. Luciferin and luciferase solutions are injected into an aqueous solution or bacterial extract containing the ATP. A multi-channel manifold was designed to monitor animal and microbial culturing processes. Cells of a mouse/mouse hybridoma strain were cultured continuously to produce Ig2a antibodies. Cells were immobilized on porous microcarrier and a fluidized bed reactor was inserted in a circulation loop. In this way, the FIA technique was used for process control of five crucial species: glucose, ammonia, glutamine, glutamate and lactate.

Finally, immobilized enzymes have also been used on various supports (cellulose, membranes) in the flow-cell of an optical detector (optosensing) for various analytical determinations including pH, glucose, gases, etc.

8

FLUORESCENCE-BASED ANALYSIS

The evolution of deoxyribonucleic acid (DNA) fragment size analysis from slab gels using radiolabeled or carcinogenic stains to capillary electrophoresis and fluorescence-based detection has provided for substantial increases in automation, accuracy, and precision. These advantages provide a cost effective, high-throughput screening method that can be utilized in a variety of pharmacogenomic investigations. The flexibility of this technique makes it a useful tool for the analysis of polymorphisms that cause an in vivo change in the size of a DNA fragment. This allows for the screening of a variety of mutational events, such as expansion or contraction of tandem repeats, insertions and deletions of varying size, or with additional manipulation of single nucleotide polymorphisms. The primary steps in a fragment size analysis protocol are the generation of the fragments containing the polymorphism of interest, the separation and detection of these fragments by capillary electrophoresis, determination of fragment size, and assignment of alleles. Fluorescence-based capillary electrophoresis requires the attachment of synthetic compounds designed to emit specific wavelengths of light upon excitation. Most high-throughput capillary electrophoresis systems use laser-induced fluorescence for excitation of these compounds and an on-line CCD camera for detection of the emitted light. The attachment of the fluorescent compounds can be done before the detection of the polymorphism by synthesizing one member of a forward and reverse primer pair with the fluorescent label attached to the 5' end. Use of these primers in a polymerase chain reaction (PCR) will generate amplicons that have incorporated the fluorescent label and will be detectable by capillary electrophoresis systems that are equipped with fluorescence detection capabilities.

MATERIALS

1. DNA samples.
2. 96-well thin wall plates suitable for thermal cycling.
3. True Allele PCR Premix.
4. Primer stocks: 2.5 μM stocks of each labeled forward and unlabeled reverse primer.
5. DNA Thermal Cycler PTC-200 or PTC-225 can be used.
6. Redistilled formamide.
7. Resin.
8. 96-well optical plates.
9. ROX400HD size standard.
10. 3100 Genetic Analyzer.
11. GeneMapper 3.0 analysis software.

Methods

PCR Amplification

1. Assemble a 15-μL reaction containing 9 μL of TrueAllele PCR Premix, 2 μL of a 2.5 *μM* stock of each forward and reverse primer, and 2 μL of DNA.

Reagent	*Volume*	*Final concentration*
True Allele PCR Premix	9 μL	1X
Labeled Forward Primer (2.5 *μM*)	2 μL	0.33 *μM*
Unlabeled Reverse Primer (2.5 *μM*)	2 μL	0.33 *μM*
DNA (2.5 ng/μL)	2 μL	5 ng

2. PCR conditions
   (a) 95°C for 10 min (hot start heat activation of the polymerase).
   (b) 30 cycles: 95°C for 1 min (Denature), 60°C for 1 min (Annealing), and 72°C for 1 min (extension)
   (c) 72°C for 10 min (final extension of products).
   (d) Hold products at 4°C until ready for processing.

Preparing PCR Products for Injection and Electrophoresis

1. Deionize Formamide: add 5 mL of redistilled formamide to 1.0 g of resin and let sit for 15 min to deionize.
2. To prepare sample for injection add 9.5 μL of deionized Formamide to 96-well optical plate, add 0.5μL of ROX400HD standard, and 1 μL of PCR product.
3. Denature mixture at 95°C for 5 min
4. Chill plate at 4°C for 2 min.
5. Briefly centrifuge sample to collect sample at the bottom of the well and to remove air bubbles.
6. Select run module for injection and electrophoresis conditions.

Data Analysis

The data analysis process begins with the identification of the primary peaks(s) from the sample electropherogram. Next is the calculation of the size, in base pairs, of the identified peak(s) followed by the assignment of alleles to complete the genotype assignment for each sample. GeneMapper 3.0 is an integrated software package that partially automates these steps with minimal user intervention.

Identification of the primary peak(s) from within the electropherogram requires the filtering of a variety of confounding information. Genemapper 3.0 software uses algorithms that are designed to look for common problems such as high background fluorescence, minimum and maximum peak height, the presence of "stutter" peaks that result from replication errors generated by polymerase slippage, and the presence of nontemplate-mediated adenosine addition generating fragments one base pair larger than expected. Problems related to peak height can often be alleviated by changing either the amount of PCR product added to the injection mixture or varying the time of the injection cycle for the electrophoresis. Polymerase slippage is a common problem in the generation of PCR fragments containing highly repetitive regions. Generation of stutter peaks in 3 and 4 bp repeat fragments is rarely a problem. The most common solution for minimizing the generation of these fragments is to increase the annealing temperature to increase the stringency of the PCR cycling.

Taq polymerase also is known to commonly add an additional Adenosine to the 3' end of an amplicon that is not present in the template. The occurrence of this +A peak can lead to the generation of multiple confounding peaks in all types of fragments, however, the most problematic cases develop

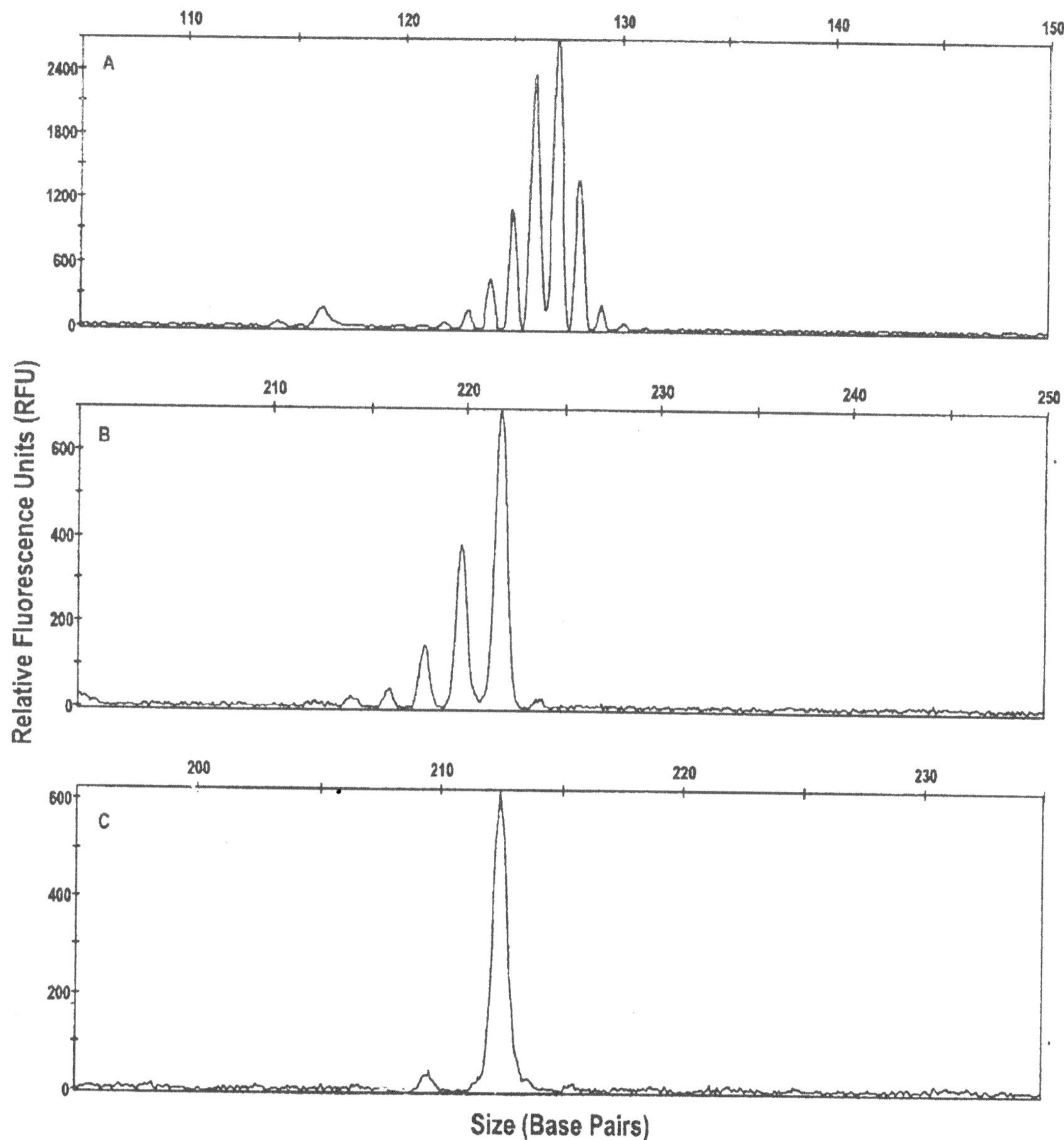

Fig. 8.1. Results of polymerase slippage in 1-, 2-, and 3- bp repeats. (A) shows the number of fragment species generated from a sample homozygous for a 26-bp pair poly-A repeat. The number of species generated by polymerase slippage in the 2-bp repeat (B) and a 3-bp repeat (C) are greatly reduced.

in shorter repeat units. It has been previously shown that different sequence motifs have varying affinities for the nontemplate-mediated adenosine addition. This work also suggested that the identification of sequence motifs that encouraged this +A addition were more effective than those that attempted to reduce its occurrence. Consequently, the synthesis of primers that contain a GTTTCT "pig-tail" of unique sequence on the 5' end can raise the affinity for the addition of adenosine. This increased affinity causes a higher proportion of the generated fragments to contain fragments of a single species, the known length plus the additional adenosine base, greatly simplifying the data analysis. Once the primary peak(s) in an electropherogram have been identified they are assigned a size in base pair by

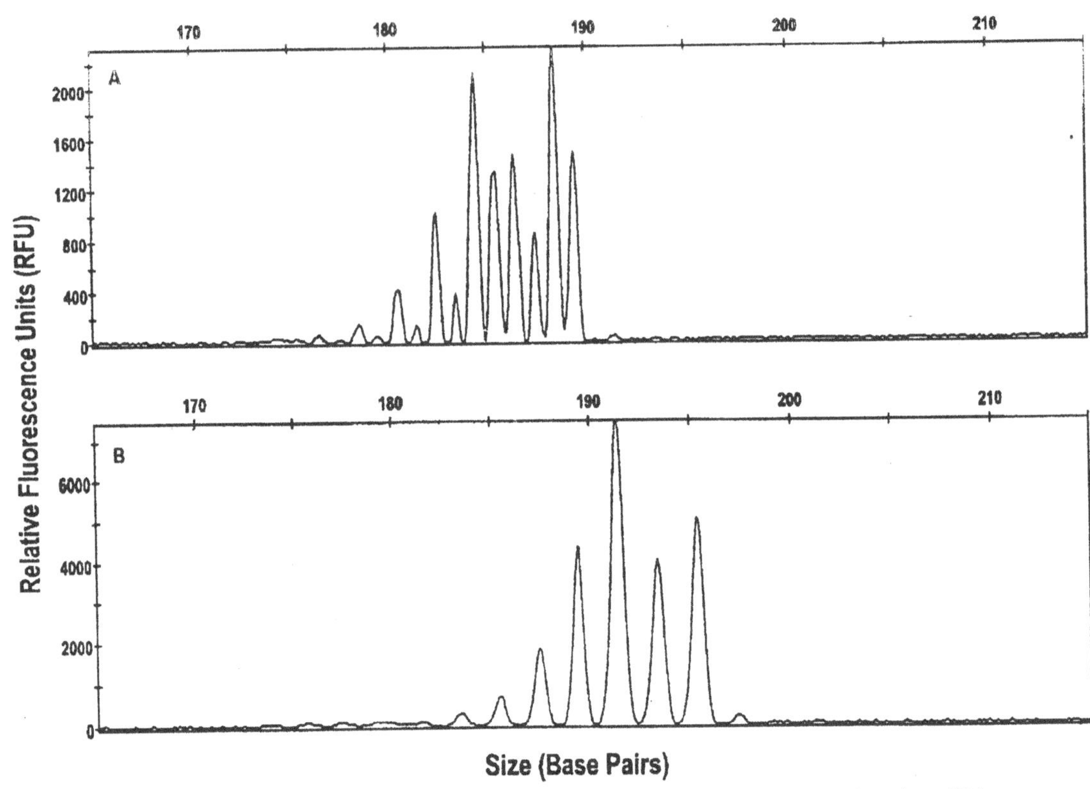

Fig. 8.2. The effects of "pig-tailing" the amplification primers to maximize the Taq adenosine addition.

the GeneMapper 3.0 software. The sizing peak sizing is done by the comparison of the detected peaks with those identified in the internal size standard, ROX400HD, that is run concurrently with the unknown sample. This size standard is run in a different color detection channel, so there is no peak overlap with the unknown sample. The peaks present in the size standard provide the algorithm with a reference for the sizing of the unknown peaks. This concurrent running of the size standard helps maintain a consistency in sizing and allele calling from run to run and allows comparison of data generated over long periods of time.

Notes

1. Synthesis of primers must take into account the addition of the proper synthetic fluorescent compound attached to the 5' end of the forward primer. This synthesis results in the accumulation of unincorporated fluor that must be removed by purification. Successful removal of both unincorporated fluor and incomplete synthesis products can be done by either high-performance liquid chromatography or reverse-phase column purification.
2. Selection of a fluorescent compound is dictated by the detection capabilities of the capillary electrophoresis instrument. The Applied Biosystems 3100 Genetic Analyzer has a variety of supported detection colors, as described in the following reference guide. Most color combinations include multiple detection channels for the detection of both samples and concurrently run standards used by the sizing algorithm.
3. An alternative to the commercial GeneMapper 3.0 genotyping software package is the freeware GeneScanView package, developed by Davide Campagna at CRIBI, University of Padova, Italy. This software is capable of reading fragment size analysis files generated by the Applied Biosystems

3100 Genetic Analyzer and generates an electropherogram for visualization and exact sizing of the data.

4. DNA template amounts from 5 to 50 ng from a variety of purification methods have been successfully used in this Fragment Size Analysis protocol. Of primary importance is the uniformity of the concentrations across all samples. This will aid in the uniformity of sample injection, providing higher quality data for downstream analysis.
5. Because of the limited amount of sample that is used in the injection procedure, smaller PCRs can be used to reduce reagent use. PCRs as small as 5 μL have been used successfully in this protocol if special care is taken to minimize evaporation of the samples during amplification. The use of 384-well plates and heat activated plate seals can help minimize this problem.

Variation in observed fluorescence can be controlled by changing the amount of PCR product that is added to the deionized formamide dilution reagent. Additionally, changes in the duration of the sample injection step of the capillary electrophoresis run module can have a stabilizing effect on the amount of sample that is loaded into the capillary. Reducing the injection time has a more profound effect on those reactions that contain excess amounts of sample than those having limited amounts. This causes a greater reduction in signal strength for those samples that may be exceeding the detection capabilities of the instrument than those exhibiting minimal signal strength. Increases in injection time can assist in recovering samples that amplify poorly. However, this often increases the amount of background fluorescence that is observed as a result of the injection of unwanted material, such as carryover PCR reagents and remnants of DNA extraction materials, which can complicate the downstream data analysis and should be used cautiously.

9

IMMUNOMODULATING AGENTS

The immune system is responsible for controlling the body's response to various types of injury and for defending the body from invading pathogens, including bacteria, viruses, and other parasites. The importance of this system in maintaining health is illustrated by the devastating effects that can occur in people who lack adequate immune function, such as patients with acquired immunodeficiency syndrome (AIDS). The use of drugs to modify immune responses, or immunomodulating agents, is therefore an important area of pharmacology. For example, it may be helpful to augment immune function if a person's immune system is not functioning adequately. By contrast, it is sometimes necessary to suppress immune function pharmacologically to prevent immune-mediated injury to certain tissues or organs. Following organ transplants and tissue grafts, the immune system may cause the rejection of tissues transplanted from other donors (*allografts*) or from other sites in the patient's body (*autografts*). Likewise, immunosuppression may be helpful when the immune system causes damage to the body's tissues. Such conditions are often referred to as *autoimmune diseases*. Clinical disorders such as rheumatoid arthritis, myasthenia gravis, and systemic lupus erythematosus are now recognized as having an autoimmune basis.

This chapter addresses immunosuppressive drugs, or *immunosuppressants*, that are currently available to prevent the rejection of transplants or to treat specific diseases caused by an autoimmune response. Clearly, these drugs must be used very cautiously because too much suppression of the immune system will increase a patient's susceptibility to infection from foreign pathogens. Likewise, these drugs are rather toxic and often cause a number of adverse effects to the kidneys, lungs, musculoskeletal system, and other tissues. Nonetheless, immunosuppressive agents are often life- saving because of their ability to prevent and treat organ rejection and to decrease immune-mediated tissue damage in other diseases.

Drugs that increase immune function, or immunostimulants, are also addressed in this chapter. This group of agents is rather small, and the clinical use of immunostimulants is limited when compared with the indications for immunosuppressive drugs. Nonetheless, the development and use of immunostimulants is an exciting area of pharmacology, and some insight into the therapeutic use of these drugs is provided.

This chapter begins with a brief overview of the immune response, followed by the drugs that are currently available to suppress or stimulate this response. Physical therapists and occupational therapists may be involved in the rehabilitation of patients who have received organ transplants, skin grafts, or similar procedures that necessitate the use of immunosuppressant drugs. Rehabilitation specialists also treat patients with autoimmune disorders or immunodeficiency syndromes that affect the musculoskeletal system; these patients are also likely to be taking immunomodulating drugs. Hence, this chapter will provide therapists with knowledge about the pharmacology of these drugs and how the drugs' effects and side effects can affect physical rehabilitation.

Overview of the Immune Response

As indicated, one of the primary responsibilities of the immune system is to protect the body from bacteria, viruses, and other foreign pathogens. The immune response consists of two primary components: innate and adaptive (acquired) immunity. Innate immunity involves specific cells (leukocytes) that are present at birth and provide a relatively rapid and nonselective defense against foreign invaders and pathogens throughout the individual's lifetime. Adaptive immunity primarily involves certain lymphocytes (T and B) that develop slowly but retain the ability to recognize specific invading microorganisms and to initiate specific steps to attack and destroy the invading cell.

The innate and adaptive branches of the immune response are both needed for optimal immune function, and the two interact extensively. The adaptive response's ability to recognize and deal with foreign pathogens likewise involves an incredibly complex interaction between various cellular and chemical (humoral) components. A detailed description of the intricacies of how these components work together is beyond the scope of this chapter. Many aspects of the immune response are still being investigated.

1. *Antigen ingestion, processing, and presentation.* An invading substance (*antigen*) is engulfed by phagocytes such as macrophages and other antigen-presenting cells (APCs). The APCs process the antigen by forming a complex between the antigen and specific membrane proteins known as major histocompatibility complex (MHC) proteins. The antigen-MHC complex is placed on the surface of the APC, where it can be presented to other lymphocytes such as the T cells. The APCs also synthesize and release chemical mediators such as interleukin-1 (IL-1) and other cytokines, which act on other immune cells (T cells) to amplify these cells' response to immune mediators.
2. *Antigen recognition and T-cell activation.* Lymphocytes derived from thymic tissues (hence the term *T cell*) recognize the antigen-MHC complex that is presented to the T cell on the macrophage surface. This recognition activates certain T cells (T-helper cells), which begin to synthesize and release a number of chemical mediators known as *lymphokines*. Lymphokines are cytokines and chemokines derived from activated T lymphocytes and include mediators such as interleukin-2 (IL-2), other interleukins, gamma interferon, B-cell growth and differentiation factors, and other chemicals that stimulate the immune system. Certain T cells (T-killer cells) are also activated by APC presentation, and directly destroy targeted antigens.
3. *Proliferation, amplification, and recruitment.* T cells continue to replicate and proliferate, thus producing more lymphokines, which further amplifies the T-cell effects. These lymphokines also recruit lymphocytes derived from bone marrow—that is, B cells. Under the direction of IL-1 and other lymphokines, B cells proliferate and differentiate into plasma cells. Plasma cells ultimately release specific antibodies known as *immunoglobulins* (IgG, IgA, IgM, and the like). Likewise, T-cell and macrophage- derived lymphokines recruit additional cellular components, including other macrophages, cytotoxic lymphocytes (natural killer, or NK, cells), and various cells that can participate in the destruction of the foreign antigen.

Clearly, the immune response is an intricate sequence of events that involves a complex interaction between a number of cellular and humoral components. The overview provided here is just a brief summary of how some of the primary components participate in mediating acquired immunity.

Pharmacologic Suppression of the Immune Response

Drugs are used to suppress the immune system for two basic reasons. First, the immune response is often attenuated pharmacologically following the transplantation of organs or tissues to prevent the rejection of these tissues. Sometimes, organs and other tissues can be attacked by the recipient's immune system, even if these tissues appear to be cross-matched between donor and recipient. This rejection is often caused by membrane proteins on the donor tissue that are recognized as antigens by the host's immune system. Hence, drugs that suppress the cellular and chemical response to these membrane proteins can help prevent them from destroying the transplanted tissues and causing additional injury to the host's tissues.

Often, several different types of immunosuppressants are used together in fairly high doses to prevent or treat transplant rejection. For instance, a glucocorticoid such as betamethasone is often administered with nonsteroidal drugs such as cyclosporine and azathioprine to provide optimal success and viability of the transplant. Of course, giving several powerful drugs at high doses often causes unpleasant or even toxic side effects. These effects must often be tolerated, however, considering the limited number of organs available for transplantation and the need to ensure the survival of the transplant as much as possible.

A second major indication for these drugs is to limit immune-mediated damage to the body's tissues— that is, suppression of an autoimmune response. Autoimmune responses occur when the immune system loses the ability to differentiate the body's own tissues from foreign or pathogenic tissues. Exactly what causes this defect in immune recognition is often unclear, but prior exposure to some pathogen such as a virus may activate the immune response in a way that causes the immune system to mistakenly attack normal tissues while trying to destroy the virus. This autoimmune activation may remain in effect even after the original pathogen has been destroyed, thus leading to chronic immune-mediated injury to the body's tissues.

Autoimmune responses seem to be the underlying basis for a number of diseases, including rheumatoid arthritis, diabetes mellitus, myasthenia gravis, systemic lupus erythematosus, scleroderma, polymyositis/dermatomyositis, and several other disorders. As indicated previously, it is not exactly clear what factors cause autoimmune responses, as well as why certain individuals are more prone to autoimmune-related diseases. Nonetheless, drugs that suppress the immune system can limit damage to various other tissues, and these drugs may produce dramatic improvements in patients with diseases that are caused by an autoimmune response.

Specific Immunosuppressive Agents

Azathioprine

Clinical use

Azathioprine (Imuran) is a cytotoxic agent that is structurally and functionally similar to certain anticancer drugs, such as mercaptopurine. Azathioprine is primarily used to prevent the rejection of transplanted organs, especially in patients with kidney transplants. Azathioprine may also be used to suppress immune responses in a wide range of other conditions, such as systemic lupus erythematosus, dermatomyositis, inflammatory myopathy, hepatic disease, myasthenia gravis, and ulcerative colitis.

Mechanism of action

Although the exact mechanism of azathioprine is unknown, this drug probably interferes with DNA synthesis in cells mediating the immune response. Azathioprine appears to act like the antimetabolite drugs used in cancer chemotherapy. The cell normally uses various endogenous substances such as purines as ingredients during DNA synthesis. Azathioprine is structurally similar to these purines, and this drug acts as a false ingredient that competes with the naturally occurring substances to slow down and disrupt DNA synthesis. Impaired nucleic acid synthesis slows down the replication of lymphocytes and other key cellular components that direct the immune response. Thus, azathioprine directly limits cellular proliferation through this inhibitory effect on DNA synthesis and ultimately limits the production of humoral components (antibodies) produced by these cells.

Adverse effects

The primary side effects of azathioprine are related to suppression of bone marrow function, including leukopenia, megaloblastic anemia, and similar blood dyscrasias. Other side effects include skin rash and gastrointestinal distress (appetite loss, nausea, vomiting); hepatic dysfunction can also occur when higher doses are used.

Cyclophosphamide

Clinical use

Cyclophosphamide (Cytoxan, Neosar) is an anticancer alkylating agent that is commonly used in a variety of neoplastic disorders. This drug may also be helpful in suppressing the immune response in certain autoimmune diseases, such as multiple sclerosis, systemic lupus erythematosus, and rheumatoid arthritis. High doses of cyclophosphamide are also used to prevent tissue rejection in patients receiving bone marrow transplants and other organ transplants.

Mechanism of action

This drug causes the formation of strong cross-links between strands of DNA and RNA, thus inhibiting DNA/RNA replication and function. Cyclophosphamide probably exerts immunosuppressant effects in a similar manner; that is, this drug inhibits DNA and RNA function in lymphocytes and other key cells, thus limiting the rapid proliferation of these cells during the immune response.

Adverse effects

Cyclophosphamide is used very cautiously as an immunosuppressant because of the possibility of severe side effects, including carcinogenic effects during long-term use. Other side effects include hematologic disorders (leukopenia, thrombocytopenia), cardiotoxicity, nephrotoxicity, and pulmonary toxicity.

Cyclosporine

Clinical use

Cyclosporine (Neoral, Sandimmune) is one of the primary medications used to suppress immune function following organ transplantation. This medication can be used alone or combined with glucocorticoids, azathioprine, and other immunosuppressants to prevent the rejection of a kidney, lung, liver, heart, pancreas, and other organ transplants.

Cyclosporine is used to a somewhat lesser extent in treating autoimmune diseases, but it may be helpful in conditions such as psoriasis, rheumatoid arthritis, inflammatory bowel disease, and glomerulonephritis. Cyclosporine has also been used in the early stages of type 1 diabetes mellitus to help control immune-mediated destruction of pancreatic beta cells, thus decreasing the severity of this disease in some patients.

Although cyclosporine is one of the most effective immunosuppressants, the traditional form of this drug is associated with unpredictable absorption from the gastrointestinal (GI) tract and potentially severe side effects, such as nephrotoxicity and neurotoxicity. In a newer form of cyclosporine (Neoral), the drug is modified into microemulsion capsules that disperse more easily within the GI tract, thereby enabling the drug to be absorbed in a more predictable fashion. The microemulsion form of cyclosporine appears to be safer because it is not as toxic to the kidneys and other tissues as is the regular formulation. Hence, this microemulsion formulation is often the optimal way to administer cyclosporine following organ transplantation or other situations requiring immunosuppression.

Mechanism of action

Cyclosporine and tacrolimus are known as calcineurin inhibitors because they inhibit a specific protein (calcineurin) in lymphoid tissues. This inhibition ultimately suppresses the production of IL-2, a cytokine that plays a critical role in immune response by promoting the growth and proliferation of activated T lymphocytes and other immune cells, such as NK cells. Thus, cyclosporine is one of the premier immunosuppressants because of its relative selectivity for T cells and its inhibition of a key mediator of the immune response (IL-2). This relatively specific inhibition is often advantageous when compared with other nonselective drugs such as azathioprine, cyclophosphamide, and glucocorticoids that inhibit virtually all the cells and chemical mediators involved in the immune response.

Adverse effects

The primary problem associated with cyclosporine is nephrotoxicity, which can range from mild, asymptomatic cases to severe kidney dysfunction, which requires discontinuation of the drug. Hypertension is also a common adverse effect, especially when cyclosporine is used for prolonged periods. Other problems include neurotoxicity, gingival hyperplasia, hair growth (hirsutism), and increased infections. These problems, however, tend to be less severe with cyclosporine than with other less-selective immunosuppressants.

Glucocorticoids

Clinical use

Glucocorticoids are powerful anti-inflammatory and immunosuppressive drugs. Glucocorticoids exert a rather nonspecific inhibition of virtually all aspects of cell- and chemical-mediated immunity, thus enabling these drugs to be used in a variety of situations when it is necessary to suppress immune function. Hence, these drugs are a mainstay in preventing transplant rejection and in treating various diseases associated with an autoimmune response.

Glucocorticoids commonly used as immunosuppressants include the following:

- betamethasone (Celestone)
- cortisone (Cortone)
- dexamethasone (Decadron, others)
- hydrocortisone (Cortef)
- methylprednisolone (Medrol)
- prednisolone (Pediapred, Prelone, others)
- prednisone (Deltasone, others)
- triamcinolone (Aristocort, others)

Mechanism of action

Although their exact mechanism of immunosuppression is unclear, glucocorticoids probably interrupt the immune response by a complex effect at the genomic level of various immune cells. These drugs enter immune system cells, where they bind to a cytoplasmic receptor. The drug-receptor complex then migrates to the cell's nucleus, where it acts directly on specific immunoregulatory genes. In particular, glucocorticoids influence the expression of cytokines and other chemicals that orchestrate the immune response; that is, glucocorticoids inhibit the transcription of messenger RNA units that are normally translated into immunostimulatory signals such as interleukin-1, gamma interferon, and other substances that activate the cells responsible for mediating the immune response. Hence, these drugs disrupt the production of chemical signals that activate and control various immune system cellular components.

Adverse effects

The immunosuppressive effects of glucocorticoids are balanced by several side effects. Glucocorticoids typically produce a catabolic effect on collagenous tissues, and breakdown of muscle, bone, skin, and various other tissues is a common adverse effect. Glucocorticoids also produce other side effects, including hypertension, adrenocortical suppression, growth retardation in children, an increased chance of infection, glaucoma, decreased glucose tolerance, and gastric ulcer. These side effects can be especially problematic when glucocorticoids are used to prevent transplant rejection because these drugs are often given in high dosages for extended periods.

Therefore, glucocorticoids are typically combined with other nonsteroidal immunosuppressants such as cyclosporine, azathioprine, or immunosuppressive antibodies so that synergistic effects can be obtained and immunosuppression can be achieved with relatively low doses of each drug. In addition, efforts are often made to progressively decrease the glucocorticoid dose so that immunosuppression is achieved by using the lowest possible dose. In some cases, the glucocorticoid may even be withdrawn during maintenance immunosuppressive therapy, and nonsteroidal drugs (cyclosporine, tacrolimus, mycophenolate mofetil) are used to provide long-term immunosuppression following organ transplantation.

Methotrexate

Clinical use

Methotrexate (Folex, Rheumatrex) was originally developed as an anticancer agent, but this drug is also used occasionally in certain noncancerous conditions that have an autoimmune component. Methotrexate is commonly used as a disease-modifying drug in rheumatoid arthritis. Methotrexate is also approved for use in psoriasis. This agent has only mild immunosuppressive effects, however, and is not typically used to treat organ transplants or other conditions that require more extensive immunosuppression.

Mechanism of action

This drug acts as an antimetabolite that interferes with the production of DNA and RNA precursors in rapidly proliferating cells. This interference produces a general inhibition of the replication of lymphocytes inherent in the immune response.

Adverse effects

The major problems associated with methotrexate include hepatic and pulmonary toxicity. These problems are dose-related, however, and serious adverse effects tend to occur less frequently at doses used for immunosuppression than at those for anticancer treatment.

Mycophenolate Mofetil

Clinical use

Mycophenolate mofetil (CellCept) is primarily used to prevent or treat organ rejection following cardiac and renal transplantation. This drug is typically combined with other immunosuppressants (cyclosporine, glucocorticoids) to provide optimal immunosuppression in patients receiving these transplant types. Mycophenolate mofetil may also be useful in suppressing the immune response associated with autoimmune conditions such as systemic lupus erythematosus.

Mechanism of action

Mycophenolate mofetil inhibits a specific enzyme (inosine monophosphate dehydrogenase) that is responsible for the synthesis of DNA precursors in T and B lymphocytes. Because these lymphocytes cannot synthesize adequate amounts of DNA, their ability to replicate and proliferate is impaired, thus blunting the immune response. This drug may also inhibit lymphocyte attraction and adhesion to the vascular endothelium, thereby impairing the lymphocytes' ability to migrate to the site of the foreign (transplanted) tissues and to infiltrate from the bloodstream into these tissues.

Adverse effects

The primary adverse effects associated with mycophenolate mofetil are blood disorders (anemia, leukopenia, neutropenia) and gastrointestinal problems (abdominal pain, nausea, vomiting, heart-burn, diarrhea, constipation). Other side effects include chest pain, cough, dyspnea, muscle pain, weakness, and cardiovascular problems (hypertension, arrhythmias).

Sulfasalazine

Clinical use

Sulfasalazine (Azulfidine, other names) has unique properties, with some antibacterial characteristics similar to sulfonamide drugs and some of anti-inflammatory characteristics similar to the salicylates. This drug is primarily used to suppress the immune response associated with rheumatoid arthritis and inflammatory bowel disease.

Mechanism of action

The exact mechanism of this drug in immune-related disorders is not fully understood. Sulfasalazine may affect key components in the immune system, including suppression of NK cells. Other effects may be related to the drug's breakdown into active metabolites, including sulfapyridine and mesalamine, which exert antibiotic and anti-inflammatory effects, respectively.

Adverse effects

Primary side effects include headache, blood dyscrasias (agranulocytosis, anemia, thrombocytopenia), increased sensitivity to ultraviolet light, and hypersensitivity reactions (fever, skin rash, itching). Hypersensitivity can be severe or even fatal in susceptible individuals.

Sirolimus

Clinical use

Sirolimus (rapamycin, Rapamune) is one of the newest immunosuppressants and is an antibiotic that also has substantial immunosuppressant effects. This drug is used primarily to prevent organ rejection in people with solid organ transplants (kidney, heart, and so forth). Sirolimus is especially helpful following kidney transplants because it helps prevent organ rejection without adversely affecting glomerular filtration and other aspects of the kidney function. Likewise, this drug is often used preferentially in patients with renal dysfunction instead of more nephrotoxic drugs (cyclosporine, tacrolimus).

To provide optimal immunosuppressant effects, sirolimus is typically combined with glucocorticoids or other immunosuppressants. Sirolimus exerts a number of other beneficial effects, including the ability to inhibit smooth muscle proliferation in blood vessel walls. For this reason, sirolimus is sometimes incorporated into drug-eluting stents; that is, a supportive tubular structure (stent) is placed in the lumen of a partially occluded artery, and the drug is released slowly from the stent to help reduce vessel occlusion.

Mechanism of action

Unlike other immunosuppressants (cyclosporine, tacrolimus), sirolimus does not interfere directly with cytokine production. Instead, sirolimus inhibits the function of a specific enzyme commonly known as the mammalian target of rapamycin (mTOR). This enzyme plays a key role in signaling pathways that promote the growth and proliferation of T and B cells. By inhibiting this enzyme, sirolimus causes cell division to stop at a specific stage (G1), thereby limiting the ability of these cells to mount an attack on transplanted tissues.

Adverse effects

Sirolimus may cause blood lipid disorders, including hypercholesterolemia and hypertriglyceridemia. Other side effects include blood disorders (anemia, leukopenia, thrombocytopenia), diarrhea, skin rash, joint and muscle pain, and hypertension.

Tacrolimus

Clinical use

Tacrolimus (Prograf) is similar to cyclosporine in structure and in immunosuppressive effects, but tacrolimus is approximately 10 to 100 times more potent than cyclosporine. Tacrolimus may be somewhat less toxic than cyclosporine and other immunosuppressants, although serious side effects may still occur at higher doses. Tacrolimus is used primarily to prevent rejection of kidney and liver transplants. This drug may also be useful in preventing or treating the rejection of other organs and tissues including heart, lung, pancreas, and bone marrow transplants. Topical preparations of tacrolimus or an analogous drug known as pimecrolimus (Elidel) can also be used to treat skin disorders such as atopic dermatitis.

Mechanism of action

Tacrolimus acts like cyclosporine by binding to a specific protein (calcineurin) in lymphoid tissues and inhibiting the production of key immune mediators such as IL-2.5 IL-2 plays a critical role in the immune response because this substance promotes the growth and proliferation of activated T lymphocytes and other immune cells, such as NK cells. This binding provides a somewhat more selective inhibition of immune function than other drugs that exert a general or nonselective inhibition of the immune response.

Adverse effects

Common side effects of tacrolimus include gastrointestinal disturbances (cramps, nausea, diarrhea, constipation), weakness, fever, and skin rashes and itching. More serious problems include renal and central nervous system (CNS) toxicity (headache, anxiety, nervousness, seizures). Tacrolimus is also associated with problems with glucose metabolism (hyperglycemia, glucose intolerance), and can cause diabetes mellitus in certain individuals.

Other Methods of Immunosuppression

Immunosuppressant antibodies

Immune function can also be suppressed by using antibodies that interact with specific immune system cells and interfere with the cell's function. These antibodies can be obtained from animal sources and cell culture techniques (monoclonal antibodies) to provide a rather selective method of suppressing immune function. For example, antibodies such as Rho(D) immunoglobulin are used routinely to suppress immune response in mothers who have been exposed to a fetus's incompatible blood type. This immunosuppression prevents the mother from developing antibodies that will be passed on to the fetus or to a fetus in a subsequent pregnancy, thus blocking the production of maternal antibodies that can attack the fetus's blood and cause a potentially fatal condition known as hemolytic anemia of the newborn.

Antibodies have also been developed that are very selective for antigens located on the surface of specific T cells and other lymphocytes; these antibodies inhibit cell function or cause destruction of the cell. Anti-T-cell antibodies are primarily used to help prevent or treat rejection of organ and bone marrow transplants.

Antibodies that block the interleukin-2 receptor, thus preventing interleukin-2 from activating T lymphocytes, have also been developed. These anti-interleukin-2 receptor agents, such as basiliximab (Simulect) and daclizumab (Zenapax), may be helpful in reducing the incidence of acute transplant rejection Antibodies seem to be especially useful in the initial (induction) phase of antirejection treatment because these drugs can delay or supplant the use of more toxic immunosuppressants such as the glucocorticoids and calcineurin inhibitors (cyclosporine and tacrolimus).

Finally, antibodies such as adalimumab (Humira) and infliximab (Remicade) have been developed that bind directly to tumor necrosis factor alpha (TNF-alpha), thereby preventing this cytokine from causing damage to joints and other tissues. These anti-TNF–alpha drugs are therefore helpful in autoimmune diseases such as rheumatoid arthritis. Immunosuppressant antibodies continue to gain acceptance as a method for preventing rejection of transplanted tissues and for treating various autoimmune diseases.

Miscellaneous Immunosuppressants

A variety of other agents with cytotoxic effects has been used to suppress the immune system. These drugs include chlorambucil (Leukeran), dactinomycin (Cosmegen), mercaptopurine (Purinethol), vinblastine (Velban), and vincristine (Oncovin, Vincasar). These agents are similar to methotrexate; they exert cytotoxic effects that interfere with the proliferation of immune system cellular components. These drugs are used primarily as anticancer agents. The use of these agents as immunosuppressants, however, has generally declined in favor of drugs that have a more selective and strategic effect on immune function. Nonetheless, these drugs may be helpful in certain autoimmune disorders, or in preventing the rejection of tissue and organ transplants in specific situations.

Finally, thalidomide can be used as an immunosuppressant in conditions such as systemic lupus erythematosus (SLE) and in preventing graft-versus-host disease following bone marrow transplant. This drug was originally developed as a sedative, but was later discovered to produce severe birth defects when administered to women during pregnancy. Nonetheless, thalidomide may help blunt immunologic responses by regulating the genes that express tumor necrosis factor-alpha. Decreased production of this factor results in diminished activation of neutrophils and other immune components, thereby reducing the severity of immunologic reactions. The effects of thalidomide on immune function appear to be very complex, however, and this drug may actually increase the production of tumor necrosis factor alpha in certain conditions such as human immunodeficiency virus (HIV) infection. Hence, thalidomide's immunomodulatory effects continue to be investigated, and use of this drug in specific diseases may be modified in the future.

Immunostimulants

A number of agents can suppress the immune system. However, there has been considerable interest in developing pharmacologic methods to modify or even stimulate immune function in specific situations. In particular, agents that have a positive immunomodulating effect could be beneficial to patients with compromised immune function (such as AIDS or certain cancers) or chronic infections. Development of immunostimulants, however, is understandably a complex and potentially dangerous proposition. Excessive or incorrect immune activation could trigger myriad problems that resemble autoimmune diseases. Likewise, it may be difficult to selectively stimulate certain aspects of the immune system to treat a specific problem without also causing a more widespread and systemic immunologic response. Nonetheless, a few strategies are currently available to modify or stimulate immune function in a limited number of situations.

Bacille Calmette-Guerin

Clinical use

Bacille Calmette-Guerin (BCG, TheraCys, others) is an active bacterial strain that can be administered systemically as a vaccine against tuberculosis. This agent may also stimulate immune function and can be administered locally within the bladder (intravesicularly) to treat certain forms of superficial bladder cancer.

Mechanism of action

The exact reason that this agent is effective in treating cancer is unknown. Some evidence suggests that it may activate macrophages locally at the site of the cancer and that these macrophages engulf and destroy tumor cells.

Adverse effects

When administered directly into the bladder, common side effects include bladder irritation and infection. Systemic administration (immunization) may also cause dermatologic reactions (peeling or scaling of the skin), allergic reactions, inflammation of lymph nodes, and local irritation or ulceration at the injection site.

Immune Globulin

Clinical use

Immune globulin (Gamimune, Gammagard, other names) is prepared by extracting immunoglobulins from donated human blood. These preparations contain all subclasses of immunoglobulin (Ig) but consist primarily of IgG. Immune globulin is administered intravenously to boost immune function in several conditions, including primary immunodeficiency syndromes (congenital agammaglobulinemia, common variable immunodeficiency, and severe combined immunodeficiency), idiopathic thrombocytopenic purpura, Kawasaki disease, chronic lymphocytic leukemia, and HIV infection in children. Other potential indications for immune globulin include dermatomyositis, Guillain-Barre syndrome, demyelinating polyneuropathies, Lambert-Eaton myasthenia syndrome, and relapsing-remitting multiple sclerosis.

Mechanism of action

Commercial preparations of immune globulin mimic the normal role of endogenous immunoglobulins. These preparations therefore directly act as antibodies against infectious agents. They can also help modulate the activity of T lymphocytes, macrophages, and other immune system cells to maintain immune system competence.

Adverse effects

Immune globulin may cause several side effects, such as joint and muscle pain, headache, general malaise, and gastrointestinal disturbances (nausea, vomiting). Although rare, allergic reactions, including anaphylaxis, can occur in some individuals. Because immune globulin is obtained from human blood, care must also be taken to prevent transmission of hepatitis and HIV from infected donors.

Levamisole

Clinical use

Levamisole (Ergamisol) is primarily used to treat colorectal carcinoma. Specifically, this drug is administered with fluorouracil to prevent recurrence of colorectal cancer after surgical removal of the primary tumor.

Mechanism of action

Although the exact effects are not known, levamisole may augment immune function by activating macrophages and immune cells that selectively engulf and destroy any residual cancerous cells.

Adverse effects

Levamisole may cause blood disorders such as agranulocytosis, leukopenia, or thrombocytopenia. Other side effects include nausea, diarrhea, and a metallic taste in the mouth.

Other Immunomodulators

Cytokines are a potential way to modify the immune system in several situations because of their ability to act as immunoregulatory chemicals. For example, cytokines such as interferon-alpha and interleukin-2 can be administered to treat certain forms of cancer. Likewise, certain interferons can help control viral infections, and interferon- beta may be helpful in autoimmune diseases such as multiple sclerosis. Researchers continue to investigate how immune function can be manipulated to treat various diseases, and additional immune system modulators will almost certainly be forthcoming.

Our knowledge of how the immune system functions in both normal and disease states has increased dramatically over the last several decades, and we now have drugs that can moderate the effects of the immune response in certain clinical situations. Immunosuppressants are a mainstay in preventing tissue rejection, and much of the current success of organ transplants is due to the judicious use of immunosuppressive drugs. These drugs are also beneficial in a number of diseases that have an autoimmune basis, and immunosuppressants can help alleviate symptoms or possibly even reverse the sequelae of certain diseases such as rheumatoid arthritis. A few agents are also available that can augment or stimulate immune function in certain situations. The use of these immunostimulants will continue to expand as more is learned about how we can enhance the immune response in conditions such as cancer and certain immunocompromised states. However, immunomodulating drugs are not without problems because many agents cause a rather nonspecific effect on immune function, which leads to serious side effects. As more is learned about the details of immune function, new drugs will be developed that are more selective in their ability to modify immune responses without causing a generalized suppression or activation of the immune system.

10

Management of Pharmacogenomic Information

There is no doubt that the sequencing and initial annotation of the human genome, completed in April 2001, is one of the great scientific advancements in history. This breakthrough in biological research was made possible by advances in high-performance computing and the use of a highly sophisticated information technology infrastructure. High-speed computers are necessary to analyze the tens of terabytes of raw sequence data and correctly order the 3.2-billion base pairs of deoxyribonucleic acid (DNA) that compose the human genome. The assembly and initial annotation is only the first step on a long road for understanding the human genome. Many companies, research institutes, universities, and government laboratories are now rapidly moving on to the next steps: comparative genomics, functional genomics, proteomics, metabolomics, pathways, systems biology, and pharmacogenomics. The latter is the study of how an individual's genetic inheritance affects the body's response to drugs. Thus, it holds the promise that drugs might one day be tailor-made for individuals and adapted to each person's own genetic makeup.

Environment, diet, age, lifestyle, and state of health all can influence a person's response to medicines, but understanding an individual's genetic makeup is thought to be the key to creating personalized drugs with greater efficacy and safety. Researchers are beginning the quest to determine exactly how each gene and protein functions and more important how they malfunction to trigger deadly illnesses such as heart disease, cancer, Alzheimer's and Parkinson's diseases.

Important prerequisites for pharmacogenomics or personalized medicine will be achieved by combining a person's clinical data sets with genome information- management systems. However, huge disparate data sources, like public or proprietary molecular biology databases, laboratory management systems, and clinical information management systems pose significant challenges to query and transform these data into valuable knowledge. The core data are collections of nucleic and amino acid sequences stored in GenBank and protein structures in the Protein Data Bank. Additionally, this core data is used to create secondary and integrated databases, such as PROSITE and InterPro. Furthermore, integrating data collected from high-throughput genomic technologies, like sequencing, microarrays, single-nucleotide polymorphism (SNP) detection, and proteomics, require the nontrivial development of information management systems. For their establishment, increasingly powerful computers and capacious data storage systems are mandatory. In the next paragraphs we will give an overview of the main and most important technologies needed for the management of pharmacogenomic information, namely database management systems (DBMS) and software and hardware architectures.

Databases and DBMS

Because pharmacogenomics deals with a great many of public and/or proprietary data, there is a need to easily store, retrieve, and exchange it. The major problem is the integration of the steadily increasing heterogeneous data sources.

The most prominent ways to manage and exchange bioinformatics data are as follows:

1. Field/value-based flat files;
2. ASN.1 files;
3. XML files; and
4. Relational databases.

Field/value-based flat files have been very commonly used in bioinformatics. Examples are the flat file libraries from GenBank, European Molecular Biology Laboratory Nucleotide Sequence Database (EMBL), DNA Data Bank of Japan, or Universal Protein Resource (UniProt). These file types are a very limited solution because they lack referencing, vocabulary control, and constraints. In addition, on the file level, there is no inherent locking mechanism that detects when a file is being used or modified. However, these file types are primarily used for reading purposes.

ASN.1 is heavily used at the National Center for Biological Information as a format for exporting GenBank data and can be seen as a means for exchanging binary data with a description of its structure. The access concurrency is like flat files just manageable at file level, there is no support for queries, and it lacks on scalability. But because ASN.1 files convey the description of its structure, it thus provides the flexibility that the client side does not necessarily need to know the structure of the data in advance.

eXtensible Markup Language (XML) documents are an emerging way to interchange data and consist of elements that are textual data structured by tags. Additionally XML documents may include a Document Type Definition (i.e., DTD) that describes the structure of the elements of an XML document. XML files are hence very flexible, human readable, and provide an open framework for defining standard specifications. For example, the MGED and Gene Ontology Consortium have adopted XML to provide and exchange data. The weaknesses of XML are the file-based locking mechanism and the large overhead of a text-based format caused by the recurrent content-describing tags. Although XML provides query mechanisms, it lacks scalability because it does not provide scalable facilities such as indexing.

A relational DBMS is a collection of programs that enables to store, modify, and extract information from a relational database. Such a relational database has a much more logical structure in the way data are stored. Tables are used to represent real world objects; with each field acting like an attribute. The set of rules for constructing queries is known as a query language. Different DBMSs support different query languages, although there is a semistandardized query language called structured query language (SQL). One major advantage of the relational model is that if a database is designed efficiently according to Codd rules, there should be no duplication of any data, which helps to maintain database integrity. DBMS do also provide powerful locking mechanisms to allow parallel reading and writing without data corruption. Needless to say, there are other ways to exchange data like the Common Object Request Broker Architecture (CORBA). This standard provides an intermediary object-oriented layer that handles access to the data between server and client. Another recently emerging way to exchange data is web services, which will be described later.

Data Warehouse and Federated Database System

Genomic management systems allow to query data assembled from different heterogeneous data sources. They are based on two different approaches:

1. Data warehouse
2. Federated database system

A data warehouse is a collection of data specifically structured for querying and reporting. Therefore, data have to be imported in regular intervals from sources of interest. These data constitute and act like a centralized repository. Applications can query these data efficaciously and create reports. Implemented data marts duplicate content in the data warehouse and allow faster responses because of a much higher granularity of the information. The drawbacks of a data warehouse are that the timeliness of the content depends on the update interval of the external data sources. These updates can be very time consuming and may result in higher storage requirements and operating costs.

Federated database systems overcome these downsides by directly accessing external data through federated database servers. Integration of external data can be complete (all data can be accessed) or partial (only information needed is available through the server). Shortcomings of federated databases are that queries spanning different data sources at different locations tend to be slow. Because of different query styles, dialects, and data formats federated database servers are quite complex.

The Sequence Retrieval System (SRS), initially developed at EMBL and the European Bioinformatics Institute, uses an interesting approach by combining the features of data warehouses and federated database systems. SRS is on the one hand heavily indexing locally stored genomic flat file databases and, on the other hand, it allows one to query DBMS on different sites. An example for a federated approach is the Mouse Federated Database of the Comparative Mouse Genomics Centers Consortium.

Software Architecture

To meet the requirements of pharmacogenomic data processing systems, a sophisticated software architecture has to be used. Less complex tasks like microarray image analysis or gene expression clustering can be performed on a commonly used workstation. In this case, applications are installed locally on a client machine on which all computational tasks are performed. Required databases are either installed locally or can be accessed via the local area network (LAN) or the Internet. This kind of direct client-server access is characteristic for two-tier systems. In a two-tier architecture the application uses the data model stored in the enterprise information system (EIS) but does not create a logical model on top of it.

All the business logic is packed into the client application and, therefore, increased workstation performance is required as soon as the applications are getting more complex or computational intensive. Furthermore, applications and database clients have to be deployed and kept up-to-date to adapt to new interfaces on the server side or to add new business logic to the system. Although there is a technology provided by Sun Microsystems called Java Web Start to automate this cumbersome task, only a few software vendors are supporting it. In general, two-tier software application design is ideal for prototyping, for applications known to have a short lifetime, or for systems where the Application Programming Interfaces will not change. Typically, this approach is used for small applications where development costs as well as development time are intended to be low.

Most of the drawbacks of two-tier architectures can be avoided by moving to a three-tier architecture with an application server as central component. In a three-tier architecture, the separation of presentation, business, and data source logic becomes the principal concept. Presentation logic is about how to handle the interaction between the user and the software. This can be as simple as a command-line or text-based menu system, a client graphical user interface (i.e., GUI), or a HTML-based browser user interface. The primary responsibility of this layer is to display information to the user and to interpret commands from the user into actions upon the business and data source logic. The business logic contains what an application needs to do for the domain it is working with. It involves calculations based on inputs and stored data, validation of data coming from the presentation layer, and figuring out exactly what data source logic to dispatch depending on commands received from the presentation layer. The data source logic, or EIS, is about communicating with other systems that carry out tasks on behalf of the application, like transaction monitors or messaging systems. But for most applications the biggest piece of data source logic is a database, which is primarily responsible for storing persistent data. The usage of a three-tier architecture leads to the following advantages:

1. Easier to modify or replace any tier without affecting the other tiers (maintenance).
2. Separating the application and database functionality leads to better load balancing and therefore supports an increasing number of users or more demanding tasks.
3. Adequate security policies can be enforced within the server tiers without hindering the clients.

The two major enterprise development platforms Java 2 Enterprise Edition (J2EE) and Microsoft.Net are supporting this kind of software architecture. They can be seen as a stack of common services, like relational database access, messaging, enterprise components, or support for web services, that each platform provides to their applications. With this knowledge in the back of one's mind, the question which platform to use can be answered based on the expertise of the team members, their preferences, and based on the existing hardware and software infrastructure.

The next step in the evolution of distributed systems is web services. The concept behind is to build applications not as monolithic systems but as an aggregation of smaller systems that work together towards a common purpose. Web services are self-contained, self-describing, modular applications that can be published, located, and invoked across the Web. Web services communicate using HTTP and XML and interact with any other web service using standards like Simple Object Access Protocol (SOAP), Web Service Description Language (WSDL), and Universal Description Discovery and Integration (UDDI) services, which are supported by major software suppliers. Web services are platform independent and can be produced or consumed regardless of the underlying programming language. The main limitations of web services are the network speed and round trip time latency. An additional limitation is the use of SOAP as protocol, since it is based on XML and HTTP, which degrades performance compared to other protocols like CORBA.

HARDWARE

Life science is becoming increasingly quantitative as new technologies facilitate collection and analysis of vast amounts of data ranging from complete genomic sequences of organisms to three-dimensional (3D) protein structure and complete biological pathways. As a consequence, biomathematics, biostatistics and computational science are crucial technologies for the study of complex models of biological processes. The quest for more insight into molecular processes in an organism poses significant challenges on the data analysis and storage infrastructure. Because of the vast amount of available information, data analysis on genomic or proteomic scale becomes impractical or even impossible to perform on commonly used workstations. Computer architecture, CPU performance, amount of addressable and available memory, and storage space are the limiting factors. Today, high-performance computing has become the third leg of traditional scientific research, along with theory and experimentation. Advances in pharmacogenomics are inextricably tied to advances in high-performance computing.

Parallel Processing Systems

The analysis of the humongous amount of available data requires parallel methods and architectures to solve the computational tasks of pharmacogenomic applications in reasonable time. State of the art technology comprises three different approaches to parallel computing:

1. Shared memory systems
2. Distributed memory systems
3. Combination of both systems

Shared memory systems

In shared memory systems multiple processors are able to access a large central memory (e.g., 16, 32, 64 GBytes) directly through a very fast bus system. This architecture enables all processors to solve numerical problems sharing the same dataset at the same time. The communication between processors is performed using the shared memory pool with efficient synchronization mechanisms making theses systems very suitable for programs with rich inter-process communication. Limiting factors are the relative low number of processors that can be combined and the high costs.

Distributed memory systems

In general, these systems consist of clusters of computers, so called nodes, which are connected via a high-performance communication network. Using commodity state-of-the-art calculation nodes and network technology, these systems provide a very cost efficient alternative to shared memory systems for dividable, numerical computational intensive problems that have a low communication/ calculation ratio. On the contrary, problems with high inter-processor communication demands can lead to network congestion, which is decreasing the overall system performance. If more performance is needed, this architecture can easily be extended by attaching additional nodes to the communication network.

Grid computing

Grid computing is an emerging technology, poised to help the life science community manage their growing need for computational resources. A compute grid is established by combining diverse heterogeneous high-performance computing systems, specialized peripheral hardware, PCs, storage, applications, services, and other resources placed over various locations into a virtual computing environment. For every numerical problem the appropriate computing facility in a worldwide resource pool can be harnessed to contribute to its solution. A computing grid differs from the earlier described cluster topology mainly by the fact that there is no central resource management system. In a grid every node can have its own resource management system and distribution policy. Grid technologies promise to change the way complex life science problems are tackled and help to make better use of existing computational resources. Soon, a life scientist will look at the grid and see essentially one large virtual computer resource built upon open protocols with everything shared: applications, data, processing power, storage, and so on, all through a network.

Partitioning

To use the parallel features of a high performance computing facility, the software has to meet parallel demands, too. A numerical problem that has to be solved in parallel must be divided into subproblems that can be subsequently delegated to different processors. This partitioning procedure can be done either with so-called *domain decomposition* or *functional decomposition*.

The term domain decomposition describes the approach to partition the input data and to process the same calculation on each available processor. Most of the parallel-implemented algorithms are based on this approach dividing the genomic databases into pieces and calculating, for instance, the sequence alignment of a given sequence on a subpart of the database. The second and simplest way to implement the domain decomposition on a parallel computing system is to take sequentially programmed applications and execute them on different nodes with different parameters. An example is to run the well-known basic local alignment search tool (BLAST) with different sequences against one database by giving every node another sequence to calculate. This form of application parallelization is called swarming and does not need any adaptation of existing programs.

On the other hand, functional decomposition is based on the decomposition of the computation process. This can be done by discovering disjoint functional units in a program or algorithm and sending these subtasks to different processors. Finally, in some parallel implementations combinations of both techniques are used, so that functional-decomposed units are calculating domain-parallelized sub-tasks.

Data Storage

Drug discovery-related data storage and information management requirements are doubling in size every 6 to 8 mo, more than twice as fast as Moore's Law predictions for microprocessor transistor counts. For life science organizations, data is necessary, but not sufficient for organizational success. They must generate information—meaningful, actionable, organized, and reusable data. Data must be stored, protected, secured, organized, distributed, and audited, all without interruption.

State-of-the-art storage architecture comprises the following solutions:

1. Directly-attached storage (DAS)
2. Network-attached storage (NAS)
3. Storage-area networks (SAN)
4. Internet SCSI (iSCSI)

Directly attached storage

This historically first and very straightforward method can be seen today in every PC: hard disks, floppy disks, CD-ROMs or DVDs are attached directly to the main host using short internal cables. Although in the mainframe arena storage devices, hard disks or tape drives are separate boxes connected to a host, this configuration is from a functional perspective equivalent to standard PC technology. DAS is optimized for single, isolated processor systems and small data volumes delivering good performance at low initial costs.

Network-attached storage

Network-attached storage (NAS) is defined as storage elements that are connected to a network providing file access services to computer systems. These devices are attached directly to the existing LAN using standard TCP/IP protocols. NAS systems have intelligent controllers built in, which are actually small servers with stripped operating systems, to exploit LAN topology and grant access to any user running any operating system. Integrated NAS appliances are discrete pooled disk storage subsystems, optimized for ease-of-management and file sharing, using lower-cost, IP-based networks.

Storage-area networks

A storage-area network (SAN) is defined as a specialized, dedicated high-speed network whose primary purpose is the transfer of data between and among computer systems and storage elements. Fibre Channel is the de facto SAN standard network protocol, although other network standards, like iSCSI, could be used. SAN is a robust storage infrastructure, optimized for high performance and enterprise-wide scalability.

Internet SCSI (iSCSI)

SCSI is a collection of standards that define I/O buses primarily intended for connecting storage subsystems or devices to hosts through host bus adapters. iSCSI is an new emerging technology and is based on the idea of the encapsulation of SCSI commands in TCP/IP (most widely used protocol to establish a connection between hosts and exchange data) packages and sending them through standard IP based networks. With this approach iSCSI storage elements can exist anywhere on the LAN and any server talking the iSCSI protocol can access them.

A pharmacogenomic DBMS has to combine public and proprietary genomic databases, clinical data sets, and results from high-throughput screening technologies. Currently, the most important public available biological databases require disk space in the magnitude of 1 terabyte (1000 gigabytes).

Considering the exponential growth of data, it can be expected that the storage requirements for proteomics will claim petabytes (1000 terabytes). Even more, systems for personalized medicine will be in the range of exabytes (1000 petabytes). Assuming that the storage capacity doubles every year it is imaginable that in 10 yr working with petabytes will be a standard procedure in many institutions. To facilitate the management, handling, and processing of this vast amount of data, such systems should comprise data-mining tools embedded in a high-performance computing environment using parallel processing systems, sophisticated storage technologies, network technologies, database and DBMS, and application services. Integration of patient information management systems with genomic databases as well as other laboratory and patient-relevant data will represent significant challenges for designers and administrators of pharmacogenomic information management systems. Unfortunately, the lack of international as well as national standards in clinical information systems will require the development of regional specific systems. Additionally all arising security issues concerning the sensitivity of certain types of information have to be solved in a proper manner. To accomplish all this stated issues, considerable endeavors have to be undertaken to provide the necessary powerful infrastructure to fully exploit the promises of the postgenomic era.

11

PHARMACOLOGIC MANAGEMENT

Rheumatoid arthritis and osteoarthritis represent the two primary pathologic conditions that affect the joints and periarticular structures. Although the causes underlying these conditions are quite different from one another, both conditions can cause severe pain and deformity in various joints in the body. Likewise, pharmacologic management plays an important role in the treatment of each disorder. Because physical therapists and other rehabilitation specialists often work with patients who have rheumatoid arthritis or osteoarthritis, an understanding of the types of drugs used to treat these diseases is important. This chapter will begin by describing the etiology of rheumatoid joint disease and the pharmacologic treatment of rheumatoid arthritis. An analogous discussion of osteoarthritis will follow. Hopefully, these descriptions will provide rehabilitation specialists with an understanding of drug therapy's role in arthritis, and the impact drugs can have on patients receiving physical therapy and occupational therapy.

RHEUMATOID ARTHRITIS

Rheumatoid arthritis is a chronic, systemic disorder that affects many different tissues in the body, but is primarily characterized by synovitis and the destruction of articular tissue. This disease is associated with pain, stiffness, and inflammation in the small synovial joints of the hands and feet, as well as in larger joints such as the knee. Although marked by periods of exacerbation and remission, rheumatoid arthritis is often progressive in nature, with advanced stages leading to severe joint destruction and bone erosion.

In addition to the adult form of this disease, there is also a form of arthritis that occurs in children known commonly as juvenile rheumatoid arthritis, or by the more recent term juvenile idiopathic arthritis (JIA). Juvenile arthritis differs from the adult form of this disease—the age of onset (younger than 16 years) and other criteria help to differentiate these two types of rheumatoid joint disease. Drug treatment of adult and juvenile rheumatoid arthritis is fairly similar, however, with the exception that children may not respond as well to certain medications (e.g., hydroxychloroquine, gold compounds, penicillamine) compared to adults. Consequently, in this chapter most of the discussion of the management of rheumatoid arthritis is directed toward the adult form.

Rheumatoid arthritis affects about 0.5 to 1.0 percent of the population worldwide. This disease occurs three times more often in women than in men, with women between the ages of 20 and 40 especially susceptible to the onset of rheumatoid joint disease. Rheumatoid arthritis often causes severe pain and suffering, frequently devastating the patient's family and social life as well as his or her job situation. The economic impact of this disease is also staggering; medical costs and loss of productivity exceed $1 billion annually in the United States. Consequently, rheumatoid arthritis is a formidable and serious problem in contemporary health care.

Immune Basis for Rheumatoid Arthritis

The initiating factor in rheumatoid arthritis is not known. It is apparent, however, that the underlying basis of this disease consists of some type of auto- immune response in genetically susceptible individuals. Some precipitating factor (possibly a virus or other infectious agent) appears to initiate the formation of antibodies that are later recognized by the host as antigens. Subsequent formation of new antibodies to these antigens then initiates a complex chain of events involving a variety of immune system components such as mononuclear phagocytes, T lymphocytes, and B lymphocytes. These cells basically interact with each other to produce a number of arthritogenic mediators, including cytokines (interleukin-1, tumor necrosis factor-alpha), eicosanoids (prostaglandins, leukotrienes), and destructive enzymes (proteases, collagenases). These substances act either directly or through other cellular components of the immune system to induce synovial cell proliferation and destruction of articular cartilage and bone. Thus, the joint destruction in rheumatoid arthritis is the culmination of a series of events resulting from an inherent defect in the immune response in patients with this disease.

Overview of Drug Therapy in Rheumatoid Arthritis

The drug treatment of rheumatoid arthritis has two goals: (1) to decrease joint inflammation and (2) to arrest the progression of this disease. Three general categories of drugs are available to accomplish these goals: (1) nonsteroidal anti-inflammatory drugs (NSAIDs), (2) glucocorticoids, and (3) a diverse group of agents known as *disease-modifying antirheumatic drugs* (*DMARDs*). NSAIDs and glucocorticoids are used primarily to decrease joint inflammation, but these agents do not necessarily halt the progression of rheumatoid arthritis. DMARDs attempt to slow or halt the advancement of this disease, usually by interfering with the immune response that seems to be the underlying factor in rheumatoid arthritis. Each of these major drug categories, as well as specific disease-modifying drugs, is discussed in the following sections.

Nonsteroidal Anti- Inflammatory Drugs

Aspirin and the other NSAIDs are usually considered the first line of defense in treating rheumatoid arthritis. Although NSAIDs are not as powerful in reducing inflammation as glucocorticoids, they are associated with fewer side effects, and they offer the added advantage of analgesia. Consequently, NSAIDs such as aspirin are often the first drugs employed in treating rheumatoid arthritis; in fact, this disease can often be controlled for short periods in some patients by solely using an NSAID. In patients who continue to experience progressive joint destruction despite NSAID therapy these drugs are often combined with disease-modifying agents. Usually, it is not advisable to use two different NSAIDs simultaneously because there is an increased risk of side effects without any appreciable increase in therapeutic benefits. Some amount of trial and error may be involved in selecting the best NSAID, and several agents may have to be given before an optimal drug is found. Aspirin appears approximately equal to the newer, more expensive NSAIDs in terms of anti-inflammatory and analgesic effects, but some of the newer drugs may produce less gastrointestinal discomfort. In particular, the cyclooxygenase-2 (COX-2) selective drugs may be especially helpful in people with a history of peptic ulcers or other risk factors for gastrointestinal problems. The choice of a specific NSAID ultimately depends on each patient's response to the therapeutic effects and side effects of any given agent.

Finally, acetaminophen (paracetamol) products may provide some temporary analgesic effects in people with rheumatoid arthritis, but these products are not optimal because they lack anti-inflammatory effects. Acetaminophen can be used to treat mild-to-moderate pain, but the lack of anti-inflammatory effects makes acetaminophen fall short of NSAIDs for conditions such as rheumatoid arthritis. Hence, patients with rheumatoid arthritis usually prefer the effects of NSAIDs to acetaminophen, and acetaminophen products are not typically used for the routine treatment of this disease.

Mechanism of action

Basically, aspirin and the other NSAIDs exert most or all of their anti-inflammatory and analgesic effects by inhibiting the synthesis of prostaglandins. Certain prostaglandins (i.e., prostaglandin E_2 [PGE_2]) are believed to participate in the inflammatory response by increasing local blood flow and vascular permeability and by exerting a chemotactic effect on leukocytes. Prostaglandins are also believed to sensitize pain receptors to the nociceptive effects of other pain mediators such as bradykinin. Aspirin and other NSAIDs prevent the production of prostaglandins by inhibiting the COX enzyme that initiates prostaglandin synthesis. Aspirin and most other NSAIDs inhibit all COX forms; that is, these drugs inhibit the COX-1 form of the enzyme that produces beneficial and protective prostaglandins in certain tissues while also inhibiting the COX-2 form that synthesizes prostaglandins in painful and inflamed tissues. Newer NSAIDs, however, are known as COX-2 inhibitors because these drugs inhibit the specific form of COX-2 that synthesizes prostaglandins during pain and inflammation. COX-2 drugs such as celecoxib (Celebrex) spare the production of normal or protective prostaglandins produced by COX-1 in the stomach, kidneys, and platelets. Hence, COX-2 selective drugs may be especially beneficial during long-term use in people with rheumatoid arthritis because they may be less toxic to the stomach and other tissues.

Adverse side effects

The most common problem with chronic use is stomach irritation, which can lead to gastric ulceration and hemorrhage. This can be resolved to some extent by taking aspirin in an enteric-coated form so that release is delayed until the drug reaches the small intestine. Other pharmacologic interventions such as prostaglandin analogs (misoprostol) and proton pump inhibitors (omeprazole [Prilosec], and so forth) can also be used if gastropathy continues to be a limiting factor during NSAID use. Chronic NSAID use can also produce bleeding problems (because of platelet inhibition) and impaired renal function, especially in an older or debilitated patient. Despite the potential for various side effects, aspirin and other NSAIDs continue to be used extensively by people with rheumatoid arthritis and are often used for extended periods without serious effects. As indicated earlier, COX-2 selective drugs may reduce the risk of toxicity to the stomach, kidneys, and other tissues because these drugs spare the production of normal or protective prostaglandins in these tissues. These drugs may cause other problems such as diarrhea, heartburn, gastrointestinal cramps, and an increased risk of upper respiratory tract infection. COX-2 drugs have also been associated with serious cardiovascular problems (heart attack, stroke), and these drugs should be avoided in people at risk for cardiac disease.

Glucocorticoids

Glucocorticoids such as prednisone are extremely effective anti-inflammatory agents, but they are associated with a number of serious side effects. Hence, these drugs (known also as *corticosteroids*) are commonly used to treat acute exacerbations in people with rheumatoid arthritis. In particular, the judicious short-term use of systemic (oral) glucocorticoids can serve as a bridge between an acute flare-up of rheumatoid joint disease and successful management by other drugs such as NSAIDs and disease-modifying agents. Glucocorticoids can often be given systemically at high doses for short periods (a week or two) to provide anti-inflammatory effects. This so-called pulse treatment may be especially helpful in managing acute exacerbations of rheumatoid arthritis without producing the severe side effects associated with long-term use.

Glucocorticoids can also be injected directly into the arthritic joint, a technique that can be invaluable in the management of acute exacerbations. There is, of course, considerable controversy about whether intra-articular glucocorticoids will produce harmful catabolic effects in joints that are already weakened by arthritic changes. At the very least, the number of injections into an arthritic joint should be limited, and a common rule of thumb is to not exceed more than four injections in one joint within one year. The long-term use of glucocorticoids, however, remains somewhat controversial. While their short-term anti-inflammatory effects can be extremely helpful, high doses of glucocorticoids for prolonged periods can cause serious musculoskeletal problems and other adverse effects. It was also believed that these drugs do not necessarily halt the progression of rheumatoid arthritis and that their short-term benefits are eventually lost during prolonged use. More recent evidence, however, suggests that glucocorticoids such as prednisone may actually have some ability to retard disease progression. That is, these drugs may have some beneficial disease-modifying properties similar to other DMARDs. Furthermore, these beneficial effects may be achieved with fairly low doses, minimizing the risk of adverse effects. Hence, the risks and benefits of long-term glucocorticoid administration continue to be investigated, and future research will help clarify how these drugs can be used most effectively alone or with other agents to manage rheumatoid arthritis.

Mechanism of action

Briefly, glucocorticoids bind to a receptor in the cytoplasm of certain cells (macrophages, leukocytes), thereby forming a glucocorticoid-receptor complex. This complex then moves to the cell's nucleus where it binds to specific genes that regulate the inflammatory process. By binding to these genes, the glucocorticoid-receptor complex increases the production of several anti-inflammatory proteins while also inhibiting the production of many pro- inflammatory substances. These agents, for example, increase the production of proteins called annexins (previously known as *lipocortins*). Annexins inhibit the phospholipase A_2 enzyme that normally liberates fatty acid precursors at the start of prostaglandin and leukotriene biosynthesis. Therefore, glucocorticoid-induced production of annexins blocks the first step in the synthesis of pro- inflammatory prostaglandins and leukotrienes. Glucocorticoids likewise increase the production of proteins such as interleukin-10, interleukin-1 receptor antagonist, and neutral endopeptidase. These other proteins contribute to anti-inflammatory effects by inhibiting, destroying, or blocking various other inflammatory chemicals, peptides, and proteins. In addition to direct effects on genes regulating inflammation, glucocorticoids also inhibit the transcription factors that initiate synthesis of pro- inflammatory cytokines (e.g., interleukin-1, tumor necrosis factor), enzymes (e.g., COX-2, nitric oxide synthase), and receptor proteins (e.g., natural killer receptors). Glucocorticoids may also exert some of their effects via a membrane-bound receptor that regulates activity of macrophages, eosinophils, T lymphocytes, and several other types of cells involved in the inflammatory response. Consequently, glucocorticoids affect many aspects of inflammation, and their powerful anti-inflammatory effects in rheumatoid arthritis result from their ability to blunt various cellular and chemical components of the inflammatory response.

Adverse side effects

The side effects of glucocorticoids are numerous. These drugs exert a general catabolic effect on all types of supportive tissue (i.e., muscle, tendon, bone). Osteoporosis is a particular a problem in the patient with arthritis because many of these patients have significant bone loss before even beginning steroid therapy. Glucocorticoids have been known to increase bone loss in patients with arthritis, especially when these drugs are used at higher doses for prolonged periods. Glucocorticoids may also cause muscle wasting and weakness, as well as hypertension, aggravation of diabetes mellitus, glaucoma, and cataracts. These side effects emphasize the need to limit glucocorticoid therapy as much as possible in patients with arthritis.

Disease-Modifying Antirheumatic Drugs

Disease-modifying antirheumatic drugs (DMARDs) are defined as "medications that retard or halt the progression of [rheumatoid] disease." These drugs comprise an eclectic group of agents that are now recognized as essential in the early treatment of rheumatoid arthritis. That is, early and aggressive use of DMARDs can slow the progression of this disease before there is extensive damage to affected joints. When used in conjunction with NSAIDs and glucocorticoids, DMARDs can help improve the long-term outcomes of patients with rheumatoid arthritis, and can contribute to substantial improvements in quality-of-life. 12

Hence, disease-modifying drugs are typically used to control synovitis and erosive changes during the active stages of rheumatoid joint disease. There is still considerable concern, however, over DMARD's safety and efficacy. Older DMARDs, such as penicillamine and oral gold, were especially problematic, and many patients who started treatment on these drugs eventually discontinued drug therapy due to side effects or lack of therapeutic benefits. Some of the newer DMARDs are substantially more effective, but these newer agents can still produce serious side effects such as hepatic and renal toxicity. Despite these limitations, there has been a definite trend toward more frequent DMARD use, and to use these drugs earlier in the course of rheumatoid arthritis before excessive joint destruction has occurred. As the name implies, DMARDs attempt to induce remission by modifying the pathologic process inherent to rheumatoid arthritis. In general, DMARDs inhibit certain aspects of the immune response thought to be underlying rheumatoid disease. For example, these drugs can inhibit the function of monocytes and T and B lymphocytes, or affect specific inflammatory mediators (e.g., cytokines) that are responsible for perpetuating joint inflammation and destruction. The pharmacology of specific DMARDs is discussed below.

Antimalarial Drugs

Originally used in the treatment of malaria, the drugs chloroquine (Aralen) and hydroxychloroquine (Plaquenil) have also been used to treat rheumatoid arthritis. In the past, these drugs have been used reluctantly because of the fear of retinal toxicity. There is now evidence, however, that these agents can be used safely, but they are only marginally effective when compared to other DMARDs. These drugs are therefore not usually the first choice, but they can be used in patients who cannot tolerate other DMARDs, or in combination with another DMARD for more comprehensive treatment.

Mechanism of action

Antimalarials exert a number of effects, although it is unclear exactly which of these contributes to their ability to halt the progression in rheumatoid arthritis. These drugs are known to increase pH within certain intracellular vacuoles in macrophages and other immune-system cells. This effect is believed to disrupt the ability of these cells to process antigenic proteins and present these antigens to T cells. Decreased T-cell stimulation results in immunosuppression and attenuation of the arthritic response. Antimalarials have also been shown to stabilize lysosomal membranes and impair DNA and RNA synthesis, although the significance of these effects in their role as antiarthritics remains unclear.

Adverse side effects

Chloroquine and hydroxychloroquine are usually considered the safest DMARDs. The major concern is that high doses of these drugs can produce irreversible retinal damage. Retinal toxicity is rare, however, when daily dosages are maintained below the levels typically used to treat rheumatoid arthritis (i.e., less than 3.5 to 4.0 mg/kg per day for chloroquine and less than 6.0 to 6.5 mg/kg per day for hydroxychloroquine). Nonetheless, ocular exams should be scheduled periodically to ensure the safe and effective use of these drugs during prolonged administration. Other side effects such as headache and gastrointestinal distress can occur, but these are relatively infrequent and usually transient.

Azathioprine

Azathioprine (Imuran) is an immunosuppressant drug that is often used to prevent tissue rejection following organ transplants. Because of its immunosuppressant properties, this drug has been employed in treating cases of severe, active rheumatoid arthritis that have not responded to other agents.

Mechanism of action

The mechanism of action of azathioprine in rheumatoid arthritis is not fully understood. This drug has been shown to impair the synthesis of DNA and RNA precursors, but it is unclear exactly how (or if) this is related to its immunosuppressant effects. Azathioprine can likewise inhibit lymphocyte proliferation, thereby impairing immune responses mediated by these cells. This action accounts for the immunosuppressant effects of this drug and for its ability to blunt the autoimmune responses that govern rheumatoid disease.

Adverse side effects

Azathioprine is relatively toxic, with more frequent and more severe side effects than other DMARDs. The primary side effects include fever, chills, sore throat, fatigue, loss of appetite, and nausea or vomiting; these effects often limit the use of this drug.

Gold therapy

Compounds containing elemental gold were among the first drugs identified as DMARDs. Specific compounds such as aurothioglucose (Sol-ganal) and gold sodium thiomalate (Myochrysine) have been used in the past and are usually administered by intramuscular injection. An orally active gold compound, auranofin (Ridaura), has also been developed and offers the advantage of oral administration. Auranofin is better tolerated than parenteral gold compounds in terms of adverse side effects. In the past, gold therapy was often used to arrest further progression of rheumatoid joint disease. Because safer and more effective agents have been developed, gold compounds are no longer used routinely in the treatment of rheumatoid arthritis, but are reserved for patients who fail to respond to other DMARDs.

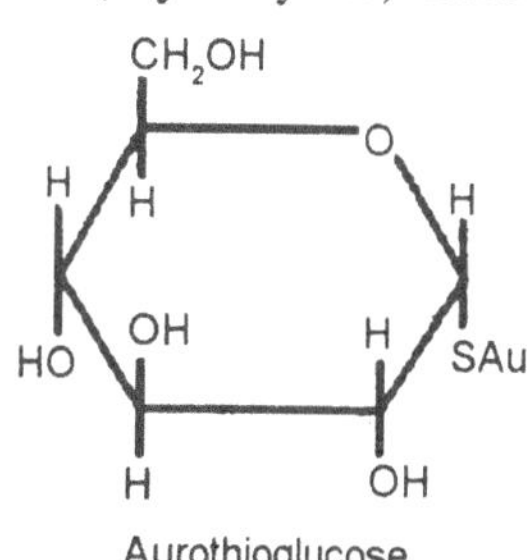

Aurothioglucose

CH_2COONa
|
AuSCHOONa

Gold Sodium Thiomalate

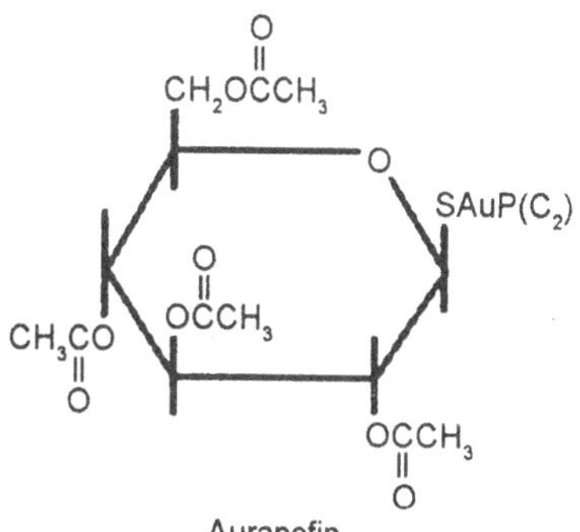

Auranofin

Fig. 11.1. Gold compounds used to treat rheumatoid arthritis.

Mechanism of action

Although the exact mechanism is not fully understood, gold compounds probably induce remission in patients with rheumatoid arthritis by inhibiting the growth and function of T cells and mononuclear phagocytes. These drugs accumulate in the lysosomes of macrophages and other synovial cells, thereby suppressing the action of key components in the cellular immune reaction inherent in this disease. A number of additional cellular effects have been noted (decreased lysosomal enzyme release, decreased prostaglandin E_2 production), and these effects may also contribute to the effectiveness of gold compounds in treating rheumatoid arthritis.

Adverse side effects

Adverse effects are relatively common with gold therapy, with approximately one third of patients experiencing some form of toxic effect. The primary side effects caused by gold compounds are gastrointestinal distress (diarrhea, indigestion), irritation of the oral mucosa, and rashes and itching of the skin. Other side effects include proteinuria, conjunctivitis, and blood dyscrasias (e.g., thrombocytopenia, leukopenia). As mentioned earlier, auranofin may be safer than parenteral gold compounds because it produces fewer cutaneous and potentially serious hematologic side effects, but auranofin tends to produce more gastrointestinal irritation than injected forms of gold.

Leflunomide

Leflunomide (Arava) is a relative newcomer to the antirheumatic drug arsenal. This drug helps decrease pain and inflammation in rheumatoid joint disease, and leflunomide has been shown to slow the formation of bone erosions in arthritic joints. Leflunomide is also fairly well tolerated by most patients and may produce beneficial effects fairly soon (1 month) after beginning treatment. This drug is therefore a potential alternative in people who have failed to respond to other DMARDs such as methotrexate.

Mechanism of action

Leflunomide acts primarily by inhibiting the synthesis of RNA precursors in lymphocytes. When stimulated, lymphocytes must radically increase their RNA synthesis to proliferate and become activated during the inflammatory response. Leflunomide blocks a key enzyme responsible for RNA synthesis, so that these lymphocytes cannot progress to a more activated state and cannot cause as much joint inflammation.

Adverse side effects

Leflunomide's primary side effects include gastrointestinal distress, allergic reactions (skin rashes), and hair loss. This drug can also affect the liver; liver function may need to be monitored periodically.

Methotrexate

Methotrexate (Folex, Rheumatrex) is an antimetabolite used frequently in the treatment of cancer. There is considerable evidence that this drug is also one of the most effective DMARDs. Methotrexate has been shown to slow the effects of rheumatoid arthritis as evidenced by decreased synovitis, decreased bone erosion, and less narrowing of the joint space. The therapeutic effects of methotrexate have also been reported to be equal to, or better than, other DMARDs such as oral gold or azathioprine, and methotrexate may offer an advantage in terms of a rapid onset. Hence, methotrexate's popularity as a DMARD has increased during the past few years, and this drug is often the first DMARD used to treat rheumatoid arthritis in both adults and children.

Mechanism of action

The ability of methotrexate and similar anticancer drugs to impair DNA and RNA synthesis is well known. Methotrexate inhibits the synthesis of folic acid, thus inhibiting the formation of nucleoproteins that serve as DNA precursors. This action inhibits cellular replication by impairing the cell's ability to produce new genetic material, an effect that helps attenuate tumor cell replication in cancer. Nonetheless, methotrexate's effects on immune function and rheumatoid arthritis are somewhat unclear. This drug could affect immune function by inhibiting folic acid metabolism, thereby limiting the proliferation of lymphocytes and other cells that cause the autoimmune responses in rheumatoid disease. Methotrexate, however, also exerts other effects, including inhibition of inflammatory cytokines and stimulation of adenosine release. The effects on adenosine release may be especially important because increased amounts of endogenous adenosine can inhibit various components of the immune response. Regardless of the exact mechanism, methotrexate has become a mainstay in the management of rheumatoid arthritis.

Adverse side effects

Methotrexate is a relatively toxic drug, and a number of adverse side effects can occur. The primary problems involve the gastrointestinal tract and include loss of appetite, nausea, and other forms of gastrointestinal distress (including intra-gastrointestinal hemorrhage). Long-term methotrexate use in patients with rheumatoid arthritis has also been associated with pulmonary problems, hematologic disorders, liver dysfunction, and hair loss. These side effects often limit the use of methotrexate with rheumatoid arthritis, and most patients who stop using this drug do so because of an adverse side effect rather than a loss of effectiveness. Methotrexate does, however, offer a favorable benefit-to-risk ratio in many patients and has become one of the most commonly used DMARDs.

Penicillamine

Penicillamine (Cuprimine), a derivative of penicillin, is officially classified as a chelating agent that is often used in the treatment of heavy metal intoxication (e.g., lead poisoning). In addition, this drug has been used in patients with severe rheumatoid arthritis, and seems to be as effective as other DMARDs such as methotrexate, sulfasalazine, and gold therapy. Penicillamine, however, tends to be substantially more toxic than other DMARDs, and is therefore used rarely in the treatment of specific patients with rheumatoid arthritis.

Mechanism of action

The basis for the antiarthritic effects of penicillamine is unknown. Reductions in serum immunoglobulin M-rheumatoid factor have been observed with penicillamine, and this drug has been shown to depress T-cell function. These and similar findings suggest that penicillamine works by suppressing the immune response in rheumatoid arthritis, but the exact mechanisms remain to be determined.

Adverse side effects

Penicillamine is considered to be fairly toxic when compared with other DMARDs. Side effects that have been reported as occurring more frequently include fever, joint pain, skin rashes and itching, and swelling of lymph glands. Other adverse effects that may occur less frequently are bloody or cloudy urine, swelling of feet and legs, unusual weight gain, sore throat, and excessive fatigue.

Tumor Necrosis Factor Inhibitors

Several agents are now available that inhibit the action of tumor necrosis factor-alpha (TNF-α). TNF-α is a small protein (cytokine) that is released from cells involved in the inflammatory response. TNF-α seems to be a key chemical mediator that promotes inflammation and joint erosion in rheumatoid arthritis. Drugs that inhibit this chemical will therefore help delay the progression of this disease by decreasing TNF-α's destructive effects.

Drugs in this group include etanercept (Enbrel), infliximab (Remicade), and adalimumab (Humira). These drugs are also referred to as "biologic" DMARDs because they affect the biologic response to a specific cytokine (TNF-α). Etanercept was the first biologic DMARD—it was created by fusing human immunoglobulin (IgG) with an amino acid sequence that mimics the binding portion of the TNF receptor. TNF-α recognizes the binding portion on the drug, attaches to this portion, and therefore cannot bind to the real TNF receptor. The two newer agents (infliximab and adalimumab) were developed using monoclonal antibody techniques. These techniques enable the drug to bind tightly to antigenic components on TNF-α, thereby forming a drug-cytokine molecule that is too large to bind to the real TNF receptor. In addition, infliximab and adalimumab can destroy cells that express TNF-α, thus further reducing the destructive effects of this cytokine.

There is substantial evidence that TNF-α inhibitors can retard the progression of inflammatory joint disease, and promote improvements in symptoms and quality-of-life with rheumatoid arthritis. These drugs are not typically used as the initial treatment, but can be used alone or added to other agents (e.g., methotrexate) if patients do not have an adequate response to other DMARDs. There is some concern about toxicity, and these drugs must be given parenterally, usually by subcutaneous injection (twice each week for etanercept; every other week for adalimumab), or by slow intravenous infusion (every eight weeks for infliximab). Nonetheless, TNF-α inhibitors represent an important breakthrough in the drug treatment of rheumatoid arthritis.

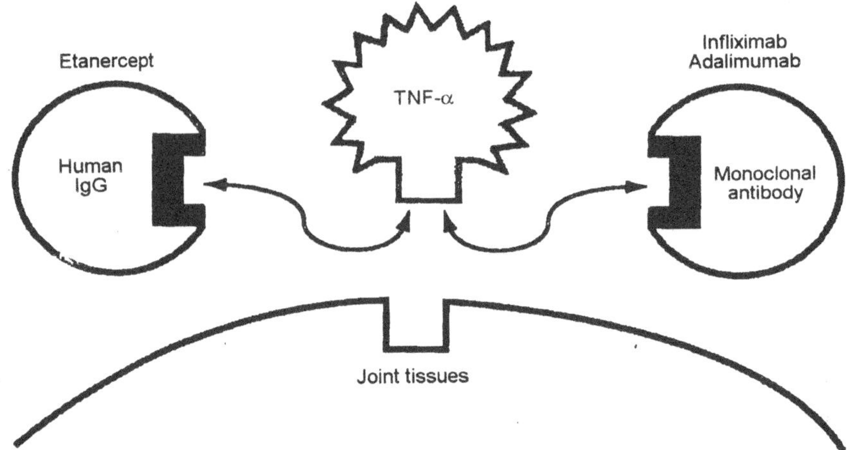

Fig. 11.2. Schematic diagram illustrating the effects of tumor necrosis factor-alpha (TNF-α) inhibitors.

Mechanism of action

As indicated, these agents bind selectively to TNF-α. This action prevents TNF-α from binding to surface receptors located on other inflammatory cells. TNF is therefore unable to activate other inflammatory cells that cause inflammation and joint destruction in rheumatoid arthritis.

Adverse side effects

Patients taking TNF-α inhibitors may be prone to upper respiratory tract infections and other serious infections, including sepsis. This increased risk of infection probably occurs because the drug inhibits a key component of the immune response—namely, TNF-α. These drugs are therefore contraindicated in people with infections, and administration should be discontinued if an infection develops. Other potential adverse responses include malignancy (e.g., lymphoma), liver disease, heart failure, lupuslike disease, irritation around the injection site, and demyelinating disorders that mimic multiple sclerosis. The incidence of these adverse effects, however, seems to be fairly low. For the most part, these drugs provide an acceptable risk-to-benefit ratio for most people with rheumatoid arthritis. Patients should, however, be screened carefully for any risk factors before beginning drug therapy, and should likewise be monitored periodically for any potential adverse reactions to these drugs.

Anakinra

Anakinra (Kineret) blocks the effects of interleukin-1 on joint tissues. Like TNF-α, interleukin-1 is a cytokine that promotes inflammation and joint destruction in rheumatoid arthritis. By blocking interleukin-1 receptors on joint tissues, anakinra prevents the destructive events mediated by this cytokine. This drug appears to be moderately effective in limiting the progression of rheumatoid arthritis, and it is generally well tolerated. Hence, anakinra is another option that can be used alone or in combination with other DMARDs such as methotrexate.

Mechanism of action

As indicated, anakinra is an antagonist (blocker) that is specific for the interleukin-1 receptor found on joint tissues, other tissues, and organs. By blocking this receptor, the drug prevents interleukin-1 from binding to this receptor and exerting destructive effects on joint tissues.

Adverse side effects

Patients receiving anakinra may be more susceptible to bacterial infections and other infectious agents. This drug is administered via subcutaneous injection, and irritation at the injection site is fairly common, but is usually not severe. More serious systemic allergic reactions may occur in a small number of patients.

Other DMARDs

Because of the autoimmune basis of rheumatoid arthritis, various other drugs that affect the immune response are used on a limited basis. For instance, cyclosporine (Sandimmune), an immunosuppressant agent that is used to prevent rejection of organ transplants, is sometimes used to treat patients with rheumatoid arthritis who have not responded to other measures. Sulfasalazine (Azulfidine), a drug that is typically used to treat inflammatory bowel disease, may also be helpful in treating rheumatoid arthritis because of its immunosuppressant effects. Cyclophosphamide (Cytoxan) is used primarily to treat cancer, but this agent can be used to suppress the immune system in severe cases of rheumatoid arthritis.

In general, these drugs are more toxic and are usually reserved for patients who have not responded to more traditional DMARDs such as methotrexate. Drugs with immunosuppressant activity may also be used in combination with more traditional DMARDs to provide optimal benefits in certain patients.

DMARD Combinations Used in Rheumatoid Arthritis

There has been a great deal of interest in using several DMARDs simultaneously to achieve optimal effects in treating rheumatoid arthritis. The strategy of com-bination therapy is to attack the underlying disease process from several pharmacologic vantage points, much in the same way that combination therapies are used in other disorders such as hypertension and cancer. Although the benefits of combining DMARDs have been questioned, most practitioners currently advocate a combination of two or more drugs so that optimal benefits can be achieved with a relatively low dose of each drug. Likewise, the best way to combine specific DMARDs is still being investigated, with various combinations of new and old DMARDs being studied for efficacy and toxicity. At present, methotrexate is typically the cornerstone of treatment, with other DMARDs added, depending on the needs of each patient. For example, a triple combination of methotrexate with hydroxychloroquine and sulfasalazine has been advocated as an effective treatment for many patients. In addition, some of the newer biologic agents such as the TNF-α inhibitors (etanercept, infliximab, adalamimab) and interleukin-1 inhibitors (anakinra) have been added to methotrexate to provide an effective combination in patients who have not responded to use of only one drug.

The drawback of combination therapy is, of course, the potential for increased toxicity and drug interactions when several DMARDs are used simultaneously. This fact is understandable, considering that many DMARDs have a relatively high risk of toxicity when used alone, and combining these drugs will certainly increase the risk of adverse drug reactions. There is, however, evidence that the incidence of side effects is not necessarily greater when DMARD combinations are used compared with a single drug such as methotrexate. Hence, combination therapy continues to gain acceptance, and the use of two or three DMARDs early in the course of the disease may provide patients with the best hope for halting the progression of rheumatoid arthritis. Continued research will hopefully lend additional insight to the best way that DMARDs can be combined to safely and effectively treat patients with rheumatoid arthritis.

Dietary Implications for Rheumatoid Arthritis

There is an ongoing search for other pharmacologic and nonpharmacologic interventions that can help arrest the progression of rheumatoid joint disease. There is some evidence, for example, that dietary manipulation can alleviate the symptoms of rheumatoid arthritis. Diets that are high in fish oil and certain fatty acids (e.g., gammalinolenic acid) have been advocated for patients with rheumatoid arthritis because these diets may supply precursors that enhance the biosynthesis of certain endogenous anti-inflammatory and immunosuppressant compounds. Foods that have antioxidant properties (e.g., fruits, vegetables) may also have beneficial effects in people with rheumatoid arthritis. On the other hand, diets that are rich in meat and protein may exacerbate rheumatoid arthritis and similar inflammatory diseases. Hence, dietary changes used in combination with drug therapy may provide additional benefits for some people with rheumatoid arthritis.

Osteoarthritis

Osteoarthritis far exceeds rheumatoid arthritis as the most common form of joint disease. The prevalence of osteoarthritis increases with age. Approximately 50 to 80 percent of people aged 65 years have osteoarthritis to some extent, and virtually everyone over 75 years has some degree of osteoarthritic joint disease. In contrast to rheumatoid joint disease, osteoarthritis does not seem to be caused by an immune response, but rather an intrinsic defect in the joint cartilage. This defect causes a slow, progressive deterioration of articular cartilage that is accompanied by degenerative bony changes, including thickening of the subchondral bone, creation of subchondral bone cysts, and formation of large bony protrusions (osteophytes) at the joint margins. Osteoarthritis typically occurs in large weight-bearing joints such as the knees and hips, as well as some of the smaller joints in the hands and feet. Patients are described as having primary osteoarthritis when there is no apparent reason for the onset of joint destruction; in secondary osteoarthritis, a factor such as previous joint trauma, infection, or metabolic disease is responsible for triggering articular changes. Obesity, genetic susceptibility, and joint vulnerability (malalignment, weakness, and so forth) have also been implicated as predisposing factors in osteoarthritis.

Clearly, osteoarthritis is a different form of joint disease than rheumatoid arthritis. Hence, treatment of these conditions also differs somewhat. As discussed previously, rheumatoid arthritis is characterized by a severe inflammatory response that is perpetuated by a cellular immune reaction. Thus, drug therapy in rheumatoid disease consists of agents that are focused on directly relieving these inflammatory symptoms (i.e., NSAIDs or glucocorticoids) or drugs that attempt to arrest the cellular immune response that causes this inflammation (DMARDs). Treatment of joint inflammation is not a major focus of drug therapy in osteoarthritis, however. A mild inflammatory synovitis does occur in osteoarthritis, but this is secondary to the articular damage inherent to this disease. Also, drug therapy represents one of the primary interventions in rheumatoid arthritis, whereas treatment of osteoarthritis should be focused more directly on nonpharmacologic measures such as physical therapy, weight loss, and joint replacement in the advanced stages of this disease.

Hence, drug therapy in osteoarthritis is focused primarily on helping patients manage their pain and maintain an active lifestyle. When joint pain begins to be a problem, simple analgesics such as acetaminophen and NSAIDs have been the major form of drug therapy. Newer pharmacologic strategies are also emerging that attempt to slow or reverse the pathologic changes in osteoarthritis. These newer strategies use disease- modifying osteoarthritic drugs (DMOADs) rather than drugs that treat only the symptoms of osteoarthritis. Two types of DMOADs will be addressed: drugs that attempt to directly improve the viscosity and function of synovial fluid (*viscosupplementation*) and agents that serve as precursors to the normal constituents of joint tissues (glucosamine and chondroitin sulfate).

Acetaminophen and NSAIDs

Acetaminophen is often the first drug used to treat osteoarthritis. Acetaminophen is as effective as NSAIDs in controlling pain, but acetaminophen does not have anti-inflammatory effects. The lack of anti-inflammatory effects is of less concern when acetaminophen is used in osteoarthritis because the inflammatory symptoms are milder. Acetaminophen is therefore successful in reducing pain, and because this drug does not cause gastric irritation, acetaminophen is often considered the drug of choice in mild-to-moderate osteoarthritis. Hence, acetaminophen provides a relatively safe and effective form of analgesia for patients with osteoarthritis, especially when this drug needs to be administered for long periods of time.

NSAIDs are also used for the symptomatic treatment of pain in osteoarthritis. These drugs are used primarily for their analgesic properties, although the anti-inflammatory effects of NSAIDs can help control the mild synovitis that typically occurs in advanced osteoarthritis secondary to joint destruction. If the primary goal is pain reduction, however, NSAIDs do not provide any advantage over acetaminophen. As indicated earlier, acetaminophen is often a better choice than traditional NSAIDs because most NSAIDs cause gastric irritation. The newer COX-2 selective NSAIDs do not appear to cause as much gastric irritation as other NSAIDs, and these COX-2 drugs may be a valuable alternative to acetaminophen and traditional NSAIDs in the longterm treatment of osteoarthritis. COX-2 drugs, however, may increase the risk of serious cardiovascular problems (heart attack, stroke), and patients should be screened carefully for cardiovascular risk factors before beginning treatment with COX-2 drugs.

Regardless of the exact drug used, there is no doubt that the analgesia produced by NSAIDs or acetaminophen plays a valuable role in the management of osteoarthritis. These drugs allow the patient to maintain a more active lifestyle and to participate in various activities, including exercise programs and other forms of physical therapy and occupational therapy. However, these drugs do not alter the progressive course of joint destruction and osteoarthritic changes. There is preliminary evidence, in fact, that some of the NSAIDs may actually impair bone healing following fractures or surgery, but their effects on cartilage formation and soft tissue repair remain unclear. At the present time, however, acetaminophen and NSAIDs remain the cornerstone of the pharmacologic treatment of joint pain in osteoarthritis.

Viscosupplementation

Viscosupplementation is a clinical procedure that is being used increasingly in the treatment of osteoarthritis. This technique uses a substance known as hyaluronan to restore the lubricating properties of synovial fluid in osteoarthritic joints. Hyaluronan is a polysaccharide that can be injected into an arthritic joint to help restore the normal viscosity of the synovial fluid. This treatment helps reduce joint stresses, thus limiting the progression of articular destruction seen in osteoarthritis. Viscosupplementation has therefore been shown to reduce pain and improve function in osteoarthritis.

When used to treat osteoarthritis, viscosupplementation typically consists of 2 to 10 weekly injections of hyaluronan Hyalgan, Synvisc, others. Patients often experience a decrease in pain within days after injection, and pain continues to diminish within the first weeks after treatment. Duration of relief is variable, but most patients who respond to visco-supplementation experience beneficial effects for 6 months to 1 year after a series of injections.

Hence, viscosupplementation may temporarily attenuate the progressive changes in joint structure and function typically seen in osteoarthritis. Although these benefits are relatively transient, viscosupplementation can delay the need for more invasive surgical treatments such as joint replacement. This intervention is also tolerated fairly well, although a pseudoseptic reaction that produces local pain and swelling may occur. Future clinical studies will be needed to determine how viscosupplementation can be used most effectively in the comprehensive treatment of people with osteoarthritis.

Glucosamine and Chondroitin Sulfate

It has been suggested that dietary supplements such as glucosamine and chondroitin sulfate may help protect articular cartilage and halt or reverse joint degeneration in osteoarthritis. These two compounds are key ingredients needed for the production of several components of articular cartilage and synovial fluid, including glycosaminoglycans, proteoglycans, and hyaluronic acid. It seems reasonable that increased amounts of these ingredients should facilitate the repair of joint tissues, improve synovial fluid viscosity, and help restore joint function in conditions like osteoarthritis. Hence, several products containing glucosamine, or glucosamine combined with chondroitin sulfate, are currently available as nonprescription dietary supplements. These supplements typically contain oral dosages of 1500 mg/d glucosamine and 1200 mg/d chondroitin sulfate.

Several recent studies suggest that chondroitin and glucosamine supplements can decrease pain and improve function in some patients with osteoarthritis. Radiographic studies also indicate that these supplements can reduce joint space narrowing in knee osteoarthritis, thus providing some protective effects on joint structure. These benefits may not occur in all patients—patients with a high rate of cartilage turnover may be more likely to experience positive effects because these supplements will provide the necessary substrates to sustain this turnover and maintain joint integrity.

Consequently, it appears that glucosamine and chondroitin supplements are certainly worth a trial for many patients with osteoarthritis. Some gastrointestinal problems may occur, but these supplements are usually well tolerated. Although these supplements are available over-the-counter in the United States, people with osteoarthritis should consult their physician and pharmacist before self-administration. Likewise, patients should be educated on the proper dosage, and should be reminded that these products may need to be consumed for several weeks or months before beneficial effects become apparent. Long-term studies on the effects of these supplements are currently being conducted, and clinicians should try to stay abreast of any new information about the potential benefits of glucosamine and chondroitin.

Rheumatoid arthritis and osteoarthritis represent two distinct forms of joint disease that can produce devastating effects on the structure and function of synovial joints. Fortunately, management of these conditions has improved substantially through advancements in drug therapy. Rheumatoid arthritis can be treated pharmacologically with NSAIDs, glucocorticoids, and various DMARDs. NSAIDs, including aspirin, represent the primary form of drug therapy in the early stages of this disease, and these drugs are often used in conjunction with other drugs as the arthritic condition increases in severity. Glucocorticoids are often effective in decreasing the joint inflammation typically found in rheumatoid arthritis, but long-term use of these agents is limited because of their toxic effects. Disease-modifying drugs can slow or halt the progressive nature of rheumatoid arthritis by suppressing the immune response inherent in this disease. Although there is some concern about the efficacy and safety of these drugs, DMARDs have been a welcome addition to the rather limited arsenal of drugs used to treat rheumatoid arthritis.

Drug treatment of osteoarthritis differs some-what from that of rheumatoid arthritis, with management of pain by using NSAIDs and acetaminophen constituting the major forms of drug therapy. A newer technique known as viscosupplementation has also been used to help restore the lubricating properties of the synovial fluid in osteoarthritic joints. Dietary supplements containing glucosamine and chondroitin sulfate may also help provide constituents that protect joint structure and function, and some people with osteoarthritis have benefited from their long-term use. In any event, drug therapy along with nonpharmacologic measures such as physical therapy can provide an effective way of dealing with the potentially devastating effects of rheumatoid arthritis and osteoarthritis.

12

DEVELOPING GOOD SPECIFICATIONS

There are varying levels of specification covering computer systems. This chapter focuses on the development of the user requirements specification (URS). As the first link in the chain between the customer and supplier, the overall quality and delivery of the final system is highly dependant on the quality, accuracy, and understanding of this key document. There are some common attributes that apply regardless of the specification type. Specifications should be defined in advance of any development activity or production of lower level specification to which they pertain. Specifications are essentially defining what you want. Where specifications are not predefined, then retrospective production is essentially a reporting activity of what you (think you) got. The intended audience for specifications should be clear, the level of detail and technical content should be consistent, and appropriate to the audience and intended specification use.

Specifications should be readable and individual requirements or functions should be clearly identified and structured in a manner that will aid traceability. Multiple requirements or functions should not be combined and certainly not defined together in long narratives. GAMP 4 recommends that individual requirement statements are no longer than 250 words. The status of the document content should be clear. For example, information that is in draft form, illustrative examples, and any assumptions should be clearly stated. The customer should write the URS, and the author must have a thorough understanding of the (business) process that the system is to support. The use of diagrams or flowcharts here can be helpful in illustrating the logic and flow of the process.

Responsibility for developing user requirements should not be delegated to technical or development staff. Technical or development staff involvement is required, indeed valuable in terms of technical review and feasibility of the requirements and advice as to available technologies, solutions or suppliers, but they are generally not experts on business processes. Where the responsibility for authoring a requirements specification is delegated to a potential systems supplier, then there is clearly potential for a conflict of interest; the requirements specification may be biased towards the suppliers products or preferred technology, and not the needs of the user.

The purpose of the URS is to clearly define what functions the user requires to support the associated business processes. Prospective system suppliers use the document to establish the adequacy of their system in meeting the requirements, and usually as the basis of cost and time estimates for implementing the system. It is essential that both the customer and prospective suppliers have a clear and common understanding of the requirements. Terminology is often a stumbling block, and the URS presents the user with the opportunity to provide clear definitions of terms to potential suppliers. The URS should not generally be written as a document specific to a particular system. It must contain sufficient detail for the customer to evaluate the suitability of proposed systems functionality against the requirements. Simply reflecting existing business processes and ways of working within the URS without challenge should be avoided. This can result in overly complex systems, replication of workarounds, expensive development of bespoke functionality (rather than utilization of standard system functions) and crucially misses a golden opportunity to make the processes more efficient.

Time spent at the outset critically analyzing, challenging, and simplifying requirements and associated processes should result in better requirements and a simpler system that is likely to take less time to implement, test, and support. Users should also consider the degree of flexibility they are prepared to accept in implementing requirements. If it is possible to make a minor change to a business process, which results in acceptance of a standard system, this may outweigh the development and support costs of bespoke system development effort. For larger projects, and particularly those involving process automation systems, the scope of the project is likely to be wider than the computer system alone, often including process equipment and facilities. Where this is the case consideration should be given to whether individual (but related) URS should be produced, or a single document. The decision is likely to be based on a number of factors. Where the project is delivering packaged equipment (i.e., process equipment with embedded computerized process control), then it makes sense to have a single specification. For a project to deliver a batch plant with a complex distributed process control system and process equipment from a variety of suppliers then individual specifications are probably more appropriate. Where multiple specifications are used, it is however, important to understand the relationship between the specifications and the impact that a change within one document may have to others.

When preparing a URS, the balance of detail must be considered. It may be tempting to include great detail on requirements that are well understood and defined. Too much detail, however, may mean that the requirements stray into defining functional requirements (i.e., delivery of a requirement rather than just defining what is to be delivered). By doing so, it is likely that the system or supplier selection will be constrained at a very early stage. This may mean that full benefit from the supplier's experience of how to most efficiently and effectively implement its solution cannot be obtained.

There may be areas where the requirements are not well understood, are poorly defined, or likely to be subject to change. It is important that such areas of ambiguity are identified as such; in many cases prospective suppliers may have sufficient experience or knowledge to assist the customer in better defining these areas. Often requirements development involves both the customer and supplier, and in such cases joint workshops, prototyping exercises, and reference site visits can contribute to gaining clear requirements definition. Where partnering type agreements are established with suppliers, then the scope for collaborative working to refine the requirements is much greater than situations where the URS is the basis for competitive tendering. Where suppliers have tendered competitive bids on the basis of the URS, then subsequent changes to the scope of requirements are almost certain to incur additional costs. The pricing of scope changes should be agreed between the customer and supplier prior to placing the order with the supplier.

The user requirements should be maintained and reflect the operational system. This document can then be used to support design and performance qualifications and the maintenance of the system in the future. Care should be taken to avoid duplication and particularly contradiction of any requirements statements. Also duplication of information contained within other project or system documentation should be avoided if possible to reduce the chances of documentation not being updated following changes made during the project, and also subsequently during the operational life of the system.

GxP Considerations

For quality related GxP applications, quality assurance or regulatory input, review and approval of the URS should be obtained. This is primarily to ensure that all quality related requirements have been identified and included, and any associated regulatory requirements addressed (for example relevance and requirements of electronic records, electronic signatures requirements). Requirements should be individually identifiable, and categorization into "must, should, and like" is worthwhile. An assessment of each requirement in terms of GxP and business criticality should also be performed, and the outcome documented. The method of recording this may be within the URS itself, or separately, for example within a requirements trace matrix.

A fundamental validation requirement is the ability to trace individual user requirements from the URS through functional or design specifications, testing, and through to user acceptance testing. This needs to be considered at an early stage in the project as the structure and style of the URS content can significantly hinder or assist subsequent efforts to provide traceability. Traceability can be achieved by means of a requirements trace matrix, these can be produced manually or with the use of computer-based tools. Computer-based tools are particularly useful for large or complex systems or projects, and generally provide electronic document management functionality in addition to requirements traceability. For smaller projects or systems often a relatively simple spreadsheet based system can be devised. Regardless of the traceability method selected, the key considerations are the complexity of the system, the likely scale of changes and the level of effort required to maintain the documentation and traceability. Within the user requirements, functions should be classified with regard to their GxP or business criticality. High, medium, low, or none are the suggested classifications. It is also recommended that records and data that the systems will collect or store should also be classified.

Systems may be direct or indirect quality impact systems. For example, manufacturing, labelling or packaging systems are direct quality impact systems, whereas document management or training systems would still be considered as GxP, but are indirect quality impact.

User Requirement Specification Sections

The following section provides an overview of some typical sections to be considered for inclusion within an URS. Provide a high level overview of the required system, its purpose and a brief summary of the key requirements. Detail the locations and departments involved in the project and the business stakeholders. Include stakeholders from the project, quality assurance, and support teams. Refer to any related projects or validation programs, provide a high level description of the overall project and background. Include a high level statement regarding required quality attributes of the system and adherence to relevant GxP pharmaceutical agency regulations. Consider including an indication of key system or supplier attributes that will influence selection such as:

1. Product maturity.
2. Installed base in pharmaceutical industry.
3. Technical support.
4. Training.
5. Staff experience.
6. Upgrade or migration strategy.
7. Product development strategy.

Include a statement to make the contractual status of the URS clear to the supplier.

System Overview

Provide an overview focusing on the key elements of the required system, including a description of the business process that the system is to support. Where possible include diagrams or flowchart representations to aid understanding. Where business processes are described ensure that people aspects (roles, responsibilities) are also included.

It is recommended that the existing systems and technology are detailed when describing the business process, and in particular indicate which of these are likely to require modifying or replacing (and hence decommissioning) as part of the project.

System Interfaces

Include a summary of any other systems with which the system must interface, if the interfaces are manual or automatic, and also highlight interfaces that include the transmission of GxP relevant information and instructions. Highlight system interfaces that will be modified, removed or decommissioned, or are new — particularly where the new interfaces are to existing systems.

Functional Requirements

Detail the operational functional requirements that the system is required to address, consider also the data and interfaces associated with required functions. It is important within this section to maintain focus on "what is required" rather than "how the function is to be delivered." Although the focus of the URS is on user requirements, also consider within this section any requirements for system administration functions. For example, system performance monitoring, user account administration, system maintenance functions, etc. Each requirement should be ranked in terms of business and GxP or quality criticality to the product or process or data. In particular records/data and functionality involving electronic signatures that are considered as GxP should be clearly identified to ensure, where applicable, compliance with pharmaceutical agency electronic record and electronic signature requirements is specified. For systems with safety, health or environmental (SHE) impact, consider whether each function needs to be individually ranked as to SHE impact.

For GxP records and signatures provide an indication of the required record retention period, and the regulation applicable to the record (i.e., GMP, GCP, GLP). As record retention periods will often be in excess of the likely system lifetime, consider requirements regarding record retrieval or migration as part of eventual system decommissioning. Note that only providing suppliers with a blanket statement regarding electronic record or electronic signature compliance is unlikely to be helpful. It is the customer, not the supplier that has the detailed understanding of the system aspects that will have direct or indirect quality or regulatory impact, and this information needs to be clearly relayed to the supplier. In some cases it may be prudent to separate out all business or quality critical requirements into separate sections of the user requirements. The following list provides some examples of areas to consider when assessing the direct or indirect GxP impact of the system requirements.

1. Product composition (manufacturing process).
2. Raw materials (identify, quantity).
3. Packaging materials.
4. Product recall.
5. Lot traceability.
6. Product labelling.
7. Environmental and storage conditions.
8. Analytical results.
9. Batch status (records, approvals).
10. Regulatory submission records.

To aid subsequent requirements traceability, each function should be individually identified and numbered. This can be facilitated by laying out the section in tabular form. This will aid identification, allows columns to be added (for example for GxP impact, criticality and electronic record or signature relevance), and deters the author from including excessive narrative and combining requirements.

The following attributes should be considered with regard to each function.

1. User access levels, login and logout, and security of interfaces to other systems.
2. Operating modes — for example manual, automatic, stop, start, hold, shutdown, action in event of hardware or software failure, etc.
3. Alarm conditions including communication of status, recovery routines, interlocks, and any associated safety requirements.
4. User interface requirements (including graphical user interface, data input, and detection of invalid input data or instructions).
5. Interfaces to other systems or functions (including detection of invalid or corrupted input data).
6. Performance, timing, and response requirements. For example, relating to input or output scanning times, report generation, fast control loops.
7. Calculations and any critical algorithms.
8. Reporting requirements — include data and description of reports, frequency of reporting and types of reports. For example standard, *ad hoc* reports, on-line or batched reports, report formats.
9. Capacity requirements (for example concurrent users, maximum number of batches in process, etc.).
10. Sequencing of process steps or transactions (and how to ensure these are enforced for systems with electronic record or signature requirements). Consider the most appropriate method of documenting these for example via flowcharts or in structured English format.

Data Requirements

The data and records requirements should be considered in conjunction with the functional requirements, and the following points should be considered.

1. Has all required data been described, including the format, required field length and precision where relevant?
2. Data and records confidentiality and security — is the status of records and data clear in terms of confidentiality, are the requirements of the Data Protection Act addressed, who should have access to records and data?
3. What are the storage and capacity requirements for data — ensure that capacity for future expansion is taken into consideration.
4. What requirements are there for data archiving and retrieval (how frequently is data likely to require restoring, what time frame is acceptable for retrieval)?
5. What requirements are there for validation or input check of data?
6. Manual data loading — what are the requirements, how will they be achieved, how will data be verified?
7. What requirements are there regarding migration of data from legacy systems — what is the expectation regarding validation of any migration tools?

System Requirements

The following sections outline some general system requirements that need to be taken into account within the URS, such as system security, electronic record or signature controls, and any environmental factors.

System Security

The following security requirements should be considered particularly for systems that include GxP electronic signatures and records. Note that there is a strong case in terms of basic good practice for applying these controls to any GxP computerized system.

1. Detection and reporting of unauthorized access attempts.
2. Configurable automatic user logouts after periods of inactivity.
3. System access must be limited to authorized users.
4. Restrictions on reuse of previously assigned user IDs and passwords.
5. System function access provided according to predefined user profiles.
6. Password expiry applied by the system according to configurable parameters.

Any corporate or local standards regarding the compatibility and installation of antivirus software or other security controls such as firewalls should be specified.

Electronic Record (ER) Controls

For systems where the requirements specify storage of GxP electronic records, the following requirements should be considered.

1. Electronic records must be accurately and completely reproducible in electronic and paper form.
2. Records must be retrievable throughout the specified retention period for the record (which may be beyond the system lifetime).
3. Include a human readable secure audit trail that includes the date and details of record or data creation, update or modification, and deletion.

Electronic Signature Requirements

For systems that include GxP electronic signature functionality, the following requirements should be considered.

1. The name of the signer, date and time stamp, and purpose of the signing must be captured and available for the signed record.
2. The signature must be applied at the time of the transaction or operation to which it relates, and the system must clearly identify the individual signing at the time of application.
3. The signature components must consist of a user identification code and password as a minimum, and must be traceable to an individual.
4. The signature must be linked to the electronic record, and must not be able to be cut, deleted, or copied either from or onto records other than by the act of signing.
5. The system must require reentry of at least one signature component for each subsequent signing within a single session.

Environmental Factors

Detail any special requirements that relate to the physical environment in which the system (or parts of the system, for example, plant-based user terminals) is to be located and used. Examples could be temperature, humidity requirements, and any applicable hazardous area (ATEX) constraints or regulations. Also consider other aspects such as sterile, dirty, wet, or dusty environments and any required ingress protection (IP) ratings for equipment. Consider any surface finish or cleaning requirements for equipment based in manufacturing facilities, and any requirements for any parts of the equipment that may be in contact with process materials.

Consider any constraints or corporate standards regarding the IT infrastructure and network environment in which the system may be installed, and in particular any standards or known compatibility issues with regard to equipment selection or use of existing infrastructure. Include any requirements where the physical layout of the equipment within the plant or workplace may be an issue. For example, with process control system there may be constraints regarding the physical length of cabling between controllers and associated input or output racks or devices. Also consider physical space limitations which may have an impact in terms of forced cooling requirements within equipment cabinets.

Operating Procedures and Training Requirements

Specify who and what are responsible for the development of operating and support procedures for the system, and the timing for their development.

Procedures must be considered for:

1. System access and security administration.
2. System backup and restoration (including disaster recovery).
3. Contingency plans for system downtime.
4. Data archive and restoration.
5. Change control.
6. Configuration management.
7. Incident reporting.

Ensure that any training requirements for technical, development, support, and operational staff are considered and where necessary included. Consider whether bespoke or standard courses are likely to be appropriate and the level of competency required.

Health and Safety

State whether the system has an impact with regard to safety, health, or environment. Describe the process to be used for detailed evaluation of the system or functions with regard to SHE. For example, HAZOP, CHAZOP, display screen evaluations, etc.

Process Equipment

Where the user requirements are a combined document for both process equipment and the associated computerized system, include details of the equipment. Include, for example, capacity, performance, maintenance, surface finishes, durability, materials of construction, cleaning requirements, etc.

System Interfaces

For each function consider and define what interfaces apply. Consider interfaces in terms of manual, end user interfaces, interfaces with other computerized systems, and those with plant or equipment. When considering interfaces consider elements such as the frequency of update, volume of information transferred, security of transfer, and compatibility with existing systems or equipment.

System Maintenance and Availability

Include the requirements for system reliability, and the expected availability. Specify maximum allowable periods of downtime, both in terms of scheduled and unscheduled maintenance and support. Consider any specific maintenance requirements, including the development or supply of relevant procedures and the requirements for any support agreements. Within the scope of support agreements consider if remote access is acceptable and what constraints the supplier would need to agree to in order to grant such access. Consider the required supplier response time to system problems, and whether 24 hour support is required.

Project Requirements

Include project-related requirements such as supplier assessment, communication, documentation, frequency of project meetings, project plan and milestones, project audits, quality systems approach, the approach to acceptance testing, and consider any specific contractual requirements. The process for performing supplier assessment should be outlined to the supplier, particularly where a detailed (site based), supplier audit is required. The fact that the scope of validation activities will be influenced by the audit results should also be made clear to suppliers.

Communication:

1. Who are the key points of contact between the supplier and customer?
2. What is the expected frequency and method of communication?
3. How will decisions be formally recorded and communicated?
4. Where there are multiple suppliers, how will they be coordinated?

Project plan:

1. How will the plan be developed, and by whom?
2. How will changes be agreed?
3. How will project delays be communicated and handled?
4. How will the project and validation plans be maintained and synchronized?

Documentation and electronic media:

1. What level of documentation is required?
2. What documentation standards are agreed?
3. Do GMP standards apply to all, some, or no system documentation?
4. How many copies are required?
5. Is documentation required in hard copy or electronic format?
6. What is the review and approval process for documentation?
7. How many copies of software will be provided, and in what format?

Acceptance testing:

1. What level of testing is expected from the supplier?
2. Will acceptance testing be performed at the supplier's premises, the customer's, or both?
3. Who will provide resources for testing?
4. Are simulation packages permitted during testing?
5. What level of documentation, witnessing, and collection of evidence is required at each stage of testing?

Quality System Requirements

State the requirements with regard to the quality management system to be used during system development. Detail and expectations with regard to the customer and supplier quality systems, in particular consider any requirements with regard to change control and configuration management during the project.

13

Technologies and Challenges of Pharmaceuticals

As the 21st century begins the field of drug discovery is filled with opportunity and challenge. The ability of the pharmaceutical industry to take advantage of the opportunities and meet the challenges while maintaining a significant growth rate will be determined by the success with which the industry makes use of the rich sources of information at its disposal. The field of pharmacogenetics is one of the many disciplines that will produce insights and avenues of opportunity for drug discovery. The facility with which the pharmaceutical industry uses this information will have a major impact on the safety, efficacy and time to market of a wide variety of therapeutic compounds in the future.

The use to which pharmacogenetics is put will be determined by how the information is collected, organized, and disseminated. The technologies brought to bear on the problems that pharmacogenetics present will be critical to the effective use of pharmacogenetics information in the therapeutic development process. The current state of technological development has permitted investigators to address an array of previously unapproachable genetic questions. This has, in turn, created an ever-growing library of DNA sequence information, cDNA clones, genes, mutations, and polymorphisms available for use in target discovery, lead identification, lead optimization, pre-clinical testing, and clinical trials. The high per patient cost of these technologies do not, however, permit the wide scale use of this information resource in large trial populations. The development of new technologies providing low cost, high throughput alternatives to genetic testing will permit the application of pharmacogenomic information across a broad range of therapeutic development. This review will endeavor to provide an overview of the current state of the art in genetic technologies along with those technologies that may facilitate the wide spread use of pharmacogenetics information.

Technology Selection

The selection of an appropriate technology is best based on the requirements of a project or area of investigation. Technologies that are appropriate for gene discovery are not universally applicable to population studies or patient group stratification. As the process moves from initial target identification through development of lead compounds the impact of genomic technology lessens while that of genetics technology increases. The impact of the limited number of technologies applicable to clinical diagnostic laboratory use is reserved for those compounds well into the development process where a genetic test is being considered as an adjunct or requirement for therapeutic selection. The selection of an appropriate technology can take two forms depending upon the state of knowledge concerning a gene, locus, or disease. In one form technology selection will be guided by a relative lack of knowledge concerning mutations and polymorphisms. The technologies selected in this manner will rely heavily on gene scanning methods and/or sequencing. In another form technology selection will be guided by a relative abundance of knowledge. The technologies selected in this environment will rely on high throughput, reliable, robust methods of identifying known mutations or polymorphisms. The driving force behind the selection of technology is the detailed knowledge of gene sequence and variation. Since the first edition of this volume a great deal of genomic and genetic information has entered the public domain. The ability of an investigator to obtain detailed DNA sequence information online has greatly facilitated the inclusion of genetic information in drug discovery.

Identification of Gene Variants

The completion of the final version of the sequence of the human genome provides an unparalleled resource for the identification of mutations and polymorphisms. The eventual knowledge of the location and sequence of genes important to the cause and treatment of disease will permit the rapid collection of sequence variations in a wide variety of potential patient populations. In advance of that a collection of governmental and commercial efforts have sought to identify as large a pool of sequence variants as possible and place them in the public domain. The SNP Consortium brought together a number of commercial entities in an effort to identify a large number of single-nucleotide polymorphisms (SNP). This effort was successful beyond its initial goal of 300,000 SNPs eventually releasing a total of over 1.2 million variants in a publicly available database. The availability of this SNP resource is a valuable starting point in any pharmacogenetics study. A limitation to these databases is the limited amount of population frequency information in the public domain. There remains a need to both identify and characterize sequence variants in patient populations. The tools used in any variant discovery fall into two categories, those technologies that are information rich but relatively costly in capital and man-hour terms (i.e., sequencing) and those technologies that are less information rich but relatively less expensive (i.e., gene scanning).

Brute Force Variant Identification

The use of DNA sequencing to identify population wide variation is, except for the largest commercial and governmental operations, a labor intensive and costly exercise. With the completion of the Human Genome Project the task of finding appropriate primer sites for both PCR and sequencing became greatly simplified. The most practical sequencing based method of variant detection is via one of the various automated DNA sequencers currently on the market. All take advantage of substantially similar sequencing chemistry while using a variety of labeling technologies. The major difference between manufacturers, marketing claims aside, is the number of different labels that can be loaded into one lane of a gel or capillary at one time and the speed with which the labeled sequence can be run by an appropriate detector. By detecting multiple labels one is able to perform all four sequencing reactions in a single tube and/or load more than one sequencing reaction into a sequencing gel lane. The throughput advantage of automated sequencers able to detect multiple labels is a strong point in their favor when variant detection on a large scale is planned.

For most laboratories, however, variant detection via sequencing remains less a completely automated collection of data and more a task composed of visually sifting through quantities of sequence data in search of variants from a "normal." Advances in DNA analysis software have automated a portion of this task but the efficiency of this process varies by sequencing chemistry and automated analyzer. The major difficulty in sequence analysis is the determination of heterozygotes and true SNPs vs. sequencing artifact. The SNP Consortium has addressed this difficulty in two ways. The genome centers that identified the sequence variants re-sequenced randomly selected SNPs for verification and, second, the consortium contracted with Orchid Biosciences (Princeton, NJ) and Celera (Rockville, MD) to verify and develop assays for randomly selected SNPs. In this way it is hoped that the accuracy level of SNPs collected by the Consortium will reach a 95% standard level.

When one looks back on the SNP discovery process in the future it is likely that the majority of sequence variants will have been identified using a brute force sequencing approach. This will no doubt be as a direct result of the amount of raw sequencing horsepower being applied to the task. There will be, however, a portion of the SNPs that will have been identified through the use of a variety of gene scanning methods. The use of such methods is appropriate for those laboratories that do not have access to large scale sequencing operations.

Gene Scanning Technologies

The identification of sequence variants in the absence of a large scale sequencing capability can be accomplished through the use of gene scanning techniques. This collection of technologies is capable, at varying degrees of precision, of comparing a "normal" DNA (and in some instances RNA) sample to a test sample. The result of this comparison is either complete identity with the standard sequence or the identification of a variant at some point within the sequence under comparison. The common weakness of virtually all such scanning technologies is the requirement for a subsequent sequencing step to characterize the variant.

The technologies that purport to identify sequence variants generally fall into two categories:

1. Gel shift assays,
2. Mismatch identification.

Gel shift assays

The mobility of DNA, either single or double stranded, through a gel matrix is determined by a number of factors. By comparing the mobility of a test DNA sample to that of a normal control sample it is possible to determine the presence of a sequence alteration in the test sample. The major factors that affect DNA mobility are listed below:

1. Sequence length,
2. Base composition,
3. Single strand secondary structure,
4. Double strand melting characteristics,
5. Double strand mobility in the presence of mismatched strands.

A variety of techniques are used to take advantage of these factors in order to discover previously unknown mutations and polymorphisms. Two excellent reviews of these technologies have been published by Cotton and Schafer and Hawkins. The following list outlines several of these techniques and a selection of their related methods.

1. Single strand conformation polymorphism (SSCP):
   - restriction endonuclease fingerprinting (REF),
   - dideoxy fingerprinting (ddF).
2. Denaturing gradient gel electrophoresis (DGGE):
   - temperature gradient gel electrophoresis (TGGE).
3. Heteroduplex analysis (HA).

Single strand conformation polymorphism

This technique is perhaps the easiest of all of the variant detection methods to establish and perform. Developed by Orita et al., PCR amplified fragments are heat denatured and then rapidly cooled to prevent reassociation of the complementary strands. The single stranded DNA is then electrophoresed through a native acrylamide gel. The rate of transit through the gel is dependent upon sequence length, and single strand secondary structure. Variations in the sequences of single stranded DNA fragments will, in theory, produce a change in the secondary structure of the DNA thereby affecting its progress through the gel matrix. It is this change in mobility that is resolved by the gel matrix producing additional or displaced bands as compared to a normal control. The resolving power of the gel matrix is affected by temperature and gel additives such as glycerol, which enhance variant detection. The detection rates for SSCP can fall into the 60–95% range depending upon the sequence context in which the variants occur. By maintaining a relatively small fragment size (~200 bp) and selecting appropriate gel conditions it is possible to routinely achieve variant detection rates of greater than 85%.

Restriction endonuclease fingerprinting

Originally described by Liu and Sommer, this technique takes advantage of the capabilities of SSCP and Restriction Fragment Length Polymorphism (RFLP) analysis to increase the amount of information available to an investigator in an alteration discovery process. A restriction fragment analysis of a normal control region of interest is completed to select a collection of restriction enzymes capable of generating a series of fragments resolvable on a standard acrylamide gel. A PCR amplified segment of DNA up to 1-2kb in length is restricted using the pre-selected enzyme set. The fragments are then radioactively or fluorescently labeled, heat denatured and run as single stranded segments on a native acrylamide gel. The electrophoretic step is identical to an SSCP gel with the resulting fragment pattern providing multiple bands whose mobility would be potentially affected by an alteration present in a fragment.

In addition, the loss or gain of a restriction site would be identified by the gain or loss of an expected fragment and the increase or decrease in length of another fragment. Thus, REF provides two concurrent methods of alteration analysis, SSCP with the advantage of multiple analyzable bands and an RFLP component. The major advantage of this technique is the increased number of bands that are available for analysis using the SSCP component. While the RFLP analysis component is useful it is not likely to provide consistently valuable information, as the statistical likelihood of an alteration creating or eliminating an enzyme site that is also a member of the REF set is low. The multiple banding patterns, however, creates several opportunities for shifts in mobility to be identified. The increased fragment size available for analysis is also a major advantage of REF over SSCP and favorably impacts throughput for this technique. The detection rate for this technique has been reported to be in the 90–95% range.

One of the difficulties in this technique is the selection of the enzyme set. It is often a difficult task of balancing informativeness, exotic enzyme expense and fragment size. A subsequent publication from the Sommer group described a computer program, which aided the enzyme selection process. As with SSCP, the detection rate is dependent upon conformation changes and their resolvability on an acrylamide gel. The read-out of the assay provides a great deal of information for analysis, which can be difficult to interpret on a routine basis. Precise localization of a variant for subsequent sequence identification is also difficult given the number of fragments, which must be analyzed.

Dideoxy fingerprinting

This technique uses a combination of SSCP and Sanger sequencing to create a larger set of bands for analysis in a native acrylamide gel. In this method an amplified fragment is sequenced using a standard Sanger protocol and primers spaced at a SSCP friendly size of approximately 200–250 bp throughout the amplified fragment. One modification to the Sanger protocol is the use of a single dideoxy nucleotide to create the banding pattern. The change in banding pattern as compared to a normal control is then indicative of a sequence alteration in that region. This technique has been adapted to fluorescence as well as using primers running in both directions to increase detection rates. Through the appropriate selection of dideoxy nucleotide, fragment size and gel running conditions a significant improvement in detection rate over SSCP can be achieved. In addition, a degree of alteration localization can be determined by noting the location of the shift in banding patterns.

The ability to perform a single PCR amplification followed by multiple Sanger reactions also reduces the overall cost of the assay. The fragment size used for variant detection remains in the SSCP range thus decreasing assay throughput. The original paper suggests that reaching the 90-95% detection rate range may be difficult for some genes and some mutation types. In this event ddF would be useful as an adjunct to SSCP rather than a subsitute.

Denaturing gradient gel electrophoresis

This technique makes use of the reduced double stranded melting characteristics inherent in heteroduplexed DNA as compared to a normal homoduplex control to identify novel sequence alterations. A key modification to DGGE was made by Myers et al. whereby a DNA sequence of interest is amplified using a specialized PCR primer pair consisting of one standard, sequence specific primer and an opposing primer containing sequence specific information at the primer's 3' end and a GC enriched sequence at the primer's 5' end. The purpose of the GC enriched sequence (often called a GC clamp) is to normalize the melting profile of the sequence of interest. The GC clamp acts as a high melting temperature region of the resulting amplicon stabilizing the melting characteristics over the entirety of the sequence. Without this normalization of amplicons containing multiple melting domains would denature at different temperatures.

The lower melting temperature domains would denature first obscuring the decrease in melting temperature contributed by sequence variants present in higher temperature melting domains. In performing DGGE the sample is heat denatured, allowed to slowly re-anneal and then electrophoresed through an acrylamide gel containing a gradient of denaturant (usually formamide). As the double stranded amplicon progresses through the gel matrix it encounters an increasing denaturant concentration and the amplicon begins to denature. This denaturation slows the progression of the amplicon through the gel. Any alteration in a heteroduplex DNA sequence will result in decreased mobility yielding a multiple banding pattern. By comparing the extent of mobility in the gradient matrix to a normal control it is possible to determine the presence of a sequence change. In theory, any sequence alteration, which changes the melting characteristics, will result in additional bands being produced on the gel. The melting profile of any sequence can be predicted using an algorithm created by Lerman and Silverstein. If the sequence under investigation is amplified as a single melting domain using the GC clamp method it is then possible to design denaturing gradient conditions under which all sequence alterations in that single domain would be identified.

The commonly accepted detection rates for DGGE are in the 90-95% range given an amplicon containing a single melting domain. The size of the routinely analyzable fragments (up to -650 bp) is greater than the 200-250 bp for SSCP. The pouring of gradient gels is a technically difficult task requiring considerable experience and patience to achieve consistent results. The cost of the clamped primers is greater than non-clamped primers due to the addition of as many as 40 or more additional bases at the 5' end of the primer to produce the clamp. Alterations closer than 40-50 bp from the 3' end of the clamped primer are unlikely to be identified due to the increase thermal stability of this region. This requires the design of a second set of clamped primers opposing the initial set of primers for each region of interest. In this manner, the region nearest to one clamp, and thus refractory to analysis, is accounted for by 3' end of the opposing clamped amplicon. This necessarily doubles the cost of the assay from the PCR step onwards.

Temperature gradient gel electrophoresis and dHPLC

These variants of DGGE make use of carefully controlled temperature gradients as a substitute for chemical denaturation. The simplest form of this method from an equipment standpoint immerses a uniform denaturant gel in a temperature controlled buffer chamber. The buffer temperature is gradually increased during the running of the gel providing the denaturing gradient range desired.

Another modification of this type of denaturing gradient methodology uses the high resolution characteristics of high performance liquid chromatography to physically separate sequences which differ in their denaturing characteristics. The main advantage is the rapid nature of HPLC coupled with the fine temperature control of HPLC resulting in an ability to resolve small differences in melting characteristics. The semi-automated manner in which the samples can be loaded into the HPLC and the potential for customizing the run characteristics is also a favorable feature for this approach. The use of dHPLC does not provide any inherent improvements over traditional DGGE other than in the area of automation, as detection for all variants must still labor under the constraints of DNA melting theory. The major advantage of dHPLC over DGGE is more one of process and throughput for the end user.

Heteroduplex analysis

This technique makes use of the change in mobility caused by mismatched heteroduplexed DNA strands as compared to perfectly homoduplexed DNA strands. In this technique a DNA sample is amplified, heat denatured and then reannealed. This results in a fraction of the single stranded DNA re-annealing with a complementary strand from an opposing allele thus forming a heteroduplex. When this mixture is subsequently electrophoresed through a non-denaturing acrylamide gel a mobility shift can be resolved indicating the presence of a sequence alteration as compared to a normal control homoduplex. The relative ease of this protocol is the major advantage to this technique. The generally accepted detection rates for a specific PCR run on an appropriate acrylamide gel ranges from the low 80% to 90–95% range. Modifications to the assay to generate heteroduplexes may increase the detection rate to a more routine 90–95%. The major difficulty with this technique is the establishment of sufficiently specific PCR amplification conditions to avoid missing important heteroduplexes or the creation of false alterations. The lack of resolution of the acrylamide matrix is another area of false negative results. In practice, the amplicon size range for routine detection is from 250 to 500 bp thus limiting the use of this technique for very large genes.

Mismatch Identification

The discovery of sequence alterations can be accomplished by the creation of mismatched base pairs, which occur when a test sample containing a sequence alteration is denatured and re-annealed witn an otherwise complementary normal control sequence. The routine and specific discovery of these mismatches and their localization to within an easily sequenced region is the goal of several techniques. There are two general methods for identification of mismatched sequences:

1. Chemical,
2. Enzymatic.

Chemical

The major method involving chemical identification of mismatched sequences is a modification of Maxam–Gilbert sequencing termed Chemical Cleavage of Mismatch (CCM). Using the C- and T-specific reactivity of hydroxylamine and osmium tetroxide, respectively, to identify mismatched bases followed by piperidine cleavage of the modified products it is possible to not only scan a genomic segment for mismatched bases but also localized the site of the mismatch. When optimized, this technique is highly efficient in alteration discovery (nearly 100%). The current practical limit of the size of a fragment suitable for analysis is in the 1–1.5 kb range. A considerable disadvantage, however, to CCM is the use of highly toxic chemicals in a clinical environment. Hydroxylamine and osmium tetroxide both require chemical grade fume hoods for use. The relatively large number of manipulations associated with the technique and the toxic nature of the chemicals render this technique a difficult choice for a clinical lab. A recent improvement on the assay has substituted potassium permangenate for osmium tetroxide making the manipulations involving these chemicals less toxic and more attractive for the routine laboratory.

Enzymatic

This set of methods makes use of specific enzymes to recognize mismatched base pairs in heteroduplexed DNA strands. In general a test sample is amplified and heat denatured in the presence of a normal control sample. This combination of test and normal control samples is allowed to slowly re- anneal forming a mixture of homo and heteroduplexes. The mixture is then exposed to any one of a number of enzymes, which recognize mismatched base pairs at various efficiencies and the sample is then analyzed for these recognized mismatches. There are several types of enzymes and assays available which purport to recognize mismatched base pairs in a heteroduplex or secondary structures formed by mismatches. A short selection of these enzymes and assays are listed below:

1. Ribonuclease cleavage,
2. T4 endonuclease VII,
3. Cleavase.

Ribonuclease cleavage

This technique, developed by Myers et al. is useful for sequence alteration discovery due to its ability to cleave double stranded RNA or RNA: DNA hybrid sequence at areas of mismatch. The mismatched areas form single stranded regions in a heteroduplex, which are then amenable to cleavage by the RNAses. A significant improvement in the assay was published by Murthy et al. whereby an amplified product is produced following a standard PCR of regions of interest. The test sample DNA is then mixed with a normal control RNA sample to produce a normal/test duplex, which creates the potential for mismatched heteroduplexes open to cleavage by RNAse. The cleaved products are then electrophoresed on a standard agarose gels (this is the most recent form of the assay which has been reduced to its simplest practice) and the banding pattern is compared to a normal control. Relative to SSCP and DGGE this technique offers slightly longer analyzable read lengths and the potential for multiple bands for analysis. The RNA handling requirements, however, are often a negative factor in a high throughput or clinical environment.

T4 endonuclease VII

Mashal et al. originally described the use of two bacteriophage resolvases to identify mismatches in heteroduplexed DNA. The current technique depends upon one of those enzymes, T4 endonuclease VII, to recognize and cleave double stranded DNA at the site of the mismatch. This technology is now incorporated in kit form by Amersham Pharmacia Biotech. The length of fragment amenable to this sort of scanning is approximately 1 kb. The assay is essentially the same as a restriction enzyme analysis with respect to ease of use. The size of the generated cleaved fragment is then used to roughly localize the site of the alteration for subsequent sequencing.

Cleavase

This enzyme cleaves secondary structure in single stranded DNA. The principle used here, as described by Brow et al., is one of secondary folding structure of single stranded DNA being altered when the underlying sequence is changed by polymorphism or mutation. Cleavase acts as a structure specific endonuclease by cutting at the 3' end of a loop structure in a single stranded DNA producing a characteristic banding pattern. When compared to a normal control sample a cleaved test sample containing a different base composition would demonstrate an altered banding pattern. This method has been developed for commercial use by Third Wave Technologies.

The main advantage of any enzyme-based gene scanning system is the relative ease of use and cost effectiveness when compared to full gene sequencing. The ability to scan through large amounts of genetic real estate identifying only those individuals demonstrating variations from a control reduces the overall amount of DNA sequencing required to characterize the panoply of genetic variation in a population. A significant disadvantage, however, is the amount and types of variations that the enzymatic methods have difficulty identifying. Depending upon the sequence context and variant type the enzyme may not recognize the mismatched base pair leading to a false negative result. This may not be a significant difficulty in the context of a large variant discovery effort where missing one polymorphism is not of great import. In a clinical diagnostic effort where each patient sample must be completely and accurately scanned enzymatic based assays must be designed with great care to reduce the false negative rate to an absolute minimum. All of the described methods are now offered commercially so it remains the consumers challenge to sort through the various detection claims and identify the enzyme which works best in their hands and for the sequence to be scanned.

Variant Identification

The technologies available to the research pharmacogenetics community are varied and numerous. The task confronting the end user in the selection of the appropriate tool set is one of overall throughput, accuracy and thoroughness.

Testing for Previously Identified Gene Variants

The development of large and publicly available SNP and mutation databases provides ample intellectual material for pharmacogenetics. The real value of this information glut will be in using it to design appropriate therapeutics and to select individuals most likely to benefit from these new treatments. The techniques and reagents, which were included in the description of variant identification methods, are not universally applicable to the task of genotyping individuals on a clinical basis. There are several technologies, which are useful to perform this type of known variant detection. Virtually all of these technologies use probes of one sort or another to detect variants. The probes in these cases are highly specific for a particular known variant and are therefore not useful for generalized gene scanning. The universe of variant detection can be broken into two categories: array based and non-array based.

Array-based systems

The use of a fixed probe system with a test sample in solution has promised to revolutionize genetic testing for nearly a decade. The promise has not entirely become a reality as of yet but the uses of arrays have increased over the decade to accommodate the potential to screen individuals for thousands of discrete polymorphisms in a single hybridization. In fixed array systems the probes are attached to a surface by a number of methods. The method pioneered by Fodor et al. uses a modification of the photolithographic system used to manufacture computer chips. In this method a mask is placed over the surface of the DNA chip covering those regions to be protected from the light activated oligonucleotide synthetic process. The process is completed and the mask realigned to uncover subsequent areas. In this manner a series of chemical reactions can take place in a defined order resulting in the building of an oligonucleotide probe of a specific design at a known location on the array. By carefully controlling the synthetic process it is possible to increase the number of probes on the array to the hundreds of thousands or greater. Other fixed array types attach fully pre-constructed probes to a number of different substrates by a variety of chemical means.

The process of analyzing a sample on fixed arrays generally takes place in several steps. The sample must first be amplified for the specific region of the genome to be probed. The sample must then be fragmented in order for optimal hybridization to a static probe. The hybridization then occurs and analysis of the hybridization pattern takes place. The number of probes able to be queried on a fixed array is not equal to the number of separate elements fixed to the substrate. Due to the detection limits of the fluorescent technology, which underlies the majority of fixed array systems multiple probe elements must hybridize to the test sample in order for a sufficient signal to be measured. The hybridization characteristics of oligonucleotide probes are often difficult to normalize when dealing with large numbers of probes. This is exacerbated when a probe must be placed in a sequence context of unfavorable hybridization characteristics due to the presence of an important sequence variant. As a result there are regions of the genome and types of variants that are not easily amenable to oligonucleotide hybridization. Nanogen has approached the hybridization problem with a methodology involving control of the hybridization and denaturation of disparate oligonucleotides by varying the electric field strength of the hybridization repelling molecules with reduced affinity for the probe.

One of the drawbacks of a fixed array system in an era where not all the relevant information concerning a biologic system may be present is the relatively inflexible nature of a fixed system. In order to add elements to a fixed array one needs to return to the chip manufacture process and redesign the array. Not all array-based systems, however, make use of a fixed solid support. Two types of arrays make use of bead technologies to permit rapid rearrangement and alteration of the components of an array. Luminex attaches oligonucleotide probes to polystyrene beads that have been colored with one of a number of colors separately identifiable by a fluorescence activated cell sorter. It is then possible to perform standard oligonucleotide hybridization to a collection of these probe bound beads using test sample material that has been labeled with another identifiable fluorescent tag. The beads are then washed and run through the cell sorter producing a profile of test sample bound and unbound beads. The colors of the bound beads are then correlated to the type of oligonucleotide previously attached to them and a positive identification of the probe is made.

This process has the advantage of speed and thus throughput as well as flexibility of array composition. In order to change the array one only needs to mix the appropriate combination of beads. A second type of non-fixed array was developed at Tufts University using beads similarly color coded with oligonucleotide probes covalently attached (29). In this method, however, the beads are deposited onto the ends of fiber optic cable following a process of etching carefully controlled pits into the end of the fiber optic. The amplified test sample is labeled with a fluorescent tag and is hybridized to the beads. The laser excitation of the fluorescent tag and the colored beads provides evidence of a positive hybridization and identification of the probe.

Non-array-based systems

Hybridization based array systems are not the only method of analyzing test samples for known genetic variants. One of the most effective methods of analyzing SNPs is a technique known as mini-sequencing or single-base extension. This technique was described in detail in the first edition of this text and is used by Orchid BioScience as well as Sequenom to type SNPs. The method takes advantage of DNA sequencing technology and the chain terminating effect of dideoxynucleotides to determine the presence of a particular nucleotide at a known position. A primer specific for a region immediately adjacent to the SNP under study is hybridized to a test sample. A dideoxynucleotide corresponding to one of the two bases indicative of the SNP is then added to the reaction. If the SNP corresponding to the particular dideoxynucleotide is present the reaction is terminated. By labeling the dideoxynucleotide with a fluorescent tag (or a mass tag for mass spectrometry based methods) it is possible to perform these assays in an automated manner increasing throughput and decreasing manpower requirements.

Another SNP detection system that does not rely on fixed arrays has been developed by Third Wave Technologies (Madison, WI). The Invader assay makes use of two probe molecules, which partially overlap a known SNP site. The probes compete for hybridization to the specified genetic sequence. When one probe binds specifically to the test sample it forces the overlapping probe to leave a portion of the overlapping region non-hybridized.

The Cleavase endonuclease described earlier in this review then cleaves the overlapping flap releasing a small fragment, which is either directly labeled or used as an "invading" oligonucleotide itself in a secondary reaction, which releases labeled sequence producing a detectable signal. This isothermal reaction is compatible with several assay formats and has been developed for a number of clinical assays. The isothermal nature of the assay and the single base discriminatory nature of the probe reactions make this system an attractive choice for those laboratories seeking an alternative to PCR-based systems.

Reduction to Practice

The construction of large-scale databases and genotype/phenotype correlations within large population groups is of great value to the future of medical care. This large-scale research effort will create opportunities for the genetic testing community previously seen as mere science fiction. For the testing community to take advantage of these opportunities a shift in technologies must take place on a scale greater than currently available. The volume of assays that might be expected over the next decade or more will be far closer to that seen in the clinical chemistry laboratories. If one considers the development of clinical chemistry testing on an industrial scale a few similarities to the challenges that pharmacogenetics will face in the future can be seen. The major development, which permitted clinical chemistry to achieve the volumes of testing that laboratories currently handle was the wide scale adoption of automation.

The modern clinical chemistry laboratory receives samples for testing, bar codes each sample and places the sample tube into an automated system. This system reads the bar code, consults a database to determine the requested testing and proceeds to perform the necessary procedures often without any human intervention. There is no currently available system for widespread genetic analysis that approaches this level of automation for even the most straightforward of test protocols. As it is unlikely that a pharmacogenetics test will involve a single SNP as the definitive predictor of therapeutic response a new generation of molecular genetic technologies and automation must be developed that can perform this highly complex testing in a clinical chemistry-like atmosphere. An example of the scale that the testing industry will have to face in the not too distant future is that presented by the volume of testing for a pharmaceutical that has a rather modest market size and a different pharmaceutical with a large market size.

One of the central assumptions often made in pharmacogenetics is that there will be a growing number of pharmaceutical products whose prescription will be linked to a genetic test. This will probably not be a safety related issue but one of selecting those patients who will benefit most from being treated by a drug or to determine an appropriate dosage level. If one creates a hypothetical drug whose market size is approximately $200 million the monthly new prescriptions can be in the range of 18,000. The market size for such a genetic test would be over 200,000 tests per year. If one increases the market for the drug to the $1 billion size the monthly new prescription rate can equal the number of prescriptions written in an entire year for the smaller market example. In this scenario the yearly testing market for a $1 billion drug with a genetic test linked to prescription would be over 2 million tests per year. To put this into context, the current number of tests for carrier status for cystic fibrosis in the United States is approximately 300,000–500,000 tests annually. The molecular genetics technology development community and the genetic testing community are only now developing the collective ability to perform that level of genetic testing. It will be some time before the level of automation seen in the clinical chemistry laboratory reaches the molecular genetics laboratory. The caveat often linked to the foregoing argument, however, is that there are unlikely to be drugs with companion diagnostics that reach the $1 billion market level. The problem becomes essentially identical to the billion-dollar drug issue, however, when one envisions multiple smaller drugs on the market that have a linked genetic test for therapeutic efficacy. This is an issue that will only increase in seriousness as more information concerning genetic markers of drug response become an increasing part of routine medical practice.

The promise of pharmacogenetics to enhance the future of pharmaceutical development and medical care has been discussed in this volume as well as a number of others. The technological task challenging the scientific community is twofold. The first challenge is identifying the relevant genetic markers that will provide significant and medically relevant information to the clinician. This effort will require the establishment of large, well- annotated databases linking information concerning disease pathogenesis, functional genomics, proteomics, and genetic variation. The most useful data will be that correlating the large databases with sub-populations of individuals particularly susceptible to severe disease, particular sequelae or in need of or obtaining a particular benefit from a specific treatment regimen significantly different from a larger population group. As the future of pharmacogenetics unfolds it will hold opportunities for the developers of novel, highly specific and efficient technologies, which provide valuable information to the medical community. Those successful in the development effort will have solved the many-layered problem of medical relevance, technologic possibility and cost effectiveness. The technologies and concepts described in this volume go a long way down this path.

14

DEVELOPMENT OF MEDICINES

Full drug development involves management of the whole project from early proof of concept to post-launch activities. The very large financial and human resource costs associated with scale up of a development project from early phase work through to Phase III and launch in major markets require that the risks associated with the investment are managed appropriately. Nevertheless, rapid progress through Phase III development will allow a longer effective patent life, which will increase the commercial return on a new medicine, and in recent years this factor alone has been a major driver for large pharmaceutical companies to project manage their product portfolios more efficiently. The changing nature of the pharmaceutical industry, with increasing numbers of small companies whose survival depends on rapid registration and successful marketing of one drug candidate, means that additional risks such as intellectual property rights, shareholder return, contractual and legal relationships are part of the risk associated with the investment. Management of business risk, which is outside the scope of this chapter, has been identified as a significant problem for small companies.

BACKGROUND

Total drug development costs are huge. It has been estimated recently that development costs are about US$350 million per drug and annual average sales are US$265 million. Currently, development costs are increasing by between 8% and 11% per annum, and soon average development costs may reach US$500 million for each major product. The majority of drug development costs are in Phase III development: these include not only the clinical trial programme itself, but significant associated regulatory and manufacturing scale-up costs. The long-forecasted consolidation in the pharmaceutical industry happened in the 1990s. The impact of this consolidation was demonstrated by an increase in of product failures and increased trial cancellations in 1999 and 2000. However, during 2001, Phase III activity increased again, albeit by a small 1·8% increase (392 to 385 projects) compared with 2000. *Pharmaprojects 2001* reports a total of 6198 R&D projects in 2001, compared with 5995 in 2000. Most of this growth has come from an 8·7% increase in Phase I projects (640 compared with 589) and a 14·3% increase in Phase II projects (1010 compared with 884). The reduction in Phase I and Phase II programmes in the early 1990s has clearly been translated into a reduction in Phase III projects in 1999 and 2000.

Senior Management Perspective

Taking into account all marketing and development failures, cost calculations demonstrate that companies have to develop more "*blockbuster*" products with annual sales over US$1 billion if they are to maintain historical rates of returns to shareholders, or they must cut significantly the development costs. Thus, the focus of management is increasingly on the high costs of Phase III programmes, and there is a need to reduce risks and costs in Phase III by:

1. Aggressive portfolio management in early phases of development
2. Life cycle management, including risk management
3. Continued spend on local trials after submission to fill gaps in the development programme such as paediatric or geriatric subjects in Phase IIIb and IV.

The biotechnology explosion has also finally arrived. Globally, the number of companies with one product in development, which is a useful proxy for biotechnology-driven or emerging pharmaceutical companies, has increased by 21% per annum, from 212 in 1998 to 373 in 2001. Moreover, the top 25 pharmaceutical companies have a significant proportion of R&D drugs in development which are licensed in, typically from smaller pharmaceutical companies or research laboratories.

Ranked by total numbers of drugs in R&D, the top five companies are GlaxoSmithKline (189 drugs in development), Pfizer (141), Aventis (140), Abbott (128), and Pharmacia (126). Of the 189 R&D drugs that GlaxoSmithKline has in development, 101 (53%) are their own drugs; Pfizer has 77 (55%), Aventis 84 (60%), Abbott 70 (55%) and Pharmacia 126 (61%). This changing picture of full drug development means that the largest pharmaceutical companies are now having to be adept at intellectual property protection, legal and contractual development and comarketing agreements, as well as accelerated drug development. The single product companies must also be adept at managing their cash flow, relationships with their shareholders, and the market place in which they need to thrive.

Recovery of costs by successful marketing of products is essential in order to maximise shareholder return. As R&D costs in the late 1990s continue to increase by between 8% and 11% per annum, and sales turnover increases by between 5% and 7% per annum, R&D takes up an increasing proportion of the pharmaceutical budget, and for the largest pharmaceutical companies is about 17% of turnover.

Clearly there is limit to how much the research costs can increase and companies are beginning to think in new ways about how to manage their R&D costs. There is an increase in the number of alliances and partnerships with academic groups, small biotechnology companies and healthcare providers who, it is hoped, will provide the entrepreneurial drug development skills that large pharmaceutical companies are currently unable to generate internally.

The International Conference on Harmonisation (ICH) and the EU GCP [Good Clinical Practice] Directive provide a unified standard for clinical trials and also facilitate mutual acceptance by the regulatory authorities in Europe, Japan and the US. Development of the guidelines has allowed companies to streamline their drug development programmes. These guidelines also provide benefits for clinical trial subjects: they are protected during studies, and they can be confident that the studies are based on good science. However, as always, increased regulation has resulted in increased costs, offset slightly by an increase in standardisation of procedures across regions of the world.

Taking Products into Later Development Phase

Clinical Perspective

This review focuses on the clinical development of drugs. This is an area where companies can plan and control much more of their activity. As more drug development projects are terminated at Phase II, companies have to be careful that the Phase II studies are particularly well designed to avoid the likelihood of a Type II error. This means that the studies do not miss a significant clinical difference or advantage for the product. Clarity of thought and detailed design considerations for Phase II studies are increasingly important in drug development. The use of external advisory boards can be especially helpful, and it can be useful to include drug development and regulatory specialists on advisory boards together with the more traditional academic staff members.

If the area of endeavour is crowded there will be significant competition for patient recruitment to clinical trials. Currently these therapy areas include diabetes, oncology and cardiovascular medicine, and it may become necessary to seek patients outside of Western Europe and the US. Investigator fees are rising and competition for patients is helping to increase fees in these geographical areas and also in some areas of Central Europe. However, even significant investigator fees may not be sufficient to encourage recruitment if there is little investigator excitement about the product. Investigators are keen to work on innovative products and may well seek increased fees to support other academic work if the product is not particularly exciting for them.

The likely effectiveness of the product, derived from the preclinical and early clinical work, will determine study design, complexity and size. It is a mistake to try to answer too many questions in a single study, despite the apparent commercial attractiveness of such a strategy. A study overburdened by many secondary objectives is more likely to fail when the design is implemented in many centres worldwide. What seems a good idea in head office can often be hard to implement in the clinic. Statistical advice is vital, and statisticians offer excellent opinions about the utility of complex study designs.

The expected adverse event profile will also determine the study design. A drug for which the prescription is to be initiated in a tertiary referral clinic by leading experts in the field, such as many oncological compounds, will have a different safety profile compared with a product which will be widely used across many different specialties in primary and secondary care. Characterisation of the risk-benefit profile is an important consideration in study design.

Consideration needs to be given to suitable clinical endpoints. It can be tempting, because of cost and speed of development, to use surrogate endpoints in a pivotal study. A surrogate endpoint is defined as an endpoint that is intended to relate to a clinically important outcome but does not, in itself, measure clinical benefit. A surrogate endpoint should be used as a primary endpoint when appropriate, for example when the surrogate endpoint is reasonably likely to, or is well known to, predict clinical outcome. However, great care needs to be taken in basing a pivotal and full development programme on the use of surrogate endpoints. Typically, these endpoints are used in early development and discussion with the regulatory authorities is advised before using such endpoints in a full development programme. The use of surrogate markers is discussed in the *ICH guideline E8: General Considerations for Clinical Trials*. The guideline makes the point that these markers are most often useful in exploratory therapeutic trials in well-defined narrow patient groups.

Regulatory Perspective

The regulatory authorities are increasingly welcoming informal or formal discussions about drug development programmes. There are differences in approach between the European Agency for the Evaluation of Medicinal Products (EMEA) and the US Food and Drug Administration (FDA) and it is wise to take regulatory advice before contacting the agencies. The FDA tends to require a formalistic approach to the development programme. This can have strengths in that the programme direction is clear, but it can be rather limiting in terms of defining a mandatory series of trials and a particular development strategy. Nevertheless, it can be particularly useful if the development programme is likely to be in a new area of medicine or unusual in any way.

The National Institute for Clinical Excellence (NICE) was set up in 1999 as a Special Health Authority for England and Wales. Its role is to provide patients, health professionals and the public with authoritative, robust and reliable guidance on current "best practice". The guidance covers individual health technologies and the clinical management of specific conditions. In practice, the pharmaceutical industry has tended to see NICE as an additional "fourth" hurdle acting after the Medicines Control Agency (MCA) or EMEA has approved the quality, safety and efficacy of a new product. Consideration has to be given in any development programme to applications to NICE and other bodies throughout the world, and companies may need to consider special and additional studies to meet any objections these bodies may have in allowing a product to be satisfactorily commercialised.

The Common Technical Document (CTD) (ICH M4) is expected to become a requirement after July 2003. The CTD is the agreed common format for the preparation of a well-structured application to the regulatory authorities. The CTD will have an impact on all organisations after this date as database integration and electronic submissions become more common. Indeed, for many companies, preparation for the CTD is currently well under way.

The ICH has played an important role in establishing guidelines for drug development. Although these are only guidelines and are not legal documents, companies would have to justify deviations from the guidelines in any application for approval. The World Health Organization (WHO) has recently stated that it expects the ICH guidelines to be adopted in non-ICH countries eventually. Interestingly, these non-ICH countries are not presently involved in the formal ICH decision-making process.

Commercial Perspective

Apart from the traditional costs associated with commercial development, the costs of selling and marketing the product will require evaluation. Decisions have to be made about whether the product will be sold by the company's own sales force or licensed to partners in some markets. The company franchise in a particular area of therapeutic endeavour may be enhanced or compromised by active patient groups. There is increasing pressure to place more development and clinical trial information in the public domain. For example in the UK, the pharmaceutical industry trade association, the Association of the British Pharmaceutical Industry (ABPI), has agreed to develop a register of Phase III trials conducted in the UK, three months after drug approval in a major market - which might not be the UK. Patients will therefore be in a position to seek entry into trials and may demand this from their physicians.

Indeed, the development of AZT (Retrovir, zidovudine), by Wellcome (now GlaxoSmithKline) is an interesting example of patient power. Patient groups obtained copies of early phase drug development protocols and some subjects demanded to be placed into these clinical trials for HIV/AIDS. The scrutiny of the protocols by patient groups resulted in improvements in clinical trial designs and the political pressure exerted by these groups ensured that the drug regulatory process became more politicised. This resulted in more rapid approval of drugs by some regulatory authorities and also pushed forward discussions about surrogate markers. It is probable that AZT did not meet fully the established principles of safety and efficacy when it was approved, and further development was required after approval. Whether this approach was beneficial to the entire community of AIDS patients remains debatable.

Other patient groups in areas as diverse as osteoporosis research, dementia and other central nervous system disorders, have learnt from the AIDS patient groups the power of politics in medicine, and these groups will have an increasing impact on drug development. Some of this impact will be positive but some is likely to be negative and may encourage a too rapid assessment of drug efficacy and safety by the authorities. Indeed, there is evidence of increased product withdrawal by the FDA. Eleven products have been withdrawn between 1997 and mid 2001, compared with eight product withdrawals in the previous ten years. Whether this is a result of more rapid early development, a more rapid assessment process or simply due to bad luck is open to conjecture. However, it is clear that a product withdrawal in either late-phase development or early post-marketing can have a devastating effect on a company's share price as a result of the expected decrease in revenue and the potential for poor public relations.

The market potential of a drug or device is clearly critical in determining the desirability of proceeding into later phase development. An increasing number of programmes are stopped at Phase

II because it is not economical for the company to develop these products. DiMasi in 2001 estimated that, compared with the 1981–86 period, where 29·8% of products were terminated because of economic reasons, between 1987 and 1992 the number of terminations was 33·8% and that this upward trend has continued.

Likely shifts in demographic factors and prescribing mean that drugs for the elderly, such as therapies for Alzheimer's disease or osteoporosis, are increasingly attractive as targets for drug development. Oncological drugs and drugs for chronic diseases also continue to be important for companies' financial health. The political environment continues to be important. All governments want to constrain healthcare costs, and an easy target is prescription drug costs. This is not necessarily the most sensible target, as improving health service management may have as important an effect on the national purse. Nonetheless, there is a continuing downwards pressure on healthcare prescribing.

The development of NICE in the UK is being watched keenly throughout the world to see if this organisation will have an indirect effect on reducing healthcare costs. There has been a perceived reduction in competitiveness in the UK pharmaceutical industry over the past few years, and to this end the ABPI and the Department of Health (DoH) established the Pharmaceutical Industry Competitiveness Task Force in April 2000. The first reports of the Task Force have established of the DoH Research Governance Framework, as well as further regulatory improvements complying with the EU GCP Directive.

Exit Strategy

Most pharmaceutical companies cannot market products by themselves in all countries of the world. This may be because, for example, there is no subsidiary in the relevant country, or because the sales forces' other commitments mean that this drug cannot be adequately marketed in one particular market. For whatever reason, all development programmes must consider an exit strategy for the product in each market. Are there to be co-licensing, co-marketing or other agreements? Is the drug to be licensed out in other markets? Such discussion is beyond the scope of this chapter, but involve important considerations for any full drug development programme.

Preparing the Plan

Structure of the Plan

The candidate drug has passed the early development hurdles. In particular, the early preclinical toxicology and commercial environments are suitable. Care must be taken regarding any intellectual property concerns, and that preliminary drug supply and manufacturing forecasts look favourable. Early evaluation and planning will take about 12 months to execute, being a complex process with many interactions and requiring the integration of many different processes. Typically, and best practice for the development of such a plan, this requires a relatively senior project manager or development scientist to take primary responsibility and ownership of the project. The "owner" must have the authority to obtain the necessary information from different departments within the organisation and from external suppliers.

The plan will eventually prescribe a likely filing date for a Marketing Authorisation Application (MAA) (product licence). This date is vital and when the plan becomes public information, any slippage in the date is likely to impact on the share price of the company. Accordingly, senior members of the company must be confident that the date can be met. There will always be pressure to bring the date forward but this has a cost in resources, and risks damaging credibility with investors if the accelerated timelines cannot be met.

Thus, a sequential plan is safe, cost effective in terms of resources, and manageable by most organisations. Unfortunately such a plan has a cost in terms of unacceptable delays to shareholders. In the early 1990s there was a vogue for massively parallel plans which ran many activities simultaneously in order to address and bring forward "stop-go" decisions and filing dates. Stop-go decisions were made aggressively and the plans were continually examined to review ways to bring the filing date forward. Such plans are now less common than they were five years ago. The principal reason cited by organisations is that such plans throw many of the company resources onto a single product. If the product fails in late stage development, other candidate compounds will have been neglected. Such plans therefore are a significant gamble for even well resourced and capitalised organisations. If they fail, a gap appears in a company's product pipeline, with serious consequences for the well-being of the organisation.

More recently, a trend within companies has been to accelerate development plans without utilising a significant part of the company's resources on any one product. Thus, it may be necessary to outsource some of the development work, but this ensures a more even pattern of portfolio management, which has benefits for the organisation. The efforts of the pharmaceutical industry have begun to be beneficial to the industry. In general, approval success rates and times increased in the first half of the 1990s to levels not seen since the 1970s. Clinical development and US approval phases by FDA therapeutic rating (priority or standard) show that priority times have decreased and standard times have been stable since 1970s until very recently.

Quite how the plan is reviewed depends on the organisation, the therapeutic class and regulatory priority rating. Large organisations will review on a 12-monthly cycle the overall shape of the drug development portfolio for, say, the next ten years, the near-term portfolio and resource requirements, say over three years, and closely review the detailed plan for the next 12 months. This allows the company to define the next 12 months in terms of budget and resource, and the next three and ten years in some detail to establish if there are likely to be gaps in the portfolio ten years hence that can be filled by in-licensing of compounds. Such a strategic review is vital for the successful integration of new compounds into the company. Furthermore, such a review allows integration of a registration package which will be acceptable to most major markets into a single dossier. This avoids fragmentation of the clinical development programme. Duplication of activities is minimised and the major, pivotal, Phase III studies and analysis are performed only once and integrated. Knowledge of the compound and likely questions from the regulatory authorities from the major markets can be centralised. This saves time and resources.

Smaller companies and venture capital funded organisations are likely to be focused on a single compound, its analogues, metabolites and differing formulations. Without the luxury of a ten-year strategic development plan, such organisations are naturally tightly focused on the success of their product. Within these companies, pressure to bring the filing date forward can be intense and if the date is missed this can have serious consequences for the market capitalisation of the company.

Therapeutic Targets

Clinical success rates and attrition rates by phase of clinical trial for new drugs are important indicators of how effectively companies are utilising drug development resources. The proficiency with which this is done reflects a complex set of regulatory, economic and company-specific factors. Success rates differ by therapeutic class, and typically vary from about 28% success rate for an anti-infective compound to 12% for respiratory drugs. It is mandatory to ensure that the therapeutic target is appropriate and commercially attractive, and to define the required product performance to ensure successful marketing. These activities demand close cooperation between discovery, development and marketing departments before embarking on a full development plan. In the treatment of herpes zoster infection, for example, there is a precedent using the speed of crusting of the vesicular lesions as a marker for the efficacy of drug treatment, with significantly more rapid crusting, associated with the active agent, permitting registration. This is hardly of major relevance to the clinical situation as a beneficial effect on the disappearance of vesicles is of minor consequence to the patient who has a painful condition. The important clinical question is the effect of treatment on pain acutely, and in the longer term, in the prevention of postherpetic neuralgia. This creates an interesting dilemma. Should the primary clinical endpoint be crusting of lesions, given that this approach will undoubtedly result in more rapid execution of studies and therefore faster registration, or should it address the real medical issue, i.e. pain, an area where the clinical evaluation of the efficacy of treatment will be more complex? The responsible clinical decision is to measure both endpoints, but the implications for marketing must be understood.

The use of the different therapeutic targets, and the implication for the organisation, surrounds competitive advantage. What may be a minor clinical advantage for a new compound can sometimes be converted into a significant commercial lever that will facilitate marketing of the compound. Many companies use the draft Summary of Product Characteristics (SPC) to establish needs and wants, allowing a useful dialogue between the drug development and marketing groups.

Draft labelling and a draft SPC are produced at the beginning of the development process and these embody the features that the marketing group regards as minimal to ensure commercial success ("needs"). These needs must be tempered by input from medical and development to ensure that the requirements are realistic. The draft would also include features that are perceived to have significant advantages over competitor agents ("wants") and those that would provide useful talking points ("nice to have").

It is always tempting to design a minimalist programme of studies, i.e. the minimum required to obtain registration for a given indication, but this approach may not even address the "needs", particularly in an area where there is relative satisfaction with available therapy and therefore intense competitor activity. For example, the development of a non-steroidal anti- inflammatory drug may include studies in relatively small numbers of patients, aiming to demonstrate less gastrointestinal blood loss than that associated with an established comparator. In such a competitive area this is likely to be insufficient without demonstrating that this translates into real clinical benefit compared with the comparator, for example, reducing the incidence of major gastrointestinal blood loss requiring transfusion. A large-scale clinical study such as this may not therefore be required for registration but would be required for launch in order to demonstrate to clinicians the place of a new agent in a crowded therapeutic area.

During this process it is necessary to establish that the marketing "wants" are indeed achievable. For example, there may be a need for an adequate therapy for delayed nausea and vomiting associated with chemotherapy. Clinicians may state that this is a clinical need. Depending on the current therapies and the early profile of the candidate drug, a good estimation of the drug's likely effectiveness in the indication can be made. However, if there are already therapies in later development or in the market place which partially address the clinical need, it might require significant therapeutic endeavour, usually through late Phase III and Phase IV clinical trials, to establish the product in the market place. It is therefore important to identify the place of an individual drug in the therapeutic armamentarium.

The prescriber will base a decision on a consideration of the relative risk–benefit, whereas the regulator will consider the drug entirely on its own merits and will tend to assess the efficacy, safety and quality of a drug in its own right. A relative judgement is straightforward in an area of high unmet medical need, when there is simply a consideration of whether it is better to have the disease treated or untreated, but much more difficult and subtle in an area where drug treatment is already available. The complexity of the decision tends to increase with an increasing number of treatment options and under these circumstances the prescriber will be more inclined to consider the options for the individual patient. For example, when treating hypertension in a middle-aged man the first choice may be a beta blocker. The choice of which beta blocker may depend on whether the particular drug has been shown to have any primary or secondary role in preventing myocardial infarction, on its effect on cholesterol, its propensity to affect adversely the peripheral vasculature, whether it limits exercise tolerance, or has undesirable effects in a patient with asthma. It is therefore important to mirror this thought process when considering the market support programme and also to take account of preclinical data that may point to establishing clinical differentiation from a competitor. Studies examining such endpoints are always attractive to marketing departments.

The use of surrogate markers is always attractive. They allow drug development timelines to be shortened and may allow particular marketing angles to be pursued, for example a cholesterol-lowering effect in a cardiovascular agent. Regulators are increasingly likely to question the use of surrogate markers for large-scale pivotal Phase III studies. Typically, at least one clinical endpoint trial is necessary. Such a trial is large and costly and it may take a considerable time to enrol and follow up subjects in the study. The large cardiovascular intervention and survival studies are examples of such studies.

Regulators may require specific studies to address specific questions, for example use of the drug in the elderly, in children or other at-risk populations. Design of these studies needs detailed consideration: the subjects might be difficult to recruit, and comparative or placebo studies may be complex, potentially unethical or unduly expensive in terms of time and resources. Drug development expertise, as well as good support from the biostatistical and biometrics groups, is vital. The ICH guidelines can be particularly helpful when conducting clinical trials in special populations. Sometimes of course the guidelines are ambiguous at best.

Safety

About 20% of new drugs will fail because of safety concerns. Nevertheless, with a clinical development programme involving an average of about 4500 patients, the potential prescriber of a new drug is faced with the absence of a large amount of safety data. The safety profile of a drug will develop over time as adverse reactions occur spontaneously in a normal clinical setting. Whilst there is no substitute for spontaneous reporting in the identification of rare side-effects, it is important to consider whether useful safety information can be generated soon after launch.

In this context, a decision on whether postmarketing surveillance studies should be built into the development programme must be taken. Such an observational study may signal the occurrence of adverse events or alternatively it may signal and quantify the frequency of adverse events. At this point in the life cycle of a new medicine, postmarketing surveillance is likely to involve cohort observational studies of 10–20 000 patients. The value of these studies is likely to be threefold:

1. To generate safety data during use of a drug in routine clinical practice, to enable a comparison to be made of the safety profile in an uncontrolled population and the controlled clinical trial population
2. To provide safety data in a defined group incompletely covered in the registration package, for example the elderly
3. To enlarge the "formal" safety database and thereby act as an insurance policy to address problems occurring at a later stage in a drug's evolution.

The possibility for such studies will depend on the disease, disease frequency and whether the prescribing setting is in primary or secondary care. The value of these studies is likely to be greatest if data are generated as soon as possible after launch, and plans for implementation must occur well in advance of submission of the regulatory dossier. Such studies might also be a condition of registration.

Postmarketing (Phase IV) studies also generate safety data, but qualitatively these are likely to be similar to those collected during the preregistration phase. In Western Europe, larger Phase IV studies that have the evaluation of clinical safety as a primary objective have been embraced by the Safety Assessment of Marketed Medicines (SAMM) guidelines, which have superseded previous guidelines on postmarketing surveillance and which are incorporated into the EMEA pharmacovigilance guidelines.

In recent years, there has been a growth in the field of mega-studies, usually clinical outcome studies involving 5000–25 000 patients, with a simple primary endpoint such as mortality and a number of secondary morbidity endpoints. The potential for studies of this magnitude to throw up less frequent side-effects than those seen in the preregistration programme is clear.

Detailed Clinical Development Plan

In this section we consider the requirements for the clinical programme leading to global registration, as well as other studies which will form part of the overall programme. Scheduling is covered elsewhere in this volume, but it must be emphasised that each activity in the clinical study programme has to be identified and an appropriate order determined. A realistic estimate of timing can thus be made and, when the sequence and timing of events has been determined, the critical path can be established. This is the chain of essential events that must be accomplished to achieve a particular goal; clearly a change to one of these events has a fundamental effect on development time.

As with any plan, well defined milestones and checkpoints must be incorporated and subsequent activity should not proceed until these have been achieved. The plan must always be sufficiently detailed to identify supporting activities such as toxicological study that must be completed to allow development to continue without interruption. Many of these activities can, and should, run in parallel.

Number of Patients

Although there are no fixed rules in devising the Phase III programme, the more subjects admitted the better in terms of a safety evaluation, but it must be kept in mind that ethical considerations demand that only sufficient patients to meet the scientific criteria of study endpoints should be randomised. For example, for a disease-modifying drug for rheumatoid arthritis, approval has been granted on a database of up to about 6000 subjects. On the other hand, a novel immunosuppressant agent has been granted an approval with fewer than 2000 subjects. Based on their experience, however, Blake and Ratcliffe suggested that about 3000 patients per indication is average for a New Drug Application (NDA) in 1991. The Tufts Institute in 2001 suggested that about 4500 subjects is average for an NDA. These two numbers are consistent with an annual compound increase in numbers of about 7%. Others have suggested that about 100 patient-years experience is satisfactory for some established drugs for well understood disease areas, such as new formulations of insulin. Much also depends on the additional supportive data that can be included in the application.

The number of subjects is likely to vary depending on the degree of unmet medical need and the seriousness of the disease indication. It is likely that a drug shown to be effective in treating stroke, a condition with a high mortality and morbidity where no effective treatment is available, will require a database of fewer than 3000 patients. Conversely, an anxiolytic, used to treat a non-life threatening condition where effective treatments already exist, may require a much larger database. However, 4500 patients represents a reasonable working total.

Number of Studies

Having established the number of patients to be included in the preregistration clinical programme, it is important to consider how these will be distributed and hence how many studies are required. This is very variable. The Tufts Institute reported that, for biopharmaceuticals, there were on average only 12 studies and 1014 subjects per NDA compared with 37 studies and 4478 subjects for a conventional pharmaceutical NDA. Generally speaking, the FDA will require placebo-controlled studies wherever possible to demonstrate efficacy at the dose to be marketed and these are termed pivotal studies. Pivotal studies do not have to be placebo- controlled, however, and in some areas, such as depression, the ICH guidelines suggest a three-arm study, with both an active comparator and a placebo control. The Declaration of Helsinki, revised in 2000, suggested that in some disease areas, placebo-controlled studies are to be examined very carefully for their ethical content. This includes areas where conventional best therapy is generally acceptable. In this case, great care needs to be taken with the choice of active comparator.

It is widely accepted that two placebo-controlled pivotal studies are necessary, although it is not clear that this is a mandatory regulation in the FDA or EMEA regulations. There is, however, a certain insurance in this approach as studies, even of drugs that are effective, can occasionally fail to show a statistically positive result if the treated population somehow deviates from the norm or if the placebo response is unexpectedly increased. In Europe the use of an active comparator in a pivotal study is more common.

Sample sizes for clinical trials are discussed more fully elsewhere in this book and should be established in discussion with a statistician. Sample sizes should, however, be sufficient to be 90% certain of detecting a statistically significant difference between treatments, based on a set of predetermined primary variables. This means that trials utilising an active control will generally be a considerably larger than placebo-controlled studies in order to exclude a Type II statistical error (i.e. the failure to demonstrate a difference where one exists). Thus, in areas where a substantial safety database is required, for example hypertension, it may be appropriate to have in the programme a preponderance of studies using a positive control.

The increasing use of active comparator studies has meant that more studies are being powered on a "non-inferiority" basis. It is essential to discuss such designs with statisticians. Other novel designs, for example initial open-label therapy followed by a randomised treatment arm following disease exacerbation, are becoming more common. These novel designs must be discussed with a statistician and with the regulatory authorities before expensive mistakes are made.

Conversely if demonstration of efficacy is more critical than establishing safety, for example in Alzheimer's disease, then placebo-controlled studies are appropriate. Although the studies may include fewer patients, the number of studies may be approximately the same as for a hypertension programme.

It is eminently sensible to aim to have the smallest number of studies in the dossier as this makes data management and analysis less complex and therefore less time consuming. It is inevitable, however, that some studies which are not universally necessary will find their way into the core dossier. In France, for example, pricing is inextricably linked to technical approval and, when granting a price, the authorities make reference to an already available treatment wherever possible. It would therefore be virtually impossible to obtain pricing approval unless a comparative study with a reference drug had been undertaken. As pricing approval is the immediate step after technical approval, the "pricing study" needs to begin at the same time as the core registration studies, hence it becomes part of the regulatory dossier.

Whilst it is desirable to avoid duplicating activity, there will undoubtedly be some duplication of studies in the clinical programme given the foregoing discussion. It is important nevertheless to ensure that *ad hoc* studies do not find their way into the plan by default. The importance of studies designed to demonstrate competitive advantage has been mentioned and whilst data from many of these studies may not find their way into the regulatory dossier, the studies are nevertheless part of the overall clinical programme. Under these circumstances, there is little point in allowing duplication of comparator drugs between studies. For example, there is a considerable variety of drugs for the treatment of depression, ranging from the old tricyclic compounds such as amitriptyline and imipramine to the more recent and less toxic compounds such as the selective monoamine and serotonin reuptake inhibitors.

In between there is a host of antidepressant drugs with distinguishing properties; some are sedative, whilst others have anxiolytic activity. The most widely used drug will also vary from country to country. This situation therefore presents an opportunity to implement an international programme to test the new agent against a variety of competitors in order to tease out differences and provide data that may be required to support registration and that will also be of major use at the time of launch and subsequent marketing in individual countries. Care must be taken at Head Office that local studies do not jeopardise the overall regulatory and marketing plan, as embodied in the draft SPC. A study in which the drug dosage is halved for local marketing reasons might have the potential to undermine the whole regulatory package unless there are clear medical reasons for such a study.

Finally, in addition to studies that may be included to address potential regulatory questions, it is important to consider whether "in-filling" is needed. In an attempt to speed drug development, a high-risk strategy is to take the decision to enter full development as early as possible. This may mean that many elements of the Phase IIb programme are not carried out sequentially and one strategy, for example, is to carry out formal dose- ranging studies as part of the large-scale Phase IIa efficacy and safety programme. "In-filling" can be used to describe any study that forms part of the essential regulatory package that is not conducted in conventional Phase I–III sequence.

Duration of Treatment

In Europe, a drug that is likely to be administered long term will require a minimum of 100 patients treated for one year to gain approval. This will vary, however, depending on the circumstances. It is likely that a new antihypertensive agent will require significantly more long-term experience than this before a licence is granted, whereas a drug that is effective in treating gastric cancer may require less. It is important to remember that data generated as a result of long-term administration will be required to support registration applications for drugs used to treat recurrent diseases, such as peptic ulcer, as well as chronic diseases such as hypertension. Most Phase III studies in a chronic disease will require one year of therapy. Most oncology studies will require 12 months' survival data.

Dose

The FDA demands, at opposite ends of the dose range, a dose that demonstrates efficacy but is associated with side-effects and a dose that is largely ineffective. A range of doses may be studied within these limits, with the aim of identifying a dose that is both effective and tolerable. In Europe, there is greater scope to justify the choice of dose in a particular set of clinical circumstances. Choice of dose should also take account of further development for new indications, for example, an antihypertensive drug may also be effective in treating angina or heart failure but the dose is likely to differ significantly.

Patient Categories

It is important to include all age ranges that are of clinical importance. Development of an anti-asthma drug, for example, should include a programme of evaluation in children as well as adults because they will form a significant portion of the database and risk–benefit considerations will be different. Development of an anti-arthritis compound, on the other hand, will be undertaken predominantly in older patients and particularly detailed information on efficacy and safety in the elderly will be required.

This raises the important question of "what is elderly"? In the average regulatory dossier, the majority of patients are likely to be less than 75 years old, yet population demographics point to the increasing importance of the "older elderly" - those aged more than 75 years. Abernethy reports, reassuringly, that there is little or no evidence to date to suggest that the toxicity of any drug is unique to the elderly and therefore it follows that the "older elderly" are probably not a discrete group. It would appear prudent, however, in a clinical situation where a drug is likely to be taken by large numbers of patients in this category for there to be an appropriate evaluation of the risks and benefits. This may not need to form part of the regulatory package but data could be generated by a cohort observational study as part of a postmarketing surveillance programme.

The FDA Modernisation Act of 1997 (FDAMA) included a number of elements that have increased the number of studies being performed in children. The FDAMA expires at the end of 2001, but is due to be reviewed by Congress and most observers agree that it is likely to be renewed. In particular, the Pediatric Rule mandates that if a drug is likely to be used in children, even if regulatory approval is not sought for the particular paediatric age group, then some paediatric information must be provided. The Patent Extension Rule allows a six-month extension on the patent if the drug can be specifically licensed in children. This can be a very valuable commercial bonus, which clearly necessitates paediatric studies. These studies may require some formulation work, for example the development of a liquid dosing formulation.

Concomitant Medical Conditions/Drug Interactions

It is important to ensure adequate collection of data in patients who have concomitant medical conditions in whom drug elimination may be reduced, particularly those with hepatic or renal impairment, as lower doses are likely to be required in these patients. It is also important to investigate potential drug interactions both clinically and pharmacologically, particularly for drugs prescribed for conditions that are likely to coexist, and specific clinical pharmacology studies must be built into the programme. For example, it is necessary to determine the effect of a new antihypertensive agent co-prescribed with an angiotensin converting enzyme (ACE) inhibitor, nitrate, calcium channel blocker, beta blocker, diuretic, in terms of both drug interactions and potentiation of antihypertensive effect. Interaction via an effect on the cytochrome P450 system must also be investigated should there be any suggestion from preclinical data that this may occur.

Dosage Form

Is the dosage form to be used for large-scale development and hence commercialisation the same as that used for earlier phase studies and is the choice underpinned by an appropriate toxicology work-up? It is common for the dosage form to change during the course of the development process. Early studies may be carried out using liquid or capsule preparations because of the ease of formulation. Almost invariably, the marketed formulation will be different and it is important to ensure that inclusion in the regulatory dossier of data obtained using the early formulations can be justified by appropriate bioavailability studies, which may be required as part of the full preregistration plan. It is highly desirable, however, that the full development programme, which will generate the largest amount of data for the registration file, utilises the formulation to be marketed in order that safety and efficacy data can be amalgamated. Phase III studies should be undertaken with the intended market formulation.

It is important to consider the impact of different formulations. The requirements for an inhaled drug, for example, will be quite different from the requirements for the same drug given orally.

Is the development of two formulations to proceed in parallel or sequentially? The size of the programme may be doubled if a second formulation is aimed at a different target group. On the other hand, it may be more cost effective to carry out a larger programme than to come back at a later date. For example, in the development of a new agent to treat inflammatory bowel disease it may be inappropriate to use an orally active formulation in a patient with disease confined to the distal end of the large bowel. Whilst this situation may account for a relatively small proportion of patients, it is nevertheless desirable to have available a range of formulations suitable for use by all patients. Under these circumstances it would substantially increase the cost of the programme to study these patients at a later date, given that during the screening process to identify patients suitable for inclusion in a trial of oral medication, these patients would be identified and would not included in the study. The length of time taken to gather data on the major formulation is unlikely to be increased as there is no competition for patients, but gathering data on the secondary formulation represents an increase in workload. The trade-off is therefore increase in workload versus a more cost-effective and clinically comprehensive programme.

Clinical Trial Supplies

This is a crucial area and one which should be given maximum attention during the planning process, as the length of time required to ensure adequate clinical trial supplies can never be underestimated. Inadequacy of clinical trial supplies can be a reason for delay in the execution of a clinical development programme. The explanation is likely to be threefold.

1. Insufficient information is provided to colleagues in pharmaceutical development early enough, so that insufficient compound has been synthesised and manufactured.
2. Insufficient time is allowed for packaging and distribution. Clinical trials packaging is becoming increasingly complex, particularly when a drug that may be a second-line treatment is being tested. For example, it would be unethical to stop an ACE inhibitor and diuretic in a patient with heart failure, therefore administration of a new drug will be against this backdrop. In order to maintain double-blind conditions, it will be necessary to employ a double-dummy technique and therefore a minimum of four different agents per patient must be packaged: the ACE inhibitor, diuretic, new agent and placebo. The situation can be hugely complex as, for example, the testing of a new antiparkinsonian agent, where packaging of more than a dozen tablets per patient per day may be necessary. Complexity is further increased if the trial is international and dosage instructions have to be supplied in a number of languages. Notwithstanding this, drug supplies have to be distributed to a number of different countries, each of which requires different documentation to satisfy local customs regulations. It is hardly surprising that this aspect of the clinical development plan sometimes does not receive the attention it warrants. The use of an interactive voice randomisation system (IVRS) becomes increasingly useful as the study design becomes more complex. IVRS also allows scarce drug supplies to be rapidly dispatched to the appropriate site.
3. Insufficient time is allowed to obtain supplies of comparator drugs. Companies are notoriously bureaucratic, or even obstructive, in dealing with requests for supplies of active drug and placebo; it therefore pays to start negotiations early. Protocols involving comparator drugs from other companies must be targeted for early drafting, particularly if they are on the critical path, as the approval process is likely to be prolonged. If adequate time is allowed then it is always possible, should there be a refusal to supply active drug and placebo, to extract the active substance from a marketed formulation, reformulate, demonstrate bioequivalence with the approved formulation, and manufacture sufficient supplies for the clinical programme, together with matching placebo. This is clearly much less efficient than negotiating successfully with another company.

Length of the Programme

The importance of taking a long-term strategic view when designing the full development programme has already be stressed, but clearly it is impossible to plan in detail studies which may or may not start some years hence. The most crucial timing in the programme is the point at which the clinical cut-off will occur to permit compilation of the clinical section of the registration dossier. From this point, the timing of submission of the dossier can be predicted and hence the timing of regulatory approval and launch. It is thus important to be able to estimate with some degree of accuracy the length of time necessary to achieve the goal of clinical cut-off and to ensure that the major pivotal studies will be finished at that point. This fact mandates that the pivotal studies should receive high priority in the execution of the plan.

As anyone involved in the conduct of clinical trials knows, it is notoriously difficult to estimate the length of time it will take to recruit patients into a study. Formal inclusion and exclusion criteria can severely restrict the numbers of patients suitable for a trial, even when common conditions are being studied. An additional and common complication is the "*overoptimistic investigator syndrome*".

It is becoming increasingly common to conduct fairly rigorous feasibility studies to determine the likelihood of patient and investigator recruitment in different countries. A complicating factor is competing studies. This is particularly so in areas of great scientific endeavour such as oncology. It is not uncommon for large oncology centres to be running upwards of 50 different studies. Competition for patients can be intense.

In more recent years, in an attempt to overcome these problems, it has become fashionable to include more centres than may be necessary in a study on the basis that some will be successful at recruiting whereas others will not. All, of course, have to be assessed to ensure that they can operate within the principles of GCP. It is important to be realistic in estimating the speed at which recruitment will occur, and even in common diseases areas it is often unreasonable to expect centres to recruit at the rate of more than one to two patients per month. Nevertheless, the geographical distribution of clinical research is of major commercial concern because involvement of influential clinicians in the evaluation of a product is vital. It necessarily follows that involvement of influential clinicians in potentially large markets is of prime importance. Studies should therefore be conducted in these areas as first choice. However, that mandates a willingness on behalf of the investigator to participate in pivotal studies, a willingness to meet development deadlines and, of course, assumes the existence of an appropriate patient population and appropriate facilities for the conduct of the study.

A further factor that will impact the speed at which the clinical programme can proceed is the human resource committed to the programme. There are some activities, however, that will not be affected by manipulation of resource such as the "in-life" phase of a two-year carcinogenicity study. On the other hand, reporting time for the study can be reduced if more resource is applied. Various models for predicting resource allocation exist but none is particularly reliable. Whilst trial monitors and data handlers may be a resource dedicated to one programme, physicians and statisticians invariably have a range of commitments and will therefore be called upon to deal with unexpected problems, which cannot be taken into account in the planning process. Blake and Ratcliffe have generated a model describing drug development, running either sequentially or in parallel. For reasons which have already been considered, the former situation generally does not exist because of time constraints, although it makes more efficient use of human resources. Blake and Ratcliffe estimated that for an average NDA of about 3000 patients, with studies proceeding in parallel, it is necessary to recruit around 200 centres. Clearly, for an NDA which requires an average of about 4500 subjects, these numbers should be extrapolated upwards. Blake and Ratcliffe estimated that the programme would require the dedicated tie-in of 25–30 staff, three- quarters of whom would be trial monitors and data processors and the remainder physicians and statisticians. This gives some idea of the level of resource commitment required to discharge a successful programme and some notion of the continued commitment of resource to market support studies.

Data Management

In many companies, data collection, handling and analysis constitute a major bottleneck and is a source of irritation to investigators and of frustration to commercial colleagues. The process of data collection begins with the protocol, which must be clear and unambiguous. If it is confusing in English it will be more so in a foreign language. There must be a flow diagram. The practical parts of the protocol, that is, those in daily use during the running of a trial, should be separate from the remainder and in a form allowing easy reference. If the protocol facilitates the study it will reduce error and hence rework.

The case report form (CRF) should be unambiguous and simple to use. Its completion should minimise the need for text. CRFs should consist of three modules. One module is common for all trials (laboratory data, etc.), one is common for all trials in the clinical programme for a given compound, and one is specific to the study in question. In this way data handlers become familiar with the forms and can therefore manage a larger number with fewer mistakes. A mechanism should be in existence to ensure that the clinician completes the CRF adequately.

Recently, significant efforts have been made in most organisations to reduce the time from last patient out to final report. As always, a balance must be struck between satisfactory resource utilisation and cost. Most companies are now be looking at an 8–12 week period from last patient out to final report. The most significant delay is in resolving final data queries at study sites and this depends principally on the clinical research associate monitoring schedules and the availability of study personal at the study site. It should be the objective of every trial monitor to produce a complete set of clean data within 1-2 weeks of the last patient completing the trial, with the target of closing the database and initiating the analysis and statistical reporting of the primary variables with the minimum of delay. Data are of little value unless they are analysed and reported; indeed, data left in an office may be potentially dangerous.

To simplify the process it is important that a single database is developed for the whole programme. This is particularly relevant to the production of safety data, not only in the interests of efficiency but also so that any safety issues will be recognised as they arise. If a particular set of adverse reactions is suggested by preclinical toxicology then they should be flagged in the database so that the monitors' attention is drawn to them.

Cost

The full clinical development plan will be a major expense, so has to be costed accurately and conducted as economically as possible. The conduct of clinical trials is being increasingly seen by investigators as a business, and grants to investigators are the largest out-of-pocket expense incurred in the clinical development phase. It is estimated that drug development costs about US$350 million per drug, on average, at 1999 prices.

Technology

Although superficially attractive, there has not been the widespread take up of technology that many have predicted for the past 15 years. The use of electronic data capture (ED C) remains in its infancy. There are many suppliers, and most companies have conducted studies with EDC. However, the difficulties in training investigators and ensuring consistent technological support 24 hours a day, 365 days a year, in many different countries remain formidable. Ss internet access improves, electronic diaries may become more widely use for some particular types of studies, such as asthma and diabetes, where patients are accustomed to keeping diaries in any event. Electronic medical records are not yet useful for significant clinical development research.

Executing the Plan

There can be no substitute for excellent planning and this is why a substantial portion of this chapter has been devoted to a consideration of the important elements of the clinical development programme. There needs to be a clear and concise map of activities leading to compilation of the clinical section of the regulatory dossier and beyond. However good the programme is, there will be a successful outcome only if it is executed in an efficient and timely manner. The important factors are:

1. Selection of sites
2. Prioritisation of trials
3. Quality assurance
4. Quality control
5. Use of contract research organisations (CROs)
6. Training - technical and process
7. Communication
8. Process improvement.

Selection of Sites

Reference to the principles of GCP has been made; only investigational centres whose personnel and facilities are capable of working to GCP should be selected to participate in the programme. The selection of an investigator is a balance between value for money and desirability of having a particular individual working within the programme.

Prioritisation

The importance of identifying pivotal studies and studies on the critical path was discussed in a previous section. It is important that these studies are given the highest priority both in execution and reporting and that provision is made to identify early if there are problems recruiting patients so that appropriate remedial action can be taken. The studies of longest duration should be started first.

Quality Assurance

Whilst quality assurance of data is rightly demanded by the FDA and EMEA, it increasingly forms an integral part of other aspects in the execution of clinical trials. Investigators must understand that this is part of the process of participating in a study and must expect to be audited and for the quality of their data recording to be monitored. Most companies now have a quality assurance function which, for management reasons, reports outside the clinical organisation. This function can also be outsourced.

Quality Control

One of the measures of the quality of the preregistration clinical programme is the total time from the decision to enter full development to the first regulatory approval in a major market. It is also important to monitor quality in other ways. One option is to assess the frequency with which predetermined milestones are achieved. More subtly, quality can be assessed by examining the number of incomplete, inaccurate or indecipherable CRFs that are returned or the number of protocol amendments made which are not based on new information. Milestones may still be achieved when quality is poor, i.e. when there is inefficiency, but this means that they were wrongly established and can be improved if efficiency improves.

Contract Research Organisations (CROs)

In a discussion on the allocation of resource and analysis of workload, the decision on whether to engage a CRO for an element of the programme should be taken during the planning stage. It is important to remember that a CRO has to be managed and this can be as much as 10% of the company resource that would otherwise be directly involved in carrying out the programme. It is important that the objectives for the CRO are clear and that the scope of the task involved, including cost and milestones, is agreed by both parties before any contractual commitment. It must also be remembered that the CRO has to be audited and quality assured.

CROs are likely to be more efficient, and on occasion can be faster. A balance has to be struck between the outsourcing costs, internal costs (which are often underestimated) and the management requirements and skill sets of the CRO and internal staff.

Training

It is obvious that appropriate technical training should be provided for anybody joining a development programme, and staff already working on the programme should be encouraged to keep abreast of developments in the therapeutic area. Equally important is process training to ensure that the principles of GCP are fully understood and applied, and that internal processes in the form of SOPs are fully documented and understood. The process, and hence the SOPs, will need to satisfy all those customers and providers who will contribute to the development programme and ensure that the many tasks involved will be performed once and once only to avoid waste. The ability of all staff to work to SOPs and therefore work between countries and disciplines with a degree of consistency is paramount in executing a successful programme and this ability should be tested by regular audit. This is a particular advantage in times of stress when personnel may become interchangeable.

Communication

All personnel involved in the programme should have the same level of knowledge of progress and this can only be achieved using a computer-based clinical trials management system, which must be constantly and accurately updated. The central monitors who have an overview of the programme must initiate remedial action should recruitment, especially into pivotal studies, be less than anticipated. Equally, information concerning adverse reactions should be disseminated promptly so that investigators can be kept closely informed and enjoy a uniform level of knowledge. Finally, in order to develop and foster teamwork, regular meetings involving internal and external staff must be arranged so that a two-way exchange of information can occur and problems solved.

Process Improvement

The importance of documenting internal processes in the form of SOPs has already been mentioned. Any activity forming part of the development plan is a process. Each SOP should be looked on as a dynamic document and opportunities for improving each process should be sought continually. For example, the time that elapses between the last patient completing a clinical trial and production of the statistical report is an activity very much on the critical path.

This activity or process can be broken down into its smallest components, each of these examined carefully for opportunities to reduce cycle time, and pieced together again, with the objective of producing a significantly quicker time overall. The implications in terms of total development time are huge and yet many companies are not attempting to harness the benefits that process improvements can bring by establishing formal process improvement initiatives.

15

PRECLINICAL AND CLINICAL DEVELOPMENT

Major advances have been made in the use of cancer chemotherapy. However, most patients, especially those diagnosed with solid tumors, fail to respond to initial treatment or relapse after an initial response. Thus, there is a need to identify factors associated with lack of response and to develop new treatment strategies that address those factors. The development of effective chemotherapeutic agents for the treatment of solid tumors depends, in part, on the ability of those agents to achieve cytotoxic drug concentrations or exposure within the tumor.

BACKGROUND

Issues Related to Drug Delivery in Solid Tumors

It is currently unclear why within a patient with solid tumors there can be a reduction in the size of some tumors while other tumors can progress during or after treatment, even though the genetic composition of the tumors is similar. Such variable antitumor responses within a single patient may be associated with inherent differences in tumor vascularity, capillary permeability, and/or tumor interstitial pressure that result in variable delivery of anticancer agents to different tumor sites. However, studies evaluating the intratumoral concentration of anticancer agents and factors affecting tumor exposure in preclinical models and patients are rare. In addition, preclinical models evaluating tumor exposure of anticancer agents and factors affecting tumor exposure may not reflect the disposition of chemotherapeutic agents in patients with solid tumors owing to differences in vascularity and lymphatic drainage. Moreover, it is logistically difficult to perform the extensive studies required to evaluate the tumor disposition of anticancer agents and factors that determine the disposition in patients with solid tumors, especially in tumors that are not easily accessible. Thus, there is an impending need to develop and implement techniques and methodologies to evaluate the disposition and exposure of anticancer agents within the tumor matrix.

The need to develop and readily gain information on the tumor disposition of agents may become more important with the increasing number of tumor targeting approaches, such as gene and antisense therapy, polyethylene glycol (PEG)-conjugated agents, and liposomal delivery. In addition, methodology and study designs used to develop classic cytotoxic anticancer agents, such as platinum, taxane, and camptothecin analogs, may not be appropriate for the new generations of anticancer therapy, such as angiogenesis inhibitors, antiproliferative agents, and signal transduction inhibitors. As these agents may not induce classic toxicities or any toxicities, it may be difficult to recommend a dose for future trials using the standard Phase I dose escalation methods and endpoints (i.e., maximum tolerable dose and dose-limiting toxicities). Alternatively, defining the dose for Phase II studies could be based on the dose that achieves exposures associated with pharmacologic modulation, optimal biological exposure, or cytotoxicity results from in vitro studies. Historically, investigators have compared in vitro IC_{50} values with plasma concentrations in patients as a means to determine if sufficient exposure has been reached in clinical studies. However, the inherent tumor characteristics that influence tumor penetration and high intra- and intertumoral variability in tumor exposure makes this comparison highly unreliable, especially when the ratio of tumor exposure to plasma exposure may be approx 0.2 to 0.5. Thus, comparing the in vitro exposures and plasma exposures in patients results in an overestimation of drug exposure in the tumor extracellular fluid (ECF), and thus the exposure required for an effect may be insufficient. The use of methodologies that measure the exposure of anticancer agents within the tumor may improve the level of information needed to make informed decisions during the drug development process.

Methods to Measure Drug Disposition in Tumors and Tissue

Until recently, drug uptake into tissues and tumors has been described indirectly based on modeling from plasma pharmacokinetics or measured directly from tissue biopsies. As stated above, modeling of tumor exposure based on plasma exposures without incorporation of factors representing tumor heterogenity is unreliable. The use of tissue or tumor biopsies is associated with several problems. Obtaining serial biopsies is most often logistically impossible, highly invasive, and associated with patient discomfort. Thus, biopsies are usually available only for a single time point or measurement. Measurements of drug concentrations from biopsies are obtained in tissue or tumor homogenates, where it may be difficult to control ex vivo catabolism and differentiate between various forms of the drug. Several new advanced techniques, such as magnetic resonance imaging (MRI), positron emission tomography (PET), and microdialysis, have been developed to quantify the concentrations of anticancer agents in vivo. However, the use of MRI and PET is complicated by the lack of ability to differentiate between different forms and metabolites of a drug, availability, chemical synthesis of effective probes, and cost. Microdialysis to evaluate the disposition of anticancer agents in tumors and surrounding tissue, on the other hand, is a methodology that has several advantages over other existing methods.

Introduction and Advantages of Microdialysis

Microdialysis is an in vivo sampling technique used to study the pharmacokinetics and drug metabolism in the blood and ECF of various tissues. The use of microdialysis methodology to evaluate the disposition of anticancer agents in tumors is relatively new. Microdialysis has been used to evaluate the tumor disposition of 5-fluorouracil and carboplatin in patients with primary breast cancer lesions and melanoma, respectively. These

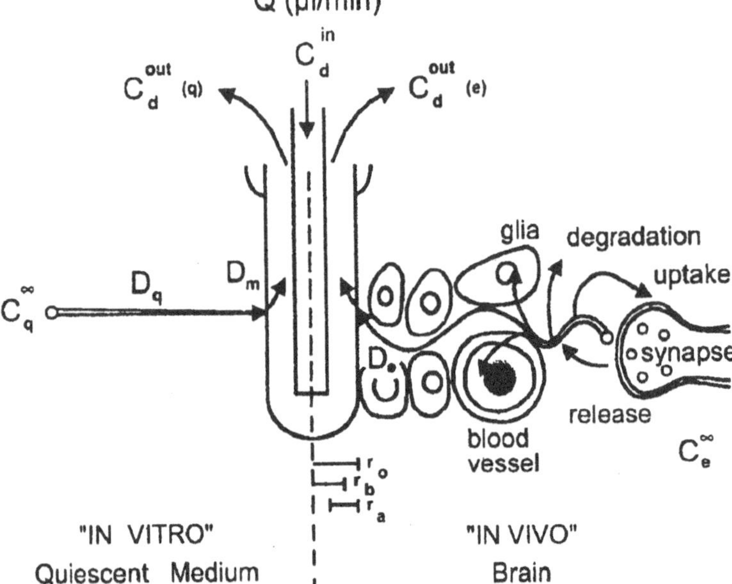

Fig. 15.1. Schematic illustration of a microdialysis probe in in vitro and in vivo (brain tissue) and the difference in diffusion paths.

studies depict the clinical utility of microdialysis in evaluating the tumor disposition of anticancer agents in patients with accessible tumors. Microdialysis is based on the diffusion of non-protein-bound drugs from interstitial fluid across the semipermeable membrane of the microdialysis probe. Microdialysis provides a means to obtain samples from tumor ECF samples from which a concentration vs time profile can be determined within a single tumor.

Microdialysis provides several advantages over autoradiographic studies of tumor biopsies as a method to evaluate anticancer drug concentrations in tumor tissue. With microdialysis techniques it is possible to obtain serial sampling of anticancer drugs from the ECF of a single tumor with minimal tissue damage or alteration of fluid balance. The microdialysis probe can remain in peripheral or central nervous system (CNS) tissue for up to 72 h without complications, such as increased risk of infection, inflammation, or alteration in probe recovery. Samples can be immediately obtained and analyzed from a single probe that allows for the real time evaluation of physiologic, pharmacologic, and pharmacokinetic changes. In addition, a single microdialysis probe can simultaneously sample several analytes of interest, thus allowing for the measurement of drug concentrations and pharmacologic endpoints that are required for pharmacodynamic studies. Furthermore, the drug concentration can be measured specifically rather than quantitating radioactivity, which may be nonspecific. Because of the pore cutoff size (20 kDa) of the semipermeable membrane, the use of microdialysis allows for the differentiation between liposomally encapsulated, conjugated drugs, protein-bound drugs, and active-unbound drug in the tumor ECF. Using microdialysis techniques, serial sampling of the non-protein-bound, active form of anticancer agents can be obtained from a single sight in a brain tumor, peripheral tumor, or surrounding tissues. In addition, multiple microdialysis probes can be placed in a single tumor to evaluate intratumoral variabiltiy of the analyte of interest. Thus, the data obtained with microdialysis techniques may more closely reflect the disposition of the active form of the drug within the tumor ECF.

Microdialysis Methodology and Study Design

Microdialysis System and Setup

In brief, a short length of hollow dialysis fiber is continuously perfused with a physiological solution. The presence of the analyte of interest in the ECF and its absence in the perfu sate leads to a concentration gradient across the dialysis membrane. The analyte diffuses through the dialysis membrane, and is collected for analysis. This process is performed in vivo through the use of a microdialysis probe that is implanted into tissue and continuously perfused with a physiologic solution at a low flow rate (0.5–10 μL/min). After the probe is implanted into tumor tissue, substances are filtered by diffusion from the extra- cellular space through the semipermeable membrane into the perfusion medium, and carried via microtubing into the collection vials.

Commercially available microdialysis probes, microperfusion pumps, and microfraction collectors are available. The type of microdialysis probe used depends on the sight or tissues of interest (e.g., subcutaneous tumor or tissue, brain, or liver), size of the tumor, and the analyte of interest. A microdialysis probe with a molecular cutoff of 20 kDa, membrane length of 4 mm, and outer diameter of 0.5 mm is the standard used for most pharmacokinetic studies of drugs in peripheral tissue and tumors. The molecular weight cutoff (i.e., 20 kDa) of the semipermeable membrane of probe prevents albumin-bound drug from crossing the membrane. However, small plasma protein, such as α_1-acid-glycoprotein, can pass through the semipermeable membrane. Thus, depending on the protein binding characteristics of a drug, the recovery may not be limited to unbound drug. The microdialysis probe is perfused by a microperfusion pump and dialysate samples are collected by the microfraction collector. Ringer's solution (USP) is the standard perfusion solution because it is similar to the makeup of ECF. Alternatively, 0.9% NaCl (USP) can be used for tissue and CNS studies.

Microdialysis Methodology and Study Design

In vitro calibration

Only a fraction (i.e., 10–50%) of the analyte can cross the probe's semipermeable membrane and the percentage that crosses can vary between probes, drug type, and flow rate. Thus, prior to in vivo studies it is standard to characterize the transfer rate, relative recovery, and the optimal flow rate of the drug and probe used in the studies. The recovery of drug across the membrane is concentration independent. The objective is to use the lowest flow rate that achieves sufficient recovery of the analyte that can be detected by the analytical system. High flow rates should be avoided owing to the propensity to alter the fluid balance in the tumors. The flow rate and collection interval are then modified to attain the needed sample volume required by the analytical system.

In vitro calibration studies are performed by placing a microdialysis probe in a beaker that contains a clinically relevant concentration of the drug or analyte of interest. The probe is perfused at various flow rates (e.g., 0.5, 1, 2, 3, 8, and 16 μL/min) and dialysate samples are collected every 10–25 min based on the required sample volume for the assay. The probe is allowed to reach equilibrium prior to sample collection at each flow rate. The time required to reach equilibrium is based on the flow rate and length of the microdialysis tubing. In vitro recovery is calculated as follows:

$$\text{In vitro recovery} = \frac{\text{Perfusate conc}_{\text{out}}}{\text{In vitro solution conc}} \qquad \ldots(1)$$

Microdialysis in vivo study design and procedures

Microdialysis probes can be placed in any accessible tumor and tissue. However, areas of the tumor with pooled blood should be avoided to prevent false results. Probe placement can be confirmed by ultrasound or after tumor or tissue removal in animal studies. Dual-probe studies can also be performed to evaluate the intratumoral disposition of the analyte or drug.

After probe placement, a short period (i.e., 45–60 min) is allowed for probe and tumor ECF equilibration prior to the start of calibration. Although use of the microdialysis technique results in less tissue damage compared to other sampling methods (e.g., biopsy), insertion of the microdialysis probe into the tumor does induce some tissue damage and immune reactivity. Thus, samples collected immediately after probe insertion may not reflect basal tumor conditions because of acute tissue damage and changes in blood flow associated with probe insertion. Therefore, it is necessary to allow time for the probe and tumor ECF to equilibrate prior to the start of the probe calibration studies.

After probe placement, calibration and washout procedures are performed. Because of variability in recovery for various probes at various sights, the calibration procedure is performed to determine the extent of recovery for each probe at each site. The washout period is performed to remove any drug introduced into the ECF during retrocalibration. The length of the washout period is determined by concentration of drug introduced in the ECF during calibration and the $t_{1/2}$ of the drug in the ECF. After the washout period the drug is administered or the procedure is started, and the sample recovery procedure is performed.

In vivo calibration and recovery

In vitro recovery may be substantially different from the in vivo (i.e., tumor ECF) recovery. In addition, recovery can vary between probes, drug type, flow rate, and tissue or tumor site. An in vivo microdialysis study is a dynamic process in which substances are continuously removed from the tumor ECF by diffusion into the probe. Consequently, the concentration of drug in the perfusate does not reach equilibrium with the tumor ECF. However, under constant conditions (i.e., perfusate flow rate) a steady-state percentage recovery, which represents a constant fraction of the ECF concentration, will be reached. Thus, the in vivo recovery value is determined for each probe in each tumor or tissue, and is specific for that single procedure. This provides the advantage of accounting for processes that affect recovery in tissues and tumors. The in vitro recovery values can be calculated by retrodialysis calibration, reference or marker compound, and point of zero net flux methods.

Retrodialysis calibration method can be used to estimate the steady-state percentage recovery. Retrodialysis quantification of in vivo recovery is based on the principle that the diffusion process across the microdialysis semipermeable membrane is equal in both directions. Therefore, the analyte of interest can be included in the perfusion medium and the disappearance from the perfusate into the tumor ECF is used as an estimation of in vivo recovery. In vivo recovery is calculated as follows:

$$\text{In vitro recovery} = \frac{\text{Perfusate conc}_{\text{in}} - \text{perfusate conc}_{\text{out}}}{\text{Perfusate conc}_{\text{in}}} \quad \ldots(2)$$

Thus, the estimated drug concentration in the tumor ECF is calculated as follows:

$$\text{Estimated tumor ECF conc} = \frac{\text{Measured microdialysis sample}}{\text{In vitro recovery}} \quad \ldots(3)$$

One limitation of the retrodialysis method is the time required to perform the calibration studies (i.e., four to five samples over 1–1.5 h) and washout (three or four samples over approx 1 h). Alternatively, if the retrodialysis calibration studies could be performed at the same time as the samples are collected, the ratio of sample number to study duration could be increased. This can be performed by using a reference or marker compound that has the same recovery characteristics as the analyte of interest. This process occurs by placing the reference compound in the dialysis solution during sampling of the analyte of interest. The analyte of interest diffuses from the ECF into the probe at the same time, rate, and extent as the reference compound diffuses out of the probe and into the ECF. The in vivo recovery of the reference compound is determined using the standard retrodialysis procedure and calculations. The in vivo recovery value for the reference compound is then used to calculate the estimated tumor concentration using Eq. (3).

The point of zero net flux is a calibration method that determines relative recovery of a drug or analyte by varying the concentrations of the drug included in the perfusate solution. This procedure is performed by perfusing four or five varying concentrations of the drug into the microdialysis probe and measuring the concentration in the outflow dialy sate. Plotting the difference between the inflow perfusate drug concentration and the outflow dialysate drug concentration as a function of the perfusate drug concentration results in a line with a slope that is equal to the relative recovery and an x-intercept that is equal to the steady-state tissue ECF concentration of the drug.

Online/Real-Time Analysis

A potential clinical implementation and advantage of microdialysis methodology is the real-time determination of drug concentration in tissue and tumors, measures of pharmacologic effect, and physiologic function. The ability to link the microdialysis sampling system directly to an analytical system allows for the measurement of pharmacokinetic and pharmacodynamic endpoints within minutes of obtaining the sample. Thus, medical and pharmacologic interventions can be performed and modifications can be made immediately.

Leggas and colleagues developed a rapid and simultaneous system that measured the inactive carboxylate and active lactone forms of topotecan using an online microdialysis system linked to a microbore high-performance liquid chromatography system. This system allowed for the continuous injection of small amounts of samples, the direct measure of both forms of the drug without loss of sensitivity, and the additional benefit of fast and automated analysis without the additional sample processing required for pharmacokinetic studies of camptothecin analogs. This system is very versatile and can be used for other camptothecin analogs and anticancer agents. The advantages of this system in pharmacokinetic studies of anticancer agents are the ability to measure the parent compound and metabolites within minutes without disrupting the fluid balance of the tissue, which is especially important in pharmacokinetic studies of drugs in the brain and cerebrospinal fluid (CSF).

Microdialysis techniques were initially developed to monitor changes in neurotransmitter levels in the brain of preclinical models. The use of microdialysis to monitor dynamic changes in glucose and lactate concentrations in the cortex of freely moving rats has accelerated the move to human studies and produced interesting methodological adaptations and results. The reduction of oxygen levels in the cage led to an immediate rise in lactate and glucose concentrations in the brain. These experiments reported the first temporal relationship between glucose and lactate changes during moderate hypoxia in unanesthetized animals. However, the inability to have the analytical instruments that are required for the detection of specific neurotransmitters, such as lactate and glucose, at the bedside in clinical studies has complicated the need for real-time results. As the function of analytical instruments increase and their size decreases, the use of these systems in clinical practice will increase. Alternatively, delivering the microdialysis sample from the bedside to the analytical laboratory, as is done with other standard laboratory studies, can produce results in a relatively short period of time.

Tolias and colleagues used microdialysis to evaluate extracellular glutamate in the brains of children with severe head injuries. A microdialysis probe was inserted next to an intracranial pressure bolt in the right frontal area of the brain. Dialysis samples were collected hourly and analyzed for glutamate, glutamine, and various structural amino acids. Clinical monitoring parameters were correlated with amino acid concentrations. A low glutamine to glutamate ratio was associated with increased morbidity. The authors concluded that glutamate metabolism may have a more significant role in the pathophysiology of pediatric head injury than had been recognized. As for the use of microdialysis to generate real-time results, the ability to obtain a sample over a relatively short period of time, send it to the clinical laboratory, and have the results sent back within hours may allow for modifications in the treatment of the patient.

Preclinical Microdialysis Studies in Tumor and Tissue

Preclinical Studies of Tumor and Tissue Distribution

Studies comparing plasma and tumor ECF exposure associated with response in pre- clinical models have used microdialysis methodology. Investigators reported a six-fold difference in dose and plasma exposure of topotecan associated with a complete response in mice bearing human neuroblastoma xenografts NB 1691 (2.0 mg/kg and 290 ng/mL·h, respectively) as compared to NB 1643 (0.36 mg/kg and 52 ng/mL·h, respectively). However, factors related to the difference in topotecan response in the two neuroblastoma xenograft lines were not identified. Moreover, macrotumor-related factors affecting sensitivity and the relationship between tumor ECF exposure to topotecan and antitumor activity in the xenograft model had not been established. As a result, the tumor ECF disposition of topotecan using microdialysis methodology was evaluated and the relationship between topotecan tumor ECF exposure and antitumor response in mice bearing the relatively resistant (NB 1691) and sensitive (NB 1643) human neuroblastoma xenografts was evaluated.

There was a 3.5-fold difference in tumor ECF exposure and penetration in NB 1643 (25.6 ± 19.6 ng/mL·h and 0.15 ± 0.11, respectively) and NB 1691 (7.3 ± 6.1 ng/mL·h and 0.04 ± 0.04, respectively) ($p < 0.05$), which was consistent with the difference in sensitivity of these xenografts based on dose and plasma exposure. These results suggest that topotecan tumor penetration may be one factor associated with neuroblastoma antitumor response. Moreover, these data suggest inherent differences in tumor vascularity, capillary permeability, and/or tumor interstitial pressure between the sensitive and resistant neuroblastoma tumor xenografts. This was the first study reporting a relationship between the exposure of an anticancer agent in tumor ECF and antitumor response. The significance of ECF as an important exposure for pharmacologic effect of anticancer agents and the inter- and intratumor variability was evaluated in preclinical studies of cisplatin using microdialysis. The relationship between unbound platinum in tumor ECF, total platinum in tumor homogenates, and the formation of platinum-DNA (Pt-DNA) adducts were evaluated after administration of cisplatin in mice bearing B 16 murine melanoma tumors. Intratumor variability in platinum disposition was evaluated by placing two probes (A and B) in the same tumor. At the end of the 2-h sample period, tumor tissue was obtained at each probe site and analyzed for total platinum, and bifunctional intrastrand DNA adducts between platinum and two adjacent guanines (Pt-GG), and platinum and adenine and guanine (Pt-AG).

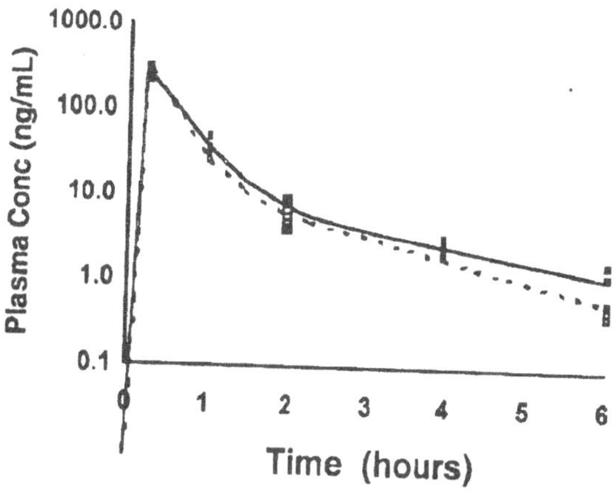

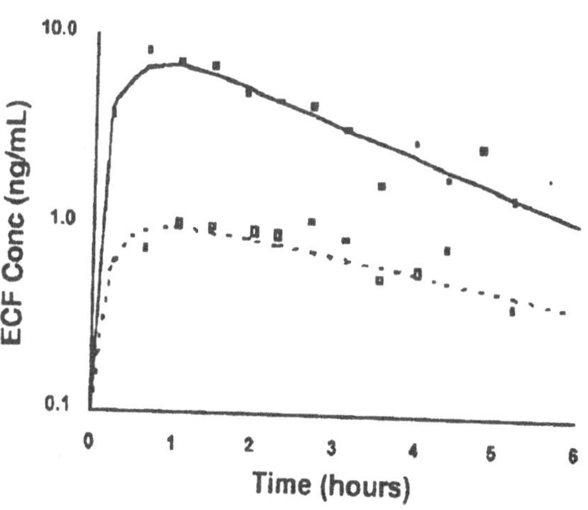

Fig. 15.2. Topotecan lactone concentration-time profiles in plasma and tumor ECF in resistant and sensitive neuroblastoma tumor xenografts.

The concentration of unbound platinum in tumor ECF of B16 tumors was detectable from 12 min to 120 min after administration. In addition, the concentration vs time profile of unbound platinum in tumor ECF did not follow the plasma concentration vs time profile, suggesting that clearance of drug from tumor may be the primary factor affecting drug accumulation within a tumor. The median (range, % CV) area under the concentration vs time curve for ECF (AUC_{ECF}) and tumor penetration were 0.42 μg/mL·h (0.05–1.57, 78%) and 0.16 (0.02–0.62, 77%), respectively. The median (range, % CV) AUC_{ECF} from probe A to probe B was 1.9 (1.3–5.5, 55%). The median (range, % CV) concentration of total platinum obtained at the end of the 2-h microdialysis procedure from probe A to probe B was 1.1 (1.0–2.0, 27%). Using an E_{max} model to describe the relationship between drug exposure and Pt-DNA adduct formation, there was a better correlation between unbound platinum AUC_{ECF} (R^2 = 0.69 and 0.63, respectively) and Pt-GG and Pt-AG compared to total platinum in tumor extracts (R^2 = 0.29 and 0.41, respectively). In addition, there was a poor correlation between unbound platinum AUC_{ECF} and total platinum in tumor extracts (R^2 = 0.26). These results suggest there is relatively high inter- (approx a 30-fold range) and low intratumor (approx a fourfold range) variability in unbound and total platinum in B 16 murine melanoma tumors, and a poor relationship between unbound and total platinum. In addition, these results suggest unbound platinum in tumor ECF is a better correlate of Pt-DNA adduct formation compared to total platinum measured in tumor extracts.

Evaluation of Angiogenesis Inhibitors

The angiogenic phenotype is associated with increased tumor neovascularization and hyperpermeability to drugs and other macromolecules. Angiogenesis inhibitors could alter the increased tumor vascularization and permeability and have an untoward effect of decreasing tumor exposures of anticancer agents when coadministered with angiogenesis inhibitors. Thus, Ma and colleagues evaluated the tumor disposition of temozolomide administered alone and in combination with the angiogenesis inhibitor TNP-470. Temozolomide was administered alone and in combination with TNP-470 to nude rats bearing tumors that differentially expressed low or high vascular endothelial growth factor (VEGF). In both the subcutaneous and intracerebral tumors with high VEGF expression, TNP-470 treatment produced significant reductions in temozolomide tumor exposure and the ratio of tumor to plasma exposures. In conclusion, the pharmacodynamic effect of angiogenesis inhibitors on tumor angiogenesis can produce a reduction in tumor concentrations of coadministered anticancer agents. It is increasingly important to understand the pharmacokinetic impact of angiogeneis inhibitors when coadministered with anticancer agents and additional studies need to be performed to determine the optimal dosing schedules for combination regimens.

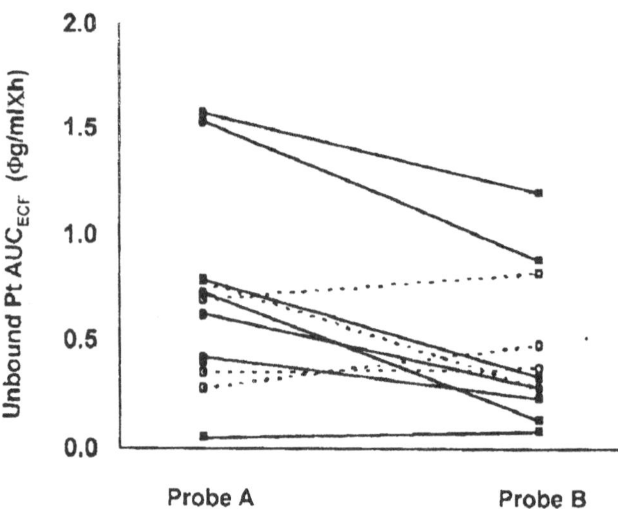

Fig. 15.3. Low intra- and high inter-tumoral disposition of cisplatin in murine melanoma tumors.

Evaluation of Liposomal Anticancer Agents

The theoretical advantages of encapsulated liposomal drugs are prolonged duration of exposure and selective delivery of entrapped drug to the site of action. Major advances in the use of liposomes as vehicles delivering encapsulated pharmacologic agents and enzymes to sites of disease have occurred over the past 10 yr. Moreover, liposomal-encapsulated drugs, such as liposomal doxorubicin (Doxil), are FDA-approved and have documented activity and decreased toxicity. Studies evaluating the disposition and tumor penetration of liposomal and nonliposomal anticancer agents suggest liposomal agents extravasate selectively into solid tumors through the capillaries of tumor neovasculature. However, the mechanisms by which liposomes enter tissue and tumors and release drug are not completely understood. In addition, the liposomes can be engineered to produce a complete spectrum of drug release rates that need to be evaluated in in vivo systems.

SPI-077 (ALZA Pharmaceuticals, Inc.) is cisplatin encapsulated in long-circulating STEALTH liposome. The disposition of liposomal-cisplatin is dependent on the liposomal vehicle. Once the cisplatin is released from the liposome, its disposition follows cisplatin pharmacology. SPI-077 has shown antitumor activity against a wide range of solid tumor xenografts, including murine colon tumors. In a study comparing SPI-077 and cisplatin tumor disposition in mice bearing murine colon tumors, the platinum exposure in tumors was several-fold higher and prolonged after SPI-077 as compared to cisplatin administration. However, because the platinum exposure was measured in tumor extracts, it is unclear whether the platinum measured was encapsulated, protein-bound platinum, or unbound platinum. In addition, it is unclear whether the platinum exposure was intracellular or extra- cellular. Thus, it is currently unclear whether SPI-077 releases cisplatin into the tumor ECF, or penetrates into the cell as the liposome and then releases the cisplatin intracellularly.

Thus, the tumor disposition of platinum after administration of liposomal formulations of cisplatin (SPI-077) and nonliposomal cisplatin was evaluated using microdialysis in mice bearing B16 murine melanoma tumors. Because of the pore cutoff size (20 kDa) of the semipermeable membrane of the microdialysis probe and the size of the liposome (100 nm), the microdialysis probe was able only to sample unbound platinum and allow the differentiation between liposomal-encapsulated cisplatin and cisplatin released into the tumor ECF.

After administration of cisplatin, the concentration of unbound platinum in tumor ECF was detectable from 12 min to 120 min after administration. However, there was no detectable unbound platinum in the tumor ECF after administration of SPI-077. The results of this study suggest SPI-077 distributes into tumors, but releases significantly less platinum into tumor ECF, which results in lower formation of Pt-DNA adducts compared to cisplatin. This was the first study using microdialysis methodology to evaluate the tumor disposition of liposomally encapsulated anticancer agents.

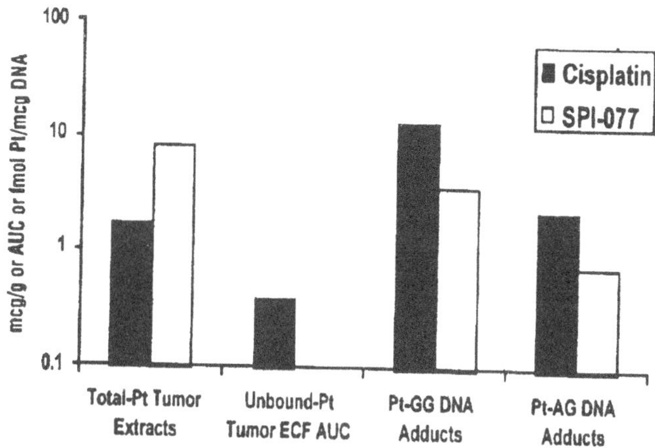

Fig. 15.4. Unbound platinum in tumor ECF, total platinum in tumor homogenates, and Pt-GG DNa adducts after administration of cisplatin and spi-077 in murine melanoma tumors.

Pharmacokinetic Brain Studies in Nonhuman Primates

Nonhuman primates are used as the standard model for the determination of drug penetration into the CNS. These models primarily evaluate the exposure of drug in the CSF of the lateral, fourth ventricle, and lumbar space after intravenous administration. This may provide important information for the evaluation of cytotoxic exposures in the treatment of embryonal CNS tumors, such as medulloblastoma, leukemia, and bacterial or viral infections that have a high propensity to disseminate throughout the subarachnoid space. However, these exposures may be irrelevant for primary brain tumors that occur in the cerebral cortex. This difference in clinically relevant exposure for primary brain tumors and tumors that spread throughout the subarachoid space is attributable to various components of the blood–brain barrier at each of these sights. Thus, there is impending need to evaluate the penetration and exposure of anticancer agents in the cerebral cortex.

Fox and colleagues evaluated the exposure of zidovudine in brain ECF as measured by microdialysis in rhesus monkeys. In vivo recovery was tissue dependent and was lower in brain than in blood or muscle. After intravenous administration, the steady-state concentrations of zidovudine in blood, temporalis muscle, and brain were 112 ± 64 μM, 105 ± 51 μM, and 14 ± 10 μM, respectively. The steady-state ultrafiltrate concentrations of zidovudine in serum and CSF were 81 ± 40 μM and 14 ± 8 μM, respectively. The authors concluded that the CSF and brain ECF concentrations were comparable at steady state. Thus, zidovudine penetration in the brain ECF and CSF is limited to a similar extent, presumably by active transport, as in other species.

Clinical Microdialysis Studies

Clinical Microdialysis Studies in Tissue

In cancer treatment it is currently unclear if it is better to dose chemotherapeutic agents based on body surface area (i.e., mg/m^2), body weight (mg/kg), or fixed doses (i.e., mg). Several studies have shown that dosing anticancer agents based on body surface area does not reduce pharmacokinetic variability. Similarly, Hollenstein and colleagues investigated whether weight-adjusted ciprofloxacin dosing results in comparable concentrations of drug in tissue ECF in obese and lean subjects. Microdialysis was used to sample ECF concentrations of ciprofloxacin in the anterior aspect of the right thigh in age- and sex-matched obese (122 ± 23 kg) and lean (59 ± 9 kg) subjects after an intravenous dose of ciprofloxacin.

The tissue penetration was significantly lower in obese patients (0.45 ± 0.27) as compared to lean patients (0.82 ± 0.36). The authors concluded that the penetration of drug into the ECF of muscle is impaired in obese patients. Therefore, antibiotic doses need not be adjusted for an increase in fat to water ratio, and weight-adjusted dosing based on actual body weight will yield adequate tissue levels of ciprofloxacin. Similar microdialysis studies evaluating the exposure of anticancer agents in tissue may help address the optimal method used to calculate doses of anticancer agents.

Clinical Microdialysis Studies in Tumors

Recently, microdialysis has been modified for use in human drug studies and has provided the opportunity to quantify drug concentrations in tissue and tumors. Microdialysis has been used to evaluate the ECF disposition of anticancer agents in patients with accessible solid tumors. The first study that demonstrated the utility of microdialysis in patients with solid tumors were studied by Blochl-Daum and colleagues. The disposition of carboplatin in blood and ECF of tumor and skin was studied in patients with cutaneous malignant melanoma metastases. Microdialysis probes were placed in cutaneous tumors and surrounding skin.

The results indicated a rapid but incomplete equilibration between blood and the tumor compartment. Similar results were reported with subcutaneous tissue. The mean ± SD AUC of total (sum of unbound and bound) carboplatin in serum, tumor, and subcutaneous tissue were 1533 ± 189 μg/mL·min, 853 ± 172 μg/mL·min, and 506 ± 87 μg/mL·min, respectively. There was also significant interpatient variability in blood, tumor, and subcutaneous tissue. However, there was greater interpatient variability in tumor and skin exposure as compared to blood. These data suggest that in addition to systemic factors that control blood exposures, there are tumor- and tissue-related factors that add to the variability in the exposure at these sites.

Muller and colleagues evaluated the relationship between 5-fluorouracil (5-FU) exposure in tumor ECF and clinical response in patients with primary breast cancer. Microdialysis probes were placed into the primary tumor and periumbilical subcutaneous adipose layer in patients with breast cancer scheduled to receive neoadjuvant chemotherapy containing 5-FU. In addition, serial blood samples were obtained. The mean ± SD AUC of 5-FU in plasma, tumor, and subcutaneous tissue were 699 ± 75 μg/mL·min, 374 ± 62 μg/mL·min, and 401 ± 151 μg/mL·min, respectively. The pharmacokinetics of 5-FU were similar in tumor and adipose tissue. A high interstitial tumor exposure of 5-FU was associated with increased tumor response and there was no association between 5-FU exposure in adipose tissue or plasma and tumor response.

The authors concluded that the exposure of 5-FU in tumor ECF may predict response in patients with breast cancer. Moreover, this information could be used to optimize dosing and administration schedules to increase the exposure of anticancer agents in tumors and thus improve response. Muller and colleagues also evaluated the interstitial disposition of methotrexate in patients with primary breast cancer lesions. Microdialysis probes were placed into the primary tumor and periumbilical subcutaneous adipose layer in patients with breast cancer receiving methotrexate as part of a three-drug regimen.

The ratio of methotrexate AUC in tumor ECF to plasma was 0.60 ± 0.20. In addition, there was no correlation between methotrexate AUC in tumor ECF and plasma. Unlike in the previous study, the exposure of methotrexate in tumor ECF was not associated with response. The lack of a relationship between methotrexate exposure in tumor ECF and response may be associated with variability in transendothelial transfer of methotrexate. This study depicts the importance of not only the disposition of drug in tumor ECF, but also the intracellular exposure of anticancer agents as cytotoxic determinants of response.

Pharmacodynamic Studies Using Microdialysis

Antibiotics

The ability of the microdialysis probe to recover any analyte that is small enough to pass through the semipermeable membrane makes it a useful technique for pharmacodyamic studies. Microdialysis methodology has been used in clinical pharmacodynamic studies of antiinfective agents, diabetes, muscle physiology, and brian neurochemistry. The specific advantage of microdialysis in the study of antiinfective agents is related to the ability of the probe to measure unbound, pharmacologically active drug in the ECF of tissue, which is the anatomically defined target site for most bacterial infections. In the study of antiinfective agents, microdialysis probes has been placed in subcutaneous tissues, brain, and lung. Microdialysis studies have demonstrated that the concentrations of antiinfective agents in the ECF of subcutaneous tissue may be subinhibitory, whereas the concentrations in the serum may be sufficient for an antimicrobial effect. Thus, the use of tissue ECF or serum concentrations as an endpoint for determining the potential efficacy of antiinfective agents may have a significant impact on clinical decision making. Microdialysis also offers unique opportunities in pharmacokinetic and pharmacodynamic research and the potential to streamline the decision process on the drug development of antiinfective agents and also anticancer agents.

Delacher and colleagues evaluated a combined in vivo pharmacokinetic and in vitro pharmacodynamic approach to simulate the target site pharmacodynamics of antibiotics in humans. This approach was based on the in vivo measurements of interstitial drug pharmacokinetics in tissue and a subsequent pharmacodynamic simulation of the drug concentration vs time profile in an in vitro setting. Individual concentration vs time profiles of ciprofloxacin were measured in the interstitial space of patients following intravenous administration. Then different isolates of *Pseudomonas aeruginosa* were exposed in vitro to the interstitial ciprofloxacin concentration vs time profile obtained from the in vivo microdialysis experiments. Significant correlations were observed between pharmacokinetic and pharmacodynamic metrics. Moreover, the data were analyzed with an integrated pharmacokinetic-pharmacodynamic model, allowing for a much more detailed evaluation of the data than possible by strictly using minimum

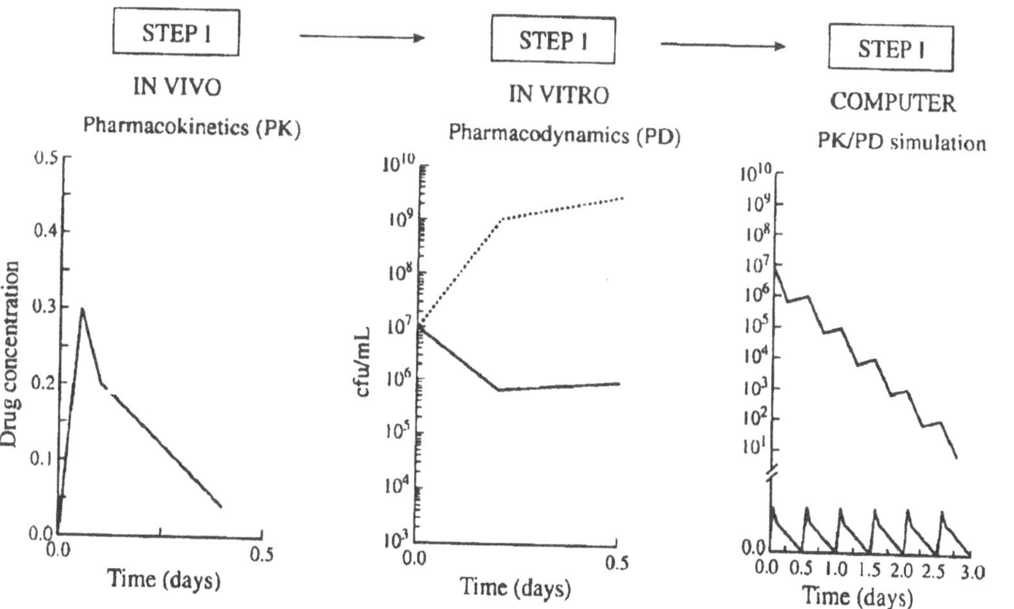

Fig. 15.5. Study design for in vivo pharmacokinetic and in vitro pharmacodynamic studies of antiinfective agents.

inhibitory concentrations. The results of these experiments showed that therapeutic success and failure in antiinfective therapy may be explained by pharmacokinetic variability at the target site, and therefore this in vivo pharmacokinetic and in vitro pharmacodynamic approach may provide valuable guidance for drug and dose selection for antiinfective agents. The use of pharmcokinetic drug exposure in the CSF of nonhuman primates to guide in vitro cytotoxcity studies has been used in the development of topotecan for the treatment of medulloblastoma. These procedures and study designs could be combined, along with microdialysis studies of anticancer agents in tumors, as described earlier, to provide information on drug and dose selection of anticancer agents as was performed for the antiinfective agents.

Brain Neurochemistry

The use of microdialysis probes in neuromonitoring is a new therapeutic opportunity for microdialysis systems. The major value of microdialysis monitoring in severe head injury has been to demonstrate different brain pathophysiologic mechanisms in the living brain and to depict the time course of these changes. Interruption of substrate delivery is a major factor of vulnerability to ischemic damage to the brain in patients with severe head injury, stroke, or subarachnoid hemorrhage. Thus, continuous monitoring of substrate levels in the brain is required to optimize therapy for critically ill patients with brain injuries. Zauner and colleagues evaluated the delivery of oxygen via residual blood as an approach to protecting the brain during ischemia. Therapy was evaluated by continuously measuring brain oxygen, brain CO_2, brain pH, and hourly glucose and lactate concentrations via a microdialysis system. There was an increase in brain tissue oxygen tension and a simultaneous decline in brain lactate during a stepwise increase in inspired oxygen. Although these new monitoring systems and methods are labor intensive and expensive, they can be readily applied in neurosurgical centers.

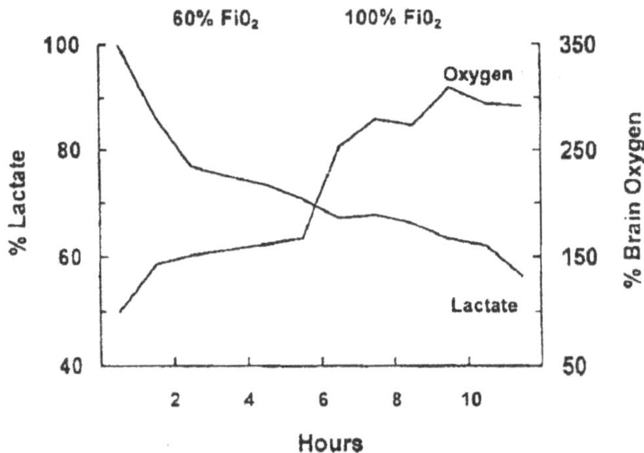

Fig. 15.6. Brain oxygenation tension and brain lactate concentration during a stepwise increase in inspired oxygen.

Disturbed ionic and neurotransmitter homeostasis are now recognized as the most important factor contributing to the development of secondary brain swelling after traumatic brain injury. Preclinical studies suggest that posttraumatic neuronal excitation by amino acids leads to an increase in extracellular potassium. Thus, Reinert and colleagues evaluated the relationship between extracellular potassium and high intracranial pressure after severe head injury. An intracranial microdialysis procedure was used to monitor potassium, glutamate, and lactate concentrations in brain ECF. Dialysate potassium concentrations were increased for more than 3 h in approx 20% of patients. Moreover, a mean dialysate potassium > 2 m*M* throughout the entire monitoring period was associated with an intracranial pressure > 30 mmHg and fatal outcome, as were progressively rising concentrations of potassium in brain ECF. These studies show that microdialysis monitoring of physiologic and pharmacologic targets can be used to predict responses in patients.

The relationship between tissue oxygenation and excitatory amino acids in peritumoral edema has also been evaluated during glioma surgery. Microdialysis was used to monitor glutamate and aspartate levels in peritumoral edema during resection of the tumor. Treatment with inspiratory oxygen led to an increase of tissue oxygenation and a decrease in glutamate and aspartate. Future microdialysis studies could evaluate the exposure of anticancer agents or pharmacologic markers of response in the ECF of a brain tumor after administration of a test dose of drug and prior to surgical resection. These studies could greatly enhance our knowledge of drug delivery and exposure in brain tumors.

Future Directions

Microdialysis has been used in the study of neurochemistry, muscle physiology, lipid metabolism, edema, diabetes, traumatic brain injury, antibiotics, and anticancer agents. The possible uses of microdialysis in the pharmacokinetic and pharmacodynamic studies of anticancer agents are virtually endless. The use of microdialysis in the development of anticancer agents is based on preclinical and clinical results suggesting that tissue and tumor exposures do not equal plasma exposure, inter- and intratumoral exposure is highly variable, and the exposures of anticancer agents in CSF and CNS lobes are not identical. The advantages of microdialysis in the study of anticancer agents are sampling drug concentrations closer to the target site, as compared to plasma pharmacokinetic studies, obtaining serial samples from a single site within tissue and tumor, measurement of the active unbound forms of drugs, differentiation between various forms and metabolites of anticancer agents, and simultaneously obtaining samples for pharmacokinetic and pharmacodynamic studies. The disadvantages of microdialysis are that it is invasive, requires in vivo calibration, and not all substances will cross the semipermeable membrane. However, as compared to other sampling instruments and methods, these disadvantages are relatively minor.

The use of microdialysis in cancer-related studies will become more important as surrogate markers for response and toxicity are determined and new therapeutic agents are developed. The use of microdialysis can be especially important when evaluating the disposition of carrier-mediated agents (e.g., liposomes and PEG conjugates), gene therapy, antisense oligonucleotides, and angiogenesis inhibitors. The disposition of carrier agents may be completely different than that of the parent compound and the release of drug systemically and in the tumor will be important in determining the antitumor effect and toxicity. The importance of microdialysis to address these issues is highlighted by the FDA's plan to inquire about methods to define and evaluate carrier systems. The pharmacokinetics and pharmacodynamics of gene therapy agents and antisense oligonucleotides may be drastically different than those of classical anticancer agents. In addition, owing to analytical assays and detection issues standard sampling strategies and processing may not be adequate for these agents. Thus, the use of methodology such as microdialysis that allows for rapid and accurate sampling and separation may become pivotal in the development of these agents. As the technology of microdialysis advances, the probe will be placed in more logistically difficult organs and tissues. Microdialysis probes can also be placed in blood vessels and obtain serial samples of unbound drug. These studies can be used to evaluate protein binding and reduce the need for repeated blood sampling and processing. Moreover, the ability to connect the mircrodialysis sampling instruments to online analytical equipment instruments allows for real-time analysis and may allow for the manipulation and modification of dosing regimens and strategies of anticancer agents.

16

Drug Development Management

The most successful new drug-development programs require competent, caring, people-oriented leaders at all levels. Overwhelming social science data show that this approach will optimize productivity, efficiency, and creativity, while fostering employee growth, enthusiasm, cooperation, and loyalty.

Drug Development Process

Before addressing the components of good management, here is a review of the basic new drug (new chemical entity or NCE) development process.

The NCE works its way through the following groups before it can be marketed:

Synthetic Chemistry → Pharmacology →

Toxicology → Pathology → Regulatory Affairs

[Investigative New Drug (IND) application] →

Product R & D → Clinical Research →

Regulatory Affairs [New Drug Application (NDA)] →

Approval by government regulatory agency

Additional Important Contributors

Other involved departments/disciplines that are equally important as the above groups include Analytical Chemistry, Biochemistry, Biopharmaceutics/Pharmacokinetics/Drug Metabolism, Chemical Pilot Plant, Experimental Engineering, Packaging Development, and Statistics. Additional significant contributors include Purchasing and Quality Assurance/Documentation.

Post-NDA Departments

After NDA approval, non-R&D functions—after being partially involved at various stages of NCE development—take over, including Chemical Manufacturing, Engineering, Marketing, Packaging, Pharmaceutical Manufacturing, Quality Control, and Sales.

Departmental Responsibilities

Companies are organized differently; for example, the various engineering responsibilities may be in one or more departments. A brief description of typical functions follows:

- Synthetic chemistry synthesizes NCE candidates for pharmacological testing.
- Pharmacology examines the in vivo activity of the NCE in animals.
  1. For economic reasons, activity is determined in animals before safety, whereas in humans, preliminary safety studies need to come first.

- Toxicology determines the "macro" negative effects of the NCE in animals.
- Pathology examines the "micro" negative effects of the NCE in animals.
- Product R&D designs a simple, preliminary dosage form for initial clinical trials.

2. Additional dosage-form development is deferred until safety/activity experiments in humans show promise. Eventually, scale-up experiments are conducted in cooperation with Pharmaceutical Manufacturing.

- Clinical research determines the safety and efficacy of the NCE in humans.
    1. Phase I examines small-dose tolerance and safety in a limited number of young adult, usually male, volunteers.
    2. Phase II, involving hundreds of patients, investigates efficacy, dosage, and prominent side effects.
    3. Phase III, utilizing thousands of patients, broadens Phase II experiments and determines safety, efficacy, and marketability.
    4. Phase IV, conducted after regulatory approval and marketing, investigates additional medical uses.
- Regulatory Affairs works closely with all relevant organizational units and is the primary contact with government regulatory agencies.
- Analytical Chemistry develops stability-indicating assays for NCEs and identifies/quantifies impurities; cooperates with Product R&D on product stability studies.
- Biochemistry determines, among other experiments, the cell-level effects of NCEs.
- Biopharmaceutics, Pharmacokinetics, and Drug Metabolism examines the absorption, distribution, metabolism, and elimination of NCEs.
- Chemical Pilot Plant produces NCEs for R&D groups.
- Experimental Engineering helps design new processes and equipment.
- Packaging Development develops containers for new products with stability and consumer issues in mind.
- Statistics is involved in planning and interpreting many R&D experiments.
- Purchasing works with R&D to ensure consistent, high-quality raw materials from vendors.
- Quality Assurance/Documentation monitors procedures and records to comply with government-regulated Good Laboratory and Manufacturing Practices.
- Chemical Manufacturing supplies the bulk NCE to Pharmaceutical Manufacturing.
- Engineering offers process/equipment services to post-NDA groups.
- Marketing, in cooperation with Sales and Advertising, determines the overall strategy for supplying NCE products to primary customers (physicians and other healthcare professionals).
- Packaging packages and labels manufactured drug products for sale.
- Pharmaceutical Manufacturing produces finished drug products for consumer use.
- Quality Control monitors the quality and stability of manufactured/marketed drug lots.
- Sales supplies products to customers.

Departmental Interactions

It's important for managers and laboratory workers to meet with colleagues from other departments to learn about interrelations and interdependencies and to use that knowledge to ensure mutual understanding, respect, support, and cooperation. Here are examples:

Sales ← → All R&D groups

R&D managers and laboratory workers should be encouraged to spend a day or two (one-on-one) with a salesperson "on the road," for two primary reasons:

1. R&D individuals can observe first hand the results of their labors.
2. Salespersons can learn important, relevant scientific facts about what they are selling and can directly inform the R&D person about problems their customers experience.

Synthetic chemistry ←→ Biopharmaceutics

Oral absorption data can help lead synthetic chemists in the most promising directions for NCE variations.

Synthetic chemistry ←→ Product R&D

Formulators usually prefer the most water-soluble form of an NCE; this can conflict with Synthetic Chemistry and Chemical Manufacturing's interest in high yields.

Biopharmaceutics ←→ Pharmacology

Interactional benefits go both ways, but Biopharmaceutics can help pharmacologists determine whether lackluster potency is attributable to inherent inactivity or poor oral absorption.

Product R&D ←→ Toxicology

True event: Product R&D helped Toxicology determine that the apparent intestinal irritation of an orally administered NCE was caused not by the drug, but by the "innocuous" solvent (glycerin).

Analytical chemistry ←→ Quality control

Analytical Chemistry develops stability-indicating assays for R&D, then transfers them to Quality Control when the product is marketed. Too often these groups are at loggerheads concerning what is an adequate, efficient assay procedure for the NCE. Management's mutual respect and cooperation, plus voluntary temporary interdepartmental transfers, can usually minimize these difficulties.

Pharmaceutical manufacturing ←→ Product R&D

1. These two groups need to interact at the appropriate stages in new drug development (especially scale-up) to ensure that a dependable, high- quality product can be consistently and economically manufactured.
2. Hands-on Manufacturing employees may feel most comfortable interacting with R&D scientists at the B.S./Associate degree level rather than at the Ph.D. level.
3. Product R&D laboratory workers at all educational levels should spend their first month or two in Pharmaceutical Manufacturing— working hands-on rather than just observing.

Marketing ←→ All R&D groups

True event: A Marketing executive was touring R&D laboratories and asked a key synthetic chemist working on antibacterials what she thought was the most important quality in an antibiotic after therapeutic activity. She replied, "lack of bacterial resistance." When the executive emphasized that Marketing was most concerned about lack of side effects, the scientist said, "No one ever told me that."

Quality assurance and documentation ←→ All R&D groups

Quality Assurance and Documentation should be thought of—and think of itself and operate accordingly—as helpful and supportive, not punitive.

Experimental engineering/product R&D ←→ Pharmaceutical manufacturing

True events:

1. Experimental engineering and Product R&D developed a computer-controlled automatic lyophilization process that was then transferred to Pharmaceutical Manufacturing.
2. Air-suspension particle/tablet coating and electronic monitoring of Pharmaceutical Manufacturing's tablet presses improved product quality and manufacturing efficiency.

Developing Line-extension Products

Once the first NCE product has been approved by the government regulatory agency, additional products (Product Line Extensions, or PLEs) are often developed. Requests for PLEs usually come from Marketing and Sales, but ideas can come from any employee/department, particularly from Product R&D. Regulatory approval of most PLEs is less demanding than for NCEs, e.g., there are fewer safety and clinical experiments.

Successful Management of Drug Development

Successful management consists of a series of thoughts, attitudes, feelings, and skilled practices, not simply (and counter productively) an "I-am-the-boss-so-do-what-I-say" culture.

Characteristics of a Fertile R&D Work Environment

Psychiatrist Abraham Maslow emphasizes that managers should not be sculptors (molding/forcing/shaping workers) but farmers who create a fertile work environment wherein all employees can learn, grow, and do their best. R&D managers can optimize group spirit, cohesiveness, innovation, and performance by looking at the team as a circle (in which everyone has a significant contribution to make), and not as the usual organizational pyramid with the boss at the top.

Here are characteristics of a fertile R&D work environment, starting with six cornerstones.

1. Ethics—This is noted first for obvious reasons.
2. Empathy—Empathy is the key to proper treatment of hands-on workers, e.g., managers should ask themselves how they would want their boss to treat them.
3. Respect—Feeling respected (valued) as a unique person and as a contributor to group success is as important as anything in the workplace.
4. Trust—This is an identical twin to respect. Without mutual trust, two or more people cannot survive a joint effort. The manager's genuine trust of employees as well intentioned, responsible adults is crucial to an efficient, productive work atmosphere.
5. Caring—Managers need to have a genuine concern for employees' personal and professional well-being.
6. Communication—Keeping employees informed fosters feelings of importance and "being in on things." Managers who listen carefully and inform abundantly will soon be surrounded by good communicators.
7. Sense of Purpose—The manager and group members need to know how their department fits into the R&D division.
8. Commitment—Everyone has a strong commitment to the long-term health of the division and to harmonized company, R&D, group, and personal goals.
9. Competence and Dedication—Group members are competent and confident in each other's ability and dedication.
10. Urgent but Well-reasoned, Goal-Focused Activity— Activity is goal-focused, with the general work pace being a healthy blend of urgency and contemplative, well reasoned, deliberate progress.
11. Involvement—Productivity, personal growth, and morale will be high if everyone feels involved in the planning, decision-making, and movement of the department toward its goals.
12. Individuality—Everyone wants to be treated as an important, unique individual.
13. Acceptance—Related to individuality, each person is valued just as they are; idiosyncrasies are tolerated, even appreciated, because variety is the "spice of life," and no one is perfect.
14. Civility—"Good management starts with good manners, society's means of ensuring consideration of others as people". . . Anonymous.

15. Agreeableness, Amiability, Friendliness—These are potent antidotes for nervous tension and anxiety and create as much tranquility in a work environment as civility.
16. Honesty, Candor, Openness—If trust is basic to all good things in human relationships, honesty, candor, and openness are basic to sustaining/ strengthening those relationships.
17. Stability, Security, Predictability—The manager needs to be ethical, fair, and consistent without being inflexible. This minimizes uncertainty and anxiety and makes employees feel safe and secure. More energy can then be focused on productive work.
18. Cooperation—When co-workers respect and care for one another and when all people feel safe and secure about their "place in the sun," the stage is set for cooperation rather than for competition, for mutual esteem and pride rather than for envy.
19. Recognition—Everyone is recognized for his or her accomplishments and value to the organization. Consequently, they feel good about themselves, their colleagues, their boss, and the corporation.
20. Thoughtfulness (Consideration for Others)—It has been said that nothing is more contagious than nervous tension, but surely thoughtfulness must run a close second. This can take many forms, but it generally involves getting outside oneself, being significantly oriented toward others rather than solely toward oneself. It means giving rather than taking.
21. Genuineness, Realness—A quality work environment helps workers feel safe, secure, and accepted, thus encouraging them to be themselves, "warts and all." This reduces facades, protectiveness, and defensiveness, and allows people to focus their energy on productive work.
22. Independence and Interdependence—When employees are valued for their basic worth and respected for their individuality, they develop a strong sense of independence. Consequently, they will have little need to "throw their weight around" or assert their individuality at the expense of others. When people feel good about themselves and receive emotional support from colleagues, they develop a strong sense of both independence and interdependence.
23. Cohesive Group Spirit—Under good management, a group develops a close, family-type working relationship in which individual members care for, trust, and respect, and have confidence in one another.
24. Deference—If the aforementioned characteristics are operative and the manager seeks advice from and defers to hands-on workers, group members will defer to one another's expertise and judgment when appropriate.
25. Pride (but not Arrogance)—Realistic pride in one-self and in the work group strengthens group cohesiveness and individual self-confidence and fosters a "can-do" attitude toward innovation and technical challenges.
26. Loyalty and Enthusiasm—When colleagues work at being civil and respectful, loyalty and enthusiasm will arise spontaneously. As Napoleon said, "An army's effectiveness depends on its size, training, experience, and morale... and morale is worth more than all the other factors combined."

Behaving Ethically

This is listed first because everything must be based on consistent ethical principles and behavior. R&D managers work in an especially complex environment: they hold great power and interact in complicated ways with hands-on workers, peers, upper management, customers, local and national government agencies, and citizen groups. R&D managers also face a unique situation because often results must be taken on faith. Most projects involve extensive experimentation and complex interpretation; some involve equivocal results. Managers must:

1. Trust the competence and honesty of laboratory workers and
2. Make honest use of the group's experimental results.

The leader is primarily responsible for the ethical attitude, behavior, and performance of the department. Here are three ways to ensure success:

1. Set a good example—The manager sets the tone for any group, acting as a role model. When employees observe that the boss is consistently ethical, they will set similar high standards for themselves.
2. Minimize unethical conformity and group-think—Peer pressure dominates most teenagers ("All·my friends do it ..."), but adults must resist the slightest unethical behavioral norms.
3. Create a safe, stable, predictable work environment—Unless they are pathological, people suffer ethical lapses out of confusion, fear, and insecurity, not out of evil. When workers are afraid of punishment or dismissal if schedules aren't met, work tends to become sloppy. When R&D vice-presidents fear their jobs are in jeopardy, they might manipulate the information going to corporate management so that their organization will look good.

In summary, leaders need to have the personal qualities of candor, genuineness, and integrity. If not, they are in danger of becoming manipulators of people and situations.

Empathizing (The Golden Rule of Management)

As one of the six cornerstones of successful management, the importance of empathy cannot be overemphasized. Before managers make decisions affecting workers (read "almost all decisions"), they need to remember the Golden Rule of Management: How would I like to be treated? This safeguard on managerial behavior is nearly infallible; here are two examples:

Promotions

Case A: An experienced laboratory scientist believes that he deserves a promotion to the next grade. He raises the issue with his supervisor; she tells him that he has potential, but she is not yet convinced that he has sufficiently proven himself. Nineteen months later he is promoted.

Case B: An experienced research scientist's manager comes into his laboratory and informs him that he has been promoted to the next grade. The scientist is delighted but surprised; he didn't expect promotion for another year. The manager says that it may be a little early, but based on his performance and obvious potential, she believes that he deserves to be promoted now. Reading this example, managers need to play the role of the laboratory scientist and ask themselves how would they would like to be treated by their boss; and would A or B elevate their spirit and incentive to work hard?

Treating employees as well-intentioned, responsible adults

Case A: Laboratory workers discover that, inadvertently, they are not in compliance with several Good Laboratory Practices regulations. When they inform the manager, he calls a department meeting, scolds all of them, orders them to shape up or else, and demands a full report within 3 days.

Case B: When the manager is informed of the GLP violations, he calls a department meeting, thanks them for alerting him to the problem, and asks them if he can be of any help; who would like to take charge of correcting the situation; and what deadline should be set so that he can reassure his boss.

Again, managers should play the role of laboratory workers and ask themselves how they would like to be treated, A or B.

Communicating

Here are two quite different definitions of communication:

1. The goal of communication is to persuade the listener to agree with the speaker. In this case, one gives little thought to the other's position. Most time and energy are spent thinking about what to say next rather than listening.

2. The purpose of communication is to create understanding. Here the emphasis is on listening, accepting differences of opinion, and freely expressing feelings.

Many sounds (street noise, small talk at a party) are assimilated through a process of hearing. This is primarily a physical phenomenon, with only a small mental element and virtually no emotional component. But when someone tries to communicate something they consider important, hearing becomes inadequate; instead, the other person needs to listen to and understand what they have to say. Now the process requires three components—physical, mental, and emotional— and becomes much more complex.

Generalizations aside, managers need to look at how communication skills apply to their job. First, the leader needs to communicate to employees the kind of person he or she is. Good working relationships, the cornerstone of good performance, depend on people getting to know one another. It is the manager's responsibility to initiate and encourage the communication process that brings about understanding. For example, he should meet at least once a year with each employee to find out:

1. How things are going, personally and on-the-job;
2. What is good and what is bad about the work environment;
3. Always refer to the department as "ours," never "mine;"
4. Always say, when introducing a group member to someone else, "she works with me," never, "she works for me;"
5. Encourage being called by his first name, because hierarchy tends to disappear when people are on a first-name basis;
6. Try to be the first one at department meetings; too many managers, for various reasons, wait until everyone else is assembled and then walk into the room. Making people wait is an inherent sign of disrespect, intended or not;
7. Keep employees informed by posting all non- confidential memos and notices on a large bulletin board under the categories of "urgent," "new," and "old." These actions are not gimmicks as long as they represent a sincere effort by the manager to communicate clearly and emphatically that everyone in the group is important.

Another valuable communication tool is seldom used—anonymous employee opinion surveys conducted by the manager, in addition to those of the Human Resources department. Annually, workers are asked to submit to the secretary their answers for three questions. The secretary then combines all responses:

1. What I like about my job;
2. What I don't like about my job; and
3. What my boss can do to make things better. Then (and most important), the manager should call a department meeting and ask the group to decide the priorities for improving the work environment.

Organizing

Hands-on laboratory workers

Experts agree that the number-one problem in any corporation is the underutilization of employees. This stems from management's failure to appreciate their intelligence and potential. Douglas McGregor says that most people enjoy working and, given the chance, prefer to exercise self-direction and self-control. They are highly motivated, seek responsibility, and can be a major positive force in company operations if management allows them.

For example, too often Ph.D.s (scientists) are informal project leaders when B.S.- level laboratory workers (associate scientists) can do that job very well, allowing the Ph.D. to act as theoretical science advisors for several project teams. Then Laboratory Assistants with high school diplomas or 2-year degrees can do most of the daily laboratory work with relatively little supervision rather than being treated as a "pair of hands." When employees feel respected and are encouraged to grow and take as much responsibility as possible, they will consult with higher-level scientists when necessary to minimize mistakes and to ensure group success.

First-line supervisors

Group Leaders/Section Heads should be responsible for approximately 15 laboratory workers and should think of themselves as supervisors, not superscientists. The non-supervisory Ph.D.s should make most of the broad scientific decisions; the Group Leader/Section Head should concentrate on becoming a successful manager of people.

Management

Most organizations have too much management; the number of supervisors at all levels should be minimized.

Supervising

Douglas McGregor says that the supervisor should act as a helper, teacher, consultant, and colleague. Rarely should she assume the role of authoritative boss. Tom Peters agrees, saying "Leaders are servants." Hands-on workers produce results; the manager's primary job is to support them and remove obstacles that prevent them from doing their best. The best supervisor will ask workers what she can do to help; rather than making sure the jobs get done, she assists the workers in doing so.

Many leaders feel this approach reduces their organizational power (using "power" in the good sense), but the exact opposite is true.

1. The manager "sees over" more clearly because discussions with employees will sharpen the view of the situation for everyone.
2. Control and communication are enhanced because employees will interact frequently with a manager who is viewed as a source of help rather than as a giver of orders.
3. Treating employees as competent, responsible adults will greatly increase her influence with them.

Controlling

Originally, controlling meant running a tight ship; the boss watched over everyone and everything, told employees what to do and when to do it, and made all the important decisions himself. But this made the leader and hands-on workers antagonists, resulting in the manager knowing relatively little about what really went on in the trenches. In contrast, appropriate (non- authoritarian) control means emphasizing employees' self-control simply because most people are trust-worthy. This is especially true in R&D organizations in which the emphasis is on high technology, creativity, and innovation.

Peter Drucker, Tom Peters, and Douglas McGregor agree:

1. Drucker says that to be productive, workers need to have control over their work; control is a tool of employees and must never be their master.
2. Peters calls this the control paradox: less is more. Less central control and more genuinely delegated self-control for those closest to the action translates into tighter overall control.
3. McGregor believes that successful supervision is largely dependent on the manager's ability to predict and control human behavior, and the essence of control is selective adaptation. People control the physical world around them, not by expecting nature to do their bidding, but by adjusting their actions to natural laws. For example, humankind does not control surface water by commanding it to flow uphill; rather, people dig channels, adjusting to the fact that water obeys the law of gravity.

Similarly, effective management control consists of channeling workers' energies, interests, and capabilities into activities that meet organizational objectives.

Management controls the work force by adjusting its decisions and actions to the realities of human nature, and not by telling people what to do and expecting blind obedience.

Delegating

Managers should delegate because employees like, want, and need to do things their own way. The wise leader assigns research projects only after consulting with laboratory workers, preferably at a department meeting, because bench scientists tend to have a much better feel than the manager concerning who has the time; who is most qualified; and how best to divide up responsibilities.

Also, employees feel more respected and involved when they are part of the work-assignment process.

Delegation, not relegation

Since the biggest waste in any organization is underutilization of employees, delegation makes sense. Unfortunately, too many leaders confuse delegation with relegation. Delegation means assigning responsibility and authority to a representative. Relegation, on the other hand, connotes consignment to an inferior position. When managers give employees narrow, menial tasks and expect them to do all "delegated" work exactly as they would, their action is relegation, not delegation.

Goals of delegation

Three primary goals of true delegation are to:

1. Relieve managers of some of their work-load so that they have more time to think, meditate, plan, learn, and grow;
2. Move work and responsibility as far down the organizational ladder as possible, increasing efficiency; and
3. Offer all employees maximum challenge and opportunities for growth, even when formal promotions are not immediately available. This increases productivity and develops future leaders.

In harmony with these goals, proper delegation has two distinguishing characteristics:

1. Most of the delegated tasks are a meaningful part of the manager's job and not just drudgery to avoid;
2. Workers are allowed, even encouraged, to perform the delegated work in their own way, with the manager helping only when asked.

Case study: In the movie Bullitt, a police lieutenant is working on a case that is of intense interest to a powerful U.S. senator. The senator is not happy with the way the lieutenant is conducting the investigation, so he pressures the lieutenant's boss to force him to proceed differently. As it happens, the captain agrees with the senator but refuses to interfere, saying "It's his case, Senator."

Monitoring

Here managers can be either authoritarian (running a tight ship) or smart. They can foolishly spend much of their valuable time monitoring their operation or they can wisely delegate most of that function to employees, thus improving productivity and orderliness, fostering growth, and freeing up more time for broader, long-range tasks.

In a good work environment, the impetus for monitoring comes from below, not from above. This places a positive focus on the process. The manager trusts group members and does not feel a need to monitor the operation closely. At the same time, employees are eager to keep managers informed because they sense that they are interested in their work and in departmental progress. They also recognize the need for management to know the general situation, to be informed of major progress or problems. On the other hand, authoritative monitoring will yield negative results.

1. Workers can't help but feel that managers don't trust them—else why would two people do one person's job? Most employees feel, correctly, that it is part of their job to monitor progress and to address problems.
2. The situation is inherently inane, and perceived management inanities contribute to employee disrespect and alienation.
3. Workers tend to lose interest in doing a careful job of monitoring when they see the boss repeating what they do.
4. Management seldom performs lower-level tasks well. Hands-on employees, to whom such tasks are often challenging, are much more motivated and equipped to do them properly.
5. Efficiency and productivity suffer, not only because of the redundancy, but because employees are forced to spend time educating the manager about the details.
6. If managers get too involved with minutia, they tend to meddle in workers' jobs, and soup is not the only brew spoiled by too many cooks.

Advocating

This management task never appears in a job description, yet it is vital to enhancing the culture, environment, and performance of an R&D operation. The world is not a fair place, and the world of work is even less fair. Why? In a free society, adults make most of their own decisions, but not in the workplace, where management and corporate rules reign supreme. Employees feel vulnerable, and "results only" oriented management practices can adversely affect their performance and well-being. In unionized organizations, the agent or steward serves as employees' advocate (although R&D scientists are seldom part of a labor union); in non-union companies, the Human Relations department usually fills that role. Seldom is management viewed as an advocate for workers, and rarely does management perceive itself that way. In fact, employees often consider the boss a powerful adversary—the very reason they need an advocate! Surely productivity, not to mention loyalty and enthusiasm, suffers when workers and management consider themselves adversaries.

Manager as advocate

In a well managed, people-oriented organization, the primary advocate for each employee is the immediate supervisor. Not only is that individual in the best position to know and help workers, but she is the major beneficiary of the increased productivity, loyalty, and enthusiasm that follow. Experience has shown that if workers believe their manager is for them and wants them to succeed, and a helper and facilitator rather than an overseer; there is little they won't do for the manager. In fact, when she is under great stress or trouble, the roles become reversed and employees will rush to her aid.

Some managers believe that they should be neither advocates nor adversaries but impartial judges. However, social science professionals have shown that managers are no more rational or impartial than anyone else, that everyone labors under a cloud of personal bias. Furthermore, strict impartiality usually results in impersonal treatment, and no one likes being regarded as a "non-person." How do managers go about becoming primary personal and organizational advocates for employees?

Personal advocacy guidelines

1. Managers should get to know each person as an individual and develop a relationship based on mutual trust, respect, and caring. Then employees will feel comfortable bringing them their concerns, and the manager will be able to give employees optimum help.
2. Managers need to be perceptive observers of employees, not to check up on them, but to pick up subtle signs of trouble. For example, if an ebullient person becomes very quiet on the job, and this persists for a week or two, the manager may want to say, "I don't want to be nosy, but is anything wrong? Anything I can do to help?" If the employee does not want to talk, the manager

should not force the issue, but observe the situation. Showing genuine interest in individuals has a positive effect, even though they may not want to confide in their supervisor. When an employee's performance starts to decline and the manager is quite sure it is not because of any action or inaction on his part, it is best not to intrude on one's privacy; treat the employee as an adult and provide her every chance to work out the difficulties.

3. If the employee's performance continues to deteriorate, there will come a time when the manager needs to meet with her and talk. But if he has built a good relationship with the employee she will most likely confide in him long before that point is reached. If the manager finds himself growing impatient with an employee during a difficulty, it's best that he wait a bit longer; it usually pays off. People appreciate a supervisor who shows patience and faith in them during times of trouble.
4. When the worker does confide in the manager, he should refrain from giving advice unless asked. Any troubled individual coming to a supervisor needs, first of all, a sympathetic ear and then appropriate reassurance.
5. Even when she presses him for advice, both individuals are best off if the manager simply outlines options and their advantages and disadvantages, leaving the ultimate decision to the employee.
6. The manager should not try to do too much. If he senses that professional help may be appropriate, a suggestion to that effect or a referral to the company's employee assistance program may be in order.

Organizational advocacy guidelines

Not all problems are highly personal or greatly troubling. Then it is best for the manager to use his administrative ingenuity to deal directly with such problems as a temporarily stalled promotion, a continuing problem with another department, tension or a disagreement with a colleague, or resentment over an ill-defined or apparently unfair company policy. The no-advice rule softens considerably when the manager has some control over the situation. Employees do not expect management to solve all their problems, but they do expect their supervisor to try when it's important to them.

The advocating manager serves as a bridge between employees and the organization. A key girder in that bridge is "loyalty up and down." Workers need to feel that the manager is truly for them, whereas the manager's boss has to be confident that the subordinate is looking out for the company's interests as well. If the manager has a reputation as a strong advocate for employees, when irreconcilable conflicts arise (assuming no violations of ethics or the law are involved), he can come down on the side of the company without straining his relationship with workers.

One of managers' primary responsibilities is to remove impediments to employees productivity. This can be viewed as advocacy as well, because such assistance improves workers' well-being.

Sheltering

Here is another managerial task that is missing from job descriptions, but it is very important, especially in these days of high-pressure, 60-h workweeks. What is sheltering? No matter what the weather outside, the roof, siding, and windows of a house provide a hospitable, safe environment for occupants. So, too, do managers need to create an optimum work atmosphere by sheltering hands-on workers. Shelter them from what? Swirling about any organization are tensions, antagonisms, organizational red tape, and inanities—unpleasant and distracting. For example, perhaps the R&D vice-president, a tense, caustic individual who is uncomfortable with the deliberate pace of research, is constantly berating department managers to speed things up and increase productivity. The strong tendency in such a situation is to translate at least some of that unpleasantness and pressure down to hands-on workers—the "kick-the-dog" syndrome. With this response, not only are managers relieving some of their own frustrations and resentments, but they are convincing themselves, and trying to convince their boss, that they are team players who are bottom-line oriented. Unfortunately, such a reaction seriously damages the group's work environment and will likely reduce, not enhance, performance, especially in R&D, in which innovation and creativity require a positive atmosphere.

To avoid such debilitating problems, managers need to prevent disruption of the group's productive, relatively tranquil work environment by absorbing as much of the pressure and unpleasantness as possible. By taking most of that burden on their own shoulders, the managers protect the department from contamination by poor management practices elsewhere in the organization. This does not mean that legitimate pressures and emergencies should not filter down; employees can and will respond with vigor and enthusiasm to them, especially when the crisis is viewed as a challenge to the entire group. But no one can do their best when they are constantly pressured to hurry! hurry! hurry! Remember, "if you don't have time to do it right, where will you find the time to do it over?"

Successful sheltering is highly dependent on the level of mutual trust, respect, and confidence within the work group. When there is a strong, caring sense of family, intense sheltering is unnecessary because intrusions from the outside have minimal effect. Quality sheltering requires that managers get out of their offices and see what's going on in the department. If they have no sense of the group's day-to-day moods, detecting rising patterns of tension or indifference becomes difficult. Also, employees are more apt to call problems to the manager's attention if they perceive her as interested, friendly, and accessible.

Five important personal qualities required for good sheltering are:

1. *Strength*. The manager needs to swim against a strong current (i.e., the system or an unreasonable, autocratic boss).
2. *Courage*. There is risk to the manager who stands up for her people against superiors or the system.
3. *Stamina*. Sheltering is a never-ending task.
4. *Ingenuity*. Deflecting a rushing stream (again, the system) usually works better than constructing a dam.
5. *Tact*. Diplomacy usually makes deflection acceptable to the system.

Managers who provide effective shelter for their employees will succeed, both with their workers and with their bosses.

Fostering Creativity

Managers contribute to creativity by:

1. Demonstrating enthusiasm and excitement for new ideas;
2. Managing with a light touch, allowing laboratory scientists the freedom to grow in their own way and at their own pace;
3. Encouraging employees to take risks and explore new territory—and being there with encouragement rather than criticism if they fail;
4. Being both flexible and secure and creating a work atmosphere with those same characteristics;
5. Being committed, not just to today's and this year's comfort and well-being, but to the long-term health of the organization and its employees; and
6. Hiring competent, innovative scientists.

Tips for encouraging creativity

1. "Two heads are better than one" is not a cliche. Ideas are often enriched through discussions with others.

2. Brain-storming sessions involving multidisciplinary groups often produce marketable ideas. The cardinal rule of brainstorming is that no expressed thought be evaluated during the session, because the threat of critique inhibits the free flow of ideas.
3. Managers should refrain from judging employees' ideas. It's best to ask workers to research their concepts with the help of their colleagues (e.g., R&D, Marketing, and Sales) and then evaluate it themselves.
4. When innovation involves replacement of old technology, management often entrusts development of the new technology to old-technology experts. At times this succeeds, but the effort often fails because these veterans have too much intellectual and emotional investment in the old way. It is usually best to assign development of new technology to competent but relevantly inexperienced scientists who will take a fresh, unencumbered approach to the problem.
5. Formal suggestion systems can be beneficial, but management must guard against calcification, by which the suggestions nourish the bureaucratic system instead of the other way around.

Motivating

When thousands of supervisors were asked to list, in descending order, what they thought motivated workers, they got it all wrong. They listed:

1. "Interesting work" as #5, but in the same questionnaire workers chose it as #1.
2. "Full appreciation for work done" as #8, whereas employees rated it #2.
3. "Feeling of being in on things" as #10 whereas workers assigned it #3.

It is clear that managers need to learn more about motivation.

Experts agree that human behavior is not random, but caused; internally motivated; and always directed toward some goal. Strictly speaking, managers do not and cannot motivate employees. The best they can do is provide the stimuli to which workers react, driven by their own internal motivation. Psychologist Abraham Maslow hypothesized a hierarchy of needs that classifies human motivation, listed in descending priority:

1. Physiological (hunger, thirst);
2. Safety (security, stability, predictability);
3. Belongingness and social integration (companionship, being part of a group);
4. Esteem (self-respect and recognition/respect from others); and
5. Self-actualization or self-fulfillment (each person's drive to move toward being the very best of which he or she is inherently capable).

The basic needs (physiological) are most important, but once satisfied, they no longer motivate, and the next set becomes operative. Because most employees are not starving nor threatened by anarchy, unless job security is a factor managers should be concerned with:

1. Belongingness or social needs;
2. Esteem; and
3. Self-fulfillment.

Fostering Employee Growth

To foster workers' growth, managers must:

1. Understand people so that their efforts will harmonize with the realities of human nature;
2. Understand the learning process to ensure the optimal rate of growth; and
3. Apply that understanding on the job with diligence and patience.

Let's examine these three components.

Understanding people

The human characteristics most relevant to the learning/ growing process are:

1. *Desire to grow.* Everyone has an inherent tendency to move toward psychological health and maturity.
2. *Personal freedom.* The more people have a say about what they do, how and when they do it, and the direction and pace of personal growth, the faster and surer they will progress.
3. *Uniqueness.* People are different from each other. Everyone is a unique individual, as varied as fingerprints. Each individual has different needs and distinct ways of satisfying those needs.

Understanding the learning process

What does an R&D manager need to know about the learning process?

- Learning can be cognitive, as in memorizing multiplication tables or reading books; or experiential, as when riding a bicycle or working effectively in groups. Most learning is a combination of the two, especially in technical organizations, in which cognitive scientific knowledge must be integrated with a wide variety of experiential skills.
- Personal growth is best achieved experientially. Carl Rogers defines the elements involved:
    1. Primarily self-initiated, involving the entire person, physically, intellectually, and emotionally. A person learns best when he is ready and wants to learn;
    2. Pervasive, making a difference in the attitudes and behavior of the learner;
    3. Self-evaluated, in that the learner is the one who decides whether the learning experience is meeting his needs; and
    4. Comprehensive, so that total (intellectual and emotional) meaning is experienced.

Application

Here are some general guidelines (keeping in mind the characteristics of a fertile work environment mentioned earlier). Leaders should:

1. Manage with a light touch;
2. Set a good example;
3. Get to know workers as individuals;
4. Involve employees as much as possible;
5. Encourage risk-taking and creative thinking;
6. Not underestimate employees' potential; and
7. Consider overall personal growth.

Recruiting

When competent workers are hired, a manager is almost guaranteed good results. However with inadequate employees even a brilliant leader is in serious trouble. Therefore, good recruiting practices are basic to a successful R&D operation.

Effective recruiting depends first on good management of the people already on hand; the motivation, enthusiasm, and loyalty of group members will be obvious to visiting prospects.

True event. Under autocratic management, a division had 18 consecutive rejections; after changing to people-centered supervision, nine of 10 candidates accepted.

Two major steps in recruiting scientific personnel are:

1. Identifying quality candidates and
2. Bringing them to the organization for in-depth interviews (including a seminar).

The best way to succeed with the first step is to visit universities for interviews with students. The ethical way to succeed with the second step is to have the candidate talk to as many hands-on workers as possible and to encourage interviewers to be honest and candid in answering questions about the organization. The more welcome and respected candidates feel, the better the chances they will accept an offer.

Recruiters should gather information about the candidate by talking with major advisors, other faculty members, former classmates, and formal references. The following personal characteristics are especially important: competence, productivity, genuineness, growth potential, flexibility, open-mindedness, cooperativeness, deference, communication, self-confidence, motivation, thoughtfulness, ethics, independence, and commitment.

Conducting Formal Performance Reviews

The typical formal performance review is similar to a trip to the dentist: There is apprehension before, pain during, and a sense of relief afterward, when the session is over.

Douglas McGregor explains why:

1. Evaluating an employee's performance is highly dependent on the manager's psychological makeup.
2. For various reasons (including managerial malfeasance), the appraisal often has little relation to reality.

True event. Roger, a first-line R&D supervisor, had always received above-average performance reviews. He made no waves, followed orders, did the required paperwork, and sleep-walked his way through corporate life for 10 years, totally ignoring employees' concerns and frustrations. When a new, highly competent department manager arrived, she quickly recognized Roger's incompetence and pressed for his demotion, transfer, or termination. This caused a great uproar because the "record"—a decade of innocuous, relatively positive performance appraisals by a variety of managers—painted an entirely different picture.

1. Experts agree that to a great extent, a worker's performance is a function of how he is managed.
2. Concerning criticism, the effectiveness in communication is inversely proportional to the employee's need to hear it. The more harsh the criticism, the less likely the person can/will accept it.
3. The manager may be able to convey negative judgments, but this will seriously damage the relationship.
4. Performance reviews accentuate the worker's dependence on the manager.
5. It's an open question if a troubled individual really wants to hear about his deficiencies.
6. Concerning amateur counselors (which managers are) Carl Rogers says that the most they can accomplish is a temporary change, which then disappears, leaving the person more than ever convinced of his inadequacy.

There's a better, well-proven, successful approach (which assumes that all employees are performing adequately; if that's not the case, then the manager needs to transfer or terminate unacceptable performers).

1. Well before the actual reviews, employees are reminded that the "system" demands a formal performance appraisal and that certain rituals must, as in the past, be followed.
2. Then the manager reminds them that she has been in close contact with each of them throughout the year, and that consequently, there will be no surprises during the formal interview.
3. The manager assures everyone that their performance review will be a pleasant experience.
4. Then the manager holds formal reviews only when in a relaxed, reassuring mood.
5. When the person first comes into her office, she reiterates the first 3 points.

6. The manager emphasizes—genuinely—what a good job the employee is doing and how glad she is to have him in the department.
7. Then the manager goes into specifics concerning what she likes about the employee and his performance over the past year; he is encouraged to add accomplishments the manager has failed to mention.
8. Next, the manager reminds the employee that the system requires that she record some negatives and asks for suggestions (e.g., he often puts things off until the last minute).
9. The manager then reassures him—genuinely— concerning any weaknesses he brings up, e.g., "If you were perfect, you'd make the rest of us look bad." "Your intentions are always good, and your strengths far outweigh your weaknesses." Any additional discussion in this area should consist exclusively of the manager asking the employee how he feels about the negatives and, most important, where she—or the work situation—is deficient in helping him do his best.
10. The manager then records—honestly—the weaknesses the employee mentions, but puts them in as positive a light as possible (e.g., "Employee tends to complete some assignments at the last minute, but has a good sense of priorities and is always on schedule").
11. Then—and this is especially important—the manager asks the employee what she can do to help him improve even more. She then sits back and listens in a non-defensive manner, thanking the employee—genuinely—for the candid feedback (and follows up on the suggestions).
12. The manager sums up by re-emphasizing— again, genuinely—an appreciation for the contributions to the group's accomplishments and her delight in having him as a member of the department.

In summary, criticism should be avoided here and in all management behavior, simply because it's counterproductive, and employees who feel accepted and valued by their supervisor will engage in self- criticism. This is, by far, more productive over the long term.

Transferring or Terminating Unproductive Employees

If, in spite of good management practices, a hands-on worker cannot do the job adequately, the manager is obliged to transfer the employee to a more suitable position elsewhere in the corporation. If that is not an option, then the employee should be terminated if legally possible and ethically acceptable.

Here's a recommended procedure to follow:

1. The manager should consult the Human Resources department personnel for official guidance. In fact, it is wise to work with them unofficially at a much earlier stage.
2. After ensuring that his actions have been consistent with company policy, the manager should bring the employee into his office for a private, candid, uninterrupted, and caring conversation.
3. He should begin by saying, "I'm sorry, but things are not working out and you are facing termination. You don't have to leave tomorrow, but if you were still here 6 months from now it would be a problem. Sometime between tomorrow and 6 months from now you need to find a job with a different company. I'll help you all I can, but in the end, that's your responsibility."
4. The person will almost certainly be upset and antagonistic toward the manager. At that point, he needs to remember that the employee is going through an ultratraumatic process and needs all the sympathy and support he can muster. The last thing the manager should do is try to defend his decision unless pressured by the employee, which usually does not occur.

Managers who recruit and manage well will seldom have to perform this unpleasant task.

Promoting

Proper selection of new supervisors is crucial to organizational success.

Promoting the wrong people

The most common mistakes made when choosing people for R&D management positions are:

1. Assuming the best laboratory worker will make the best supervisor (management is an entirely different world than laboratory research);
2. Choosing autocratic, results-oriented people rather than person-centered individuals; and
3. Going outside the company instead of promoting from within, which lowers employee morale and motivation.

Promoting the right people

A key element in promoting the right people is having the right people to promote; thus, recruiting the best candidates and creating a growth-fostering environment are crucial. It is also important to recognize the personal qualities needed to make a good supervisor. Managers should avoid promoting people with little talent for or interest in management. The best way to prevent this is to provide potential supervisors with temporary responsibilities and then evaluate their performance.

Organizing Project Teams

There are two common ways to organize project teams:

1. Informal (in which team members belong to scientific discipline-oriented departments with the leader's role being coordinator, not boss).
2. Formal (in which the project leader has organizational authority over team members).

In pharmaceutical R&D, it seems best to have informal project teams because:

1. Everyone needs an organizational "home" for emotional stability and security reasons, and formal project teams tend to make scientists migrant workers, e.g., when the project is completed, they are often assigned to another project with a new boss.
2. Formal project teams tend to inhibit intergroup cooperation and create unhealthy competition among teams (we should have the highest priority regarding limited joint resources and we want to make sure that our project comes out first in upper management's rating).

International R&D

Domestic R&D managers face special challenges in a multinational corporation; in general, they need to do the following:

1. Know the organizational specifics of their company's international operations;
2. Learn as much as possible about the cultural, economic, technical, and governmental differences among the various countries;
3. Establish close ties with their international R&D colleagues.

A multilingual R&D manager is especially valuable.

R&D Management and Corporate Management

R&D management needs to:

1. Understand and appreciate the views and concerns of corporate management;
2. Develop a broad vision for R&D that is harmonious with long-range corporate plans; and
3. Decide, with workers' help, what is in the best interests of the corporation.

Corporate management must learn enough about the world of R&D to:

1. Appreciate R&D's point of view;
2. Understand the R&D process so that funding is steady, not sporadic; and
3. Recognize the danger signals (confusion, aimlessness, consistently poor decisions, laboratory worker malaise) of poor R&D management to distinguish them from bad-luck cycles inherent to all R&D.

Industry and Academia

Interactions between industry and academia have mutual benefits.

Advantages for academia

1. Educational benefits:
   - Encourages the cross-fertilization of ideas;
   - Offers temporary, education-focused work in industry for faculty, undergraduates, and graduate students; and
   - Develops joint projects for increased knowledge.
2. Financial and other benefits:
   - Support for research.
   - Possible employment opportunities for students after graduation.
   - Consultantships for faculty.
   - Rapid commercialization of academic research.

Advantages for industry

1. An increased knowledge base for:
   - Cross-fertilization of ideas.
   - More options for new and better products.
   - More flexibility in R&D spending (academic support can be enlisted for an urgent but speculative project without making long-term internal commitments).
2. Greater professional development of employees through:
   - Teaching and lecturing opportunities in academia.
   - Research sabbaticals.
   - Internal short courses given by academic consultants.
3. Successful recruiting of new personnel owing to:
   - More thorough evaluation of potential job candidates via summer employment of students.
   - Improved corporate image among students and faculty.

17

Microbiologic Monitoring

Microbiologic monitoring of controlled pharmaceutical and medical device manufacturing, and pharmacy compounding processes, is mandated in numerous standards and guidelines, although procedures, limits, and frequencies are not well defined. Because many characteristics of microbiologic sampling limit its value as a monitoring method, efforts to detect contamination in controlled environments require carefully developed and executed sampling plans to produce reliable data that confirm the acceptability of operating conditions.

Monitoring of any controlled process is a component of an outcome-producing, closed-loop system for assuring continued operation of critical processes in accordance with validated design conditions. To achieve this goal, a monitoring plan must be developed, conducted, and evaluated within the context of a Validation and Monitoring protocol. All results must be related to the original validated process, either as evidence that it continues to operate within acceptable limits, or as a means of detecting shifts in the process that might impinge on product quality. Ideally, monitoring results will also provide information that will be useful in determining the cause of such shifts. The objectives of the monitoring plan within the validation and monitoring system for quality management must be clearly defined so that the information collected will be relevant to system goals. The limitations of sampling equipment and methods must be taken into consideration when developing the sampling plan and interpreting results. The underlying causes for shifts in various monitoring results must be understood in order to facilitate development of effective corrective action plans.

Validation and Monitoring Rationale

The regulatory requirements for validation of pharmaceutical aseptic processes are clear. Generally accepted quality assurance principles require initial demonstration of the efficacy of any process (*validation*), followed by regular, periodic observation to demonstrate that the process continues to operate in accordance with validation conditions (*monitoring*).

Validation usually consists of a series of "worst-case" process simulations, wherein a sterile growth medium is substituted for product to demonstrate that processing consistently yields products of acceptable quality. During this Process Qualification (PQ) phase, variable conditions that might effect product quality are carefully defined, controlled, monitored, and documented, and the assumption is reasonably made that the process will then yield the same product quality achieved during the PQ, so long as all variable factors are controlled to duplicate validation conditions. This assumption is based upon the results of monitoring data obtained from a variety of sources. The validity of the assumption of acceptable quality is, therefore, dependent upon the reliability of the monitoring data as a measure of control of process variables.

Validation Protocol

The validation protocol should define the manufacturing or compounding process, its purpose in terms of the desired positive impact on product quality, and how that impact will be demonstrated. The protocol should include the following components:

1. A description of the product, and applicable release criteria including AOQL/ROQL;
2. The facility design rationale for maintaining process integrity, including identification and elimination of inaccessible areas that may be difficult to decontaminate, enumeration of the clean-space engineering controls, and how these controls will be applied, tested, and monitored;
3. A schematic description of the aseptic process and the critical work surfaces, work zones, and support areas, including the designation of particulate cleanliness class, microbial target values, and engineering control equipment validation methods;
4. The selection and justification of gowning and barrier techniques to ensure adequate isolation of personnel, based upon industry standards and process requirements;
5. A definition of the aseptic techniques and work practices of operative personnel, and a report of findings based upon videotaped observation of the actual work stream during prequalification runs for identification and elimination of personnel-generated contamination sources, identification of susceptible areas including critical sites and steps, and indicator sites;
6. A description of sanitizing methods and sanitizing compound validation;
7. A definition of the equipment and methods to be used in assuring reliable test data; and
8. All test data, including instrument calibrations, testing and certification reports, and statistical justification.

Monitoring Plan

Following evaluation of all environmental monitoring data collected during the PQ, a monitoring plan defining ongoing monitoring procedures, locations, and frequency should be implemented. The PQ data from product testing should be compared to environmental and process monitoring results to determine the monitoring sites and methods that best correlate with shifts in product quality. The plan should

1. Assure specified, periodic monitoring of critical manufacturing or compounding process parameters at critical points during periods of peak activity, and establish the circumstances and frequency with which monitoring is to be carried out to assure a reliable basis for claiming process control.
2. Provide for standardized, quantitative microbiologic sampling of process air, environmental surfaces, and personnel barriers, as well as sampling of other, related parameters.
3. Include sampling location maps, sample sizes, probe heights, methods, equipment, and frequency during manufacturing operations, and a method for statistical justification of results.
4. Include alert and action limit criteria for acting upon ongoing monitoring information.
5. Include a system for evaluating and modifying the monitoring plan to assure collection of reliable, useful data, and
6. Include a corrective action plan, and methods of verifying the efficacy of any corrective actions taken.

Limitations of Microbiologic Monitoring

The minimum media-fill validation requirement of not more than one sterility failure per thousand units, representing the minimum sterility assurance level of 10^{-3} (>99.9%) is the only microbiologic limit in the validation and monitoring scheme that is based upon demonstrated product quality. Achievement of this sterility assurance level represents the aggregate impact of all process design and control factors, including sampling and attendant laboratory procedures. (This limit, however, probably does not reflect the true integrity of a valid aseptic process.) All other limits are indices, which are used indirectly to demonstrate that the process is under control as validated. Because all environmental monitoring is necessarily performed at some point downstream and apart from the product, no absolute evaluation of product quality is obtainable through monitoring procedures, however intensive. In addition, testing and monitoring methods do not always parallel or identify the pathways through which contaminants are introduced into the product.

Difficulty in validating microbiologic monitoring methods results from a lack of comprehensive testing standards, reliable test equipment, and reliable methods for correlating sample data to predictions of product quality. Several characteristics and qualities of both contamination events and sampling methods limit the usefulness of microbiologic monitoring as a method of determining the acceptability of a specific product batch:

1. Microbiologic contamination events in controlled facilities are usually not randomly distributed in time, space, or by type of organism;
2. No single sampling method repeatedly recovers a known and consistent percentage of all types of organisms;
3. For most types of contamination detected, there are usually many possible sources, not the least of which are the sampling personnel, equipment, and lab processing; and
4. An extended interval is required for development of results.

Perspectives

These considerations underscore recent concerns that regulatory groups may require that unreliable environmental monitoring data be used as release criteria. Current industry standards and regulatory guidelines do not, and should not be interpreted to condone the rejection of batches on the basis of absolute environmental counts alone. Microbiologic monitoring is employed for practical reasons, not because it is ideal or unique in detecting shifts in process conditions.

Regulatory agencies and auditors understandably seek easy-to-interpret data as a basis for decisions regarding product acceptability, and are becoming increasingly hesitant to accept product release in the absence of demonstrable levels of microbiologic control. Conversely, industry is justifiably reluctant to set microbiologic monitoring limits because regulators may misinterpret their meaning in a quality assurance (QA) context. The failure to meet process control limits is quite different from the failure to meet product specifications. Failure to meet a monitoring limit means only that monitoring data can no longer demonstrate validation conditions, and product quality may be adversely affected. Enhanced product testing or other corrective actions may be indicated, but batch rejection should not be extrapolated from QA monitoring results, alone.

Setting Limits

In the QA context, limits are established to trigger specific actions, or outcomes. The alert (warning) limit is the point at which the operator should become alerted to the possibility of a deteriorating trend. When an action limit is exceeded, the operator must take action to identify and correct the condition(s) that are causing a verified trend before a "fail" limit is reached and the data fail to indicate process control and support continued production. In a well-designed and executed process, however, such a fail limit should never be exceeded, except in the event of a sudden and catastrophic breakdown of a critical process control component.

Akers noted that values presented in the current U.S.P. are target values. Given this designation, it is reasonable to consider these values to be operational target levels, rather than product quality control limits. There are several models for setting alert, action and fail limits, although many only establish alert and action limits (other terminology may be used). Extending one current model, the alert limit might be considered to be the 95th percentile. Analysis and trending of actual data allow the calculation of this limit, as well as the 97th percentile for the action limit, and the 99th percentile as the fail limit. Regardless of the model used initially to set limits, they should be based upon both historical data, and an evaluation of correlations between monitoring results and product quality. Data analysis should include a mechanism for evaluation and modification of the monitoring program and limits.

It is expected that results will fall within normally anticipated operating levels with 95% confidence, if randomness in critical environments and operations is sufficiently controlled. If data from successful PQ runs (when the process is demonstrated to be under control) do not meet this criterion, the monitoring methods may not measure a phenomenon that relates directly to process control, may not be sufficiently reproducible to provide useful information, or may have been incorrectly conducted. Every effort should be made to develop monitoring methods that comply with this performance expectation so that data will be useful.

Initial limits may be calculated and compared to results of any unsuccessful trials. These limits should eventually be adjusted based on historical data. When evaluating data to adjust limits, Wilson noted, "Including data taken from a period of unusually high counts, where the process was out of control, will lead to inappropriately high alert/action limits."

Conduct of Sampling

Quality management and sampling personnel require both an in-depth understanding of the environmental sampling rationale, and a complete understanding of commonly available equipment, materials, sampling techniques, and development methods. Reporting forms should be carefully designed to convey all relevant information including identification of the technician, sample location (from a standardized sample map), date and time, media (including lot, expiration, and validation date), method, duration of sampling, and equipment (including calibration date and serial number). In addition, information such as the product batch, number and names of personnel, line throughput rate, number and nature of line interventions, and other available monitoring data such as room pressure and other engineering control status readings should be recorded. Any observed deviations from standard operating procedures (SOPs) should be noted and communicated to the individuals responsible for training and management of operative personnel. It is essential to repeat samples when such deviations occur in order to evaluate the impact they may have on results.

Sampling and laboratory personnel must be highly competent on both philosophical and functional levels, and must develop and exercise perfect aseptic technique. A training program and operating procedures should be established defining all monitoring steps, including gowning, preparation of samplers, aseptic sampling techniques, sample recovery, handling and transport, and laboratory techniques for aseptic sample development. A laboratory QA program should assure that monitoring personnel conform to operating procedures and that technician skills are periodically tested and validated for high competence and flawless technique.

Sample Handling

Sampling, sample transport, and sample development should be conducted in a way that does not affect results. For example, if agar plates are improperly transported, condensate may form on the lid and drip onto the agar surface, redistributing microorganisms over the surface and around the edges of the plate, causing false readings. Agar plates should, therefore, be kept inverted and oriented horizontally during storage and transport. They should be handled gently, and transferred to the incubator as quickly as possible after exposure. With sieve impactors, false positives can usually be identified as colony

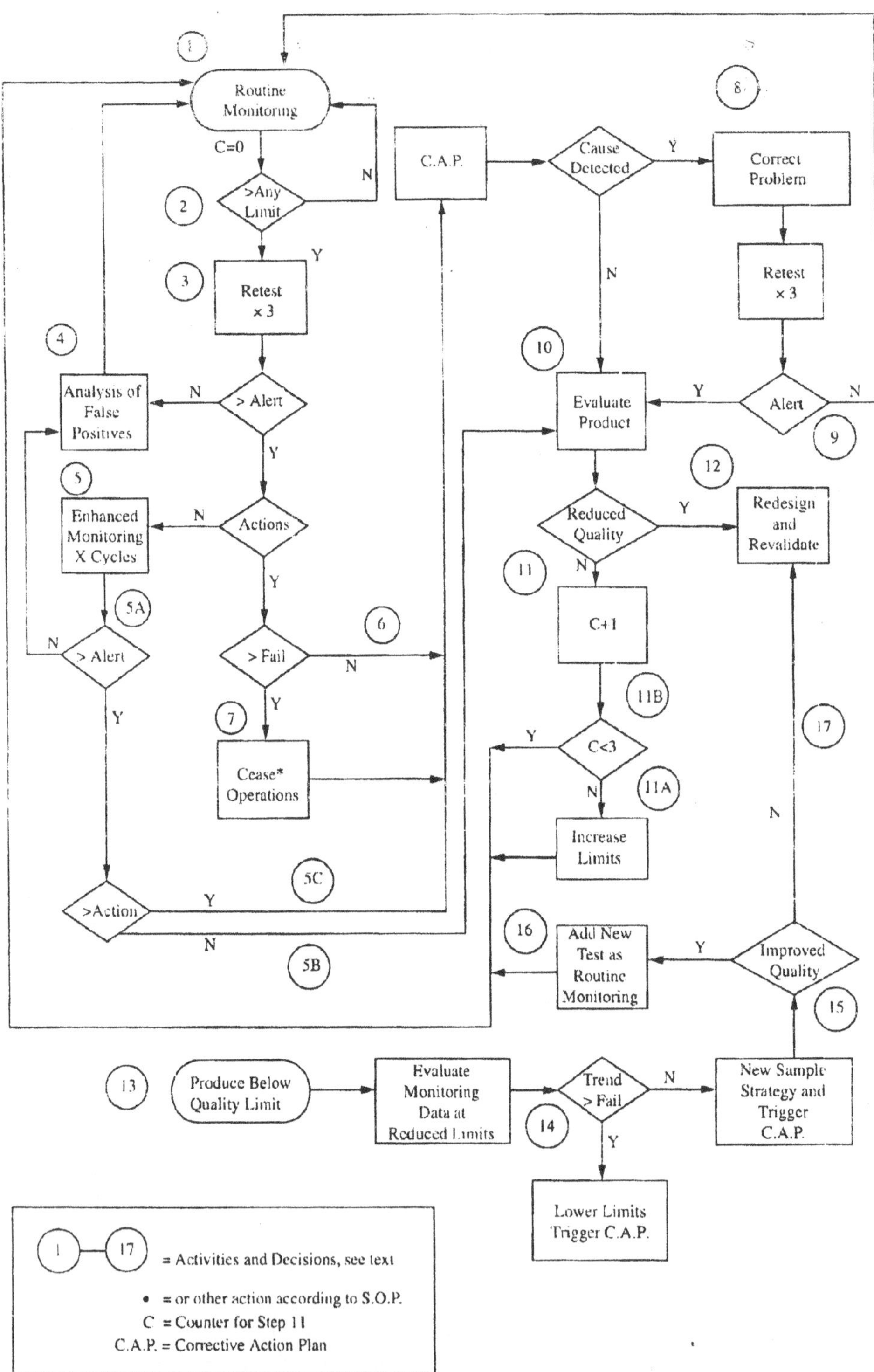

Fig. 17.1. Evaluation of monitoring plan and limits.

forming units (CFUs) that fall outside the star pattern of jet indentations in the agar surface below the holes. Counts >20 CFUs may also be statistically corrected for increased accuracy by using the positive-hole correction table.

It is recommended that colony counts be made at several points in the incubation process, with separate tallies for bacterial and fungal colonies that tend to merge at a critical point during incubation, when fungal colonies may overgrow and obscure bacterial colonies. For this reason, any bacterial subcultures should be made prior to the onset of rapid fungal growth. Whenever possible, optical electronic colony counters with sufficient backlighting and magnification to enhance contrast and enumeration should be employed to increase accuracy. In the presence of known or potentially high counts, the microscope enumeration method should be used to closely differentiate and count microcolonies in impact areas on sample plates following a short incubation period.

Developing A Monitoring Plan

Site Selection

A critical site is a point at which the product is exposed to the environment, when something is added to the product or product pathway, or a point at which unprotected product is manipulated. Any intervention into the process line increases the potential for contamination. (Examples of line interventions include the introduction, removal, or manipulation of materials and product, equipment adjustments, and sampling activities.) Particular attention should be given to these sites and events in the development of the monitoring plans.

Analysis of a videotape of repetitive prequalification should be studied for behavior and practices that may produce or harbor environmental contamination, leading to the refinement and optimization of work practices, and development of the formalized process to be instituted for the PQ validation run. The videotape may be used for identifying indicator sites, which should be incorporated into the monitoring plans, and intensively sampled during the validation run. These tapes should be retained and edited for both training and informational purposes.

For critical processes, it is important to select noninvasive sampling methods that have high collection efficiency for a broad range of organisms. To select the most suitable monitoring methods and equipment, the probable route of contamination for each critical site or process should be identified. For example, when the most likely route of potential contamination is touch, select surface sampling techniques for personnel barriers. When the most likely route is transfer from contaminated work surfaces, sampling of these surfaces is most useful. At sites where unprotected product is exposed to the environment, aerobiological monitoring is indicated, and, in unidirectional airflow, must be carried out isokinetically and isoaxially in the manner of non-viable particle-count testing. Some processing steps may require multiple sampling methods.

Controlled support areas adjacent to critical areas are the essential interfaces in the transition from the general environment to the aseptic processing core. These areas should be adequately pressurized, facilitating a gradient flow of contaminants from cleaner to dirtier areas. Controlled staging, support, material storage areas, and work practices should be examined and indicator sites identified. Controlled areas should be maintained and monitored in accordance with guidelines and industry standards.

Personnel, Equipment, and Facility

Validation and monitoring of a process are normally divided into three main areas of concern: personnel, equipment, and facility.

The human factor is the greatest potential variable in any process. Uncontrolled variation in personal health and hygiene, barrier techniques, and aseptic technique may cause wide variation in contamination of controlled support areas and process materials during staging and preparation, as well as adventitious contamination of the aseptic process core and product. A suitable aseptic process, defining appropriate and standardized personal hygiene expectations, scrubbing and preparation techniques, barrier techniques, and operator techniques should be developed and challenged intensively during the PQ exercise. Personnel should periodically take both written and media-fill skill tests.

Ongoing monitoring for compliance with pertinent SOPs should then be conducted. Sampling of personnel barriers, such as gloves, shoe covers, hair cover, and gowns facilitates detection of potential "fallout" contaminants shed from personnel for evaluation of both barrier and aseptic techniques. This information may be useful in establishing required garb-change intervals, based upon measured garb-penetration times by endogenous contaminants. All accumulated data should be used periodically to develop a facility trend analysis which, in turn, modifies training and work practices as necessary.

All equipment used in controlled manufacturing or compounding processes should be designed, staged, and sanitized in a manner that facilitates unvarying routine operation, with minimal human intervention. This reduces the potential for random cross- contamination by operative personnel. Improperly sanitized or sterilized equipment or components are also a possible source of contamination. Monitoring of representative surfaces of process equipment should be carried out and documented.

Facility sampling should be carried out under both as-built and at-rest conditions during initial installation qualification (IQ) and operational qualification (OQ) of the facility, in order to baseline and "bracket" performance of the engineering controls, and to identify the normal background flora present in the manufacturing environment. Sampling should then be conducted in-process under operational conditions during the PQ, to identify the impact of the process and personnel on the product and environment. It is important to monitor the validation process during all shifts and throughout the shift. Sites should be standardized and selected by statistical models or grid profiling, based upon testing and monitoring requirements appropriate to the specific process.

Surface sampling is useful in verifying the effectiveness of housekeeping and sanitizing procedures. It may also provide an alert to poor materials preparation prior to introduction into the controlled environment, or to lapses in personnel technique or barrier use. Aerobiologic sampling is most useful when conducted in conjunction with a complete program for testing of the engineering control system. Recommended tests include the following:

1. Facility pressurization, which should be routinely monitored at recommended intervals;
2. High efficiency particulate air (HEPA) filter velocity anduniformity testing for laminar airflow, and volume in cubic ft/min (CFM) for conventional flow, including a determination of room installation air changes;
3. HEPA filter leak-integrity testing;
4. Non-viable particulate cleanliness testing; and
5. Smoke-tracer visualization for establishing the integrity of unidirectional-flow areas.

Periodic retesting of challenges 1–4 is required by some regulatory groups, with the interval determined by the nature of the process and product in a given area. Repeating Test 5 may be useful in evaluating failures and can be an extremely valuable training tool. Concomitant particle count testing may be useful in identifying contamination indicator sites.

Monitoring of laminar airflow workstations (LAFWs) requires a complete understanding of HEPA filtration system performance, and is frequently conducted in ways that do not yield useful information. When properly validated in accordance with Federal Standard 209, LAFWs provide air at the entrance plane which is far cleaner than Class 100. Testing to this cleanliness level would permit particulate contamination levels two orders of magnitude greater than during filter OQ validation testing. More important, the use of any apparatus that samples discrete locations in a unidirectional slip stream is unlikely to detect filter leakage because isoaxial and isokinetic sampling at the exact point of leakage would be required. Therefore, placement of a sampling probe upstream from the product is unreliable and an unnecessary threat to sterility. The only practical, in-process use of these instruments is to detect shifts in the amount of particles and microbiologic contaminants caused by the process at some point adjacent to or downstream from the product. Such a shift might signal a lapse in personnel technique, barrier use, or prestaging material preparation, or be caused by HEPA filter loading, which reduces airflow velocity.

Avoiding Sampling-Induced False Positives

Line interventions for sampling purposes must be balanced carefully against the total number of interventions necessary for production purposes. Sampling should present the minimum risk of contamination, which is theoretically the same for every line intervention. Because sampling-induced positives should not exceed 10% of total positives ($10^{-1}N_p$), the number of sampling interventions should be significantly lower than the number of production line interventions. In isolators or other isolated critical processes, where no line interventions occur during production, not more than one, carefully controlled, aseptic sampling intervention is recommended.

Surface sampling the exterior of finished products, as indicator sites, assembled from purportedly sterile components as they exit the process while still under aseptic conditions, may be a more efficacious method of estimating microbiologic contamination potential than invading the critical production site. This method allows sampling the most critical site adjacen to the product, and more sites may be non-invasively sampled over a longer interval. In addition, this method may substantially reduce the incidence of sampling- induced contamination.

Monitoring Frequency

The frequency of monitoring should be determined by the maximum interval acceptable for an over-limit condition to remain undetected. This depends upon the critical nature of the process within the monitored area. In general, the minimum frequency should be consistent with applicable regulatory guidelines. Although it has been suggested that monitoring frequency can be reduced if no over-limit condition is detected within a predetermined number of monitoring cycles, this practice is inconsistent with basic monitoring rationale. Monitoring is conducted to detect a breakdown in process controls, which may occur at any time. Even if no control component has failed for a prolonged period, it must be assumed that a failure will occur eventually and must be detected within the predetermined interval. In addition, lack of over- limit test results may be due to the fact that monitoring method(s) are not sufficiently sensitive, or that limits are too high.

Evaluation of the Monitoring Plan and Limits

Most discussions of microbiologic monitoring recommend that the monitoring plan and limits be based on historical data, but offer little guidance on how this can be accomplished. An in-depth evaluation may be triggered by over-limit results from monitoring or by adverse product testing results without detection of any over- limit condition through routine monitoring.

Entry point 1

1. Conduct routine monitoring. A counter (C) is used for Step 11. $C \leftarrow 0$ at the beginning of the routine monitoring program.
2. If the results do not exceed any limit, then continue routine monitoring.
3. If the results exceed any limit, then perform retesting in triplicate to verify the accuracy of results. Retest under the same conditions noted on the sampling form (i.e., same time of day, same location and operator, same type of production).

4. If triplicate retest results are not over-limit, it is assumed that the original over-limit result was due to a non-assignable cause (*NAC*). Determine the probable cause of the over-limit count (i.e., unusual activities noted on test documentation, sampling, lab error, etc.). A record of positive NACs should be kept and analyzed to determine ways to improve affected processes and sampling procedures. Return to routine monitoring.
5. If results are over an alert limit, but not over the action limit, then enhance monitoring frequency for X cycles. (X is determined by the critical level of the area and process where the over-limit event occurred but should provide an adequate interval to assure detection of a continued deterioration of process control.)
   (a) If the alert limit is not exceeded again within X cycles, then return to Step 4.
   (b) If the alert limit is exceeded but the action limit is not, then proceed to Step 10.
   (c) If the action limit is exceeded, then go to the corrective action plan (CAP).
6. If results following the triplicate retesting are over the action limit, but not the fail limit, then go to the CAP.
7. If the results following the triplicate resting are over the fail limit, traditional QA protocols usually require that operations cease. However, the appropriate action taken should depend on the critical nature of the monitored step and other conditions. An alternative to operation shut down may be to segregate and hold the product for enhanced testing for adverse effect; go to the CAP.
8. If implementation of the CAP results in the determination of the cause of the over-limit condition, then correct the condition, and retest in triplicate to verify that the problem was corrected. If no cause was found, then proceed to Step 10.
9. If test results following corrective action are within limits, then return to routine monitoring.
10. If test results following corrective action are still over-limit, or if no cause of the over-limit condition can be identified, then evaluate the product for adverse effects.
11. If no adverse impact on product quality can be detected, add 1 to the counter (*C*). The result may indicate that limits are too low, but one event is not sufficient to support a decision to increase limits.
    (a) If C = 3, then the limits are too sensitive, and should be increased.
    (b) If C = <3, return to routine monitoring, Because the results are over-limit at this point, a repeat investigation of the cause of over-limit results will be triggered. Limits should be increased judiciously, and it is important to be thorough in attempting to resolve any cause of over-limit testing with reasonable certainty before increasing limits. For example, if the cause of the over-limit result is sampling mistakes or lab error, there will be no detectable cause in the production facility, the process or engineering control evaluations, and probably no adverse effect on product quality. This should not, however, be interpreted to mean that limits are too sensitive.
12. If product is adversely affected, and no cause can be detected following implementation of the CAP, the monitoring plan and/or the process should be redesigned and revalidated.

Entry point 2:

13. If product quality is below limits, but monitoring data did not detect the shift, then reevaluate monitoring data using lower limits to determine whether or not the process shift could have been detected. If the data have been graphically represented, this should be quite simple; increasing the amplitude of the graph may be useful.
14. If lower limits would have detected the shift, then lower the limits and institute the CAP

15. If lower limits would not have detected the shift, then evaluate the cause of the failure, and develop a new sampling strategy for the key step(s) where failure occurred. Institute the CAP and verify that corrective actions taken were effective in improving product quality.
16. If product quality improves, then add the new sampling method to the routine monitoring program.
17. If it does not, return to Step 12.

Selection of Monitoring Methods, Materials, and Equipment

Effective microbiologic monitoring of controlled processes usually includes sampling of process air for aerobiologic contamination, and facility, equipment, and operative personnel barriers for surface contamination. Equipment and methods used in monitoring procedures must be carefully considered for attributes and limitations and must be matched to sampling objectives to ensure that methods and techniques are non-invasive, and to facilitate development of well- organized sampling plans, techniques, data, and data trending analysis.

Surface Sampling

Surface sampling may be performed at the conclusion of critical operations to minimize disruption of these processes and prior to sanitizing procedures to estimate cumulative, inprocess contaminant burden. In addition, presanitization surface sampling is beneficial in detecting operations-induced bioburden and cross-contamination between environmental and equipment surfaces. Postsanitization surface sampling is useful for evaluating sanitizing methods and in retrieving sanitization-resistant isolates for identification and trend analysis in demonstrating sanitizing compound efficacy. The two most common types of surface sampling are swab-sampling, and surface contact sampling.

Swab-sampling

Swab-sampling is normally used for flat or irregular, non-absorbent surfaces with qualitative development by inoculation of the swab matrix directly into nutrient broth, observed for growth/no growth. Quantitative development is also possible. The main advantage of the swab method is accessibility to difficult-to-reach equipment surfaces and areas of the production environment. Limitations are excessive time consumption, increased potential for adventitious contamination due to the cumbersome nature of the procedure, and failure of enumeration processes to correlate to full recovery of organisms.

Contact plates

Surface contact plates are normally used for sampling flat or irregular, absorbent or non-absorbent surfaces. The surface contact plate consists of a clear plastic base housing a convex protrusion of nutrient agar with a plastic cover. Sampling is accomplished by pressing the agar against the site.

The covered plate is then incubated for development, and the CFUs per square centimeter enumerated. Advantages of surface contact plates are reproducibility, speed, simplicity of collection mechanism, and minimized potential for adventitious contamination; collection and correlation to recovery of organisms are superior to swab-sampling.

Aerobiologic Sampling

Aerobiologic sampling is conducted in critical and controlled areas to detect airborne viable contaminants present during manufacturing operations. Aerobiologic sampling procedures, frequency, and limits should be established based upon environmental conditions required to maintain product quality, and established for each processing step. Aerobiologic sampling employs two basic methodologies:

1. The gravity settle plate, which provides passive measurement of microorganisms likely to deposit by sedimentation at critical and controlled sites within a given period, and
2. The volumetric air sampler, which provides active measurement of viable contaminants by mechanical aspiration and dynamic inoculation of process air.

Gravity settle plates

The gravity settle plate measures microorganisms settling from the air onto a known surface area in a known time. Settle plates may be positioned within the critical area at indicator sites where the product may become exposed to airborne contamination, and in controlled areas at locations identified as likely sources or areas of "fallout" aerobiologic contamination. Settle plates are not appropriate aerobiologic sampling method for monitoring the efficiency of unidirectional (laminar) airflow or other air-cleaning devices. This is based upon studies, and the general assumption that "...the settling velocity of contaminants (in unidirectional airflow) is negligible, which implies that gravitation plays an inferior role. With the assumption of a constant value of the diffusion coefficient, the diffusion equation in a velocity field within rectangular coordinates becomes

$$\frac{\partial_c}{\partial_t} + \upsilon_X \frac{\partial_c}{\partial_X} + \upsilon_y \frac{\partial_c}{\partial_Y} + \upsilon_z \frac{\partial_c}{\partial_Z} = D\left(\frac{\partial_c^2}{\partial_X^2} + \frac{\partial_c^2}{\partial_Y^2} + \frac{\partial_c^2}{\partial_Z^2}\right) \quad \text{...(1)}$$

where c is concentration: υ_x, υ_y, υ_z are velocities in the x, y, and z directions: and D is diffusion coefficient.

This gives the simplest possible mathematical model which describes a system with regard to transport of contaminants emitted in a source of an arbitrary position...,'' demonstrating that particle dispersion in undisturbed streamlines is primarily a function of streamline uniformity and velocity. Disruptions of the parallel (laminar) airflow streamlines caused by equipment, personnel movement, and product result in turbulent flow, creating small and temporary vortices and eddies. It is only turbulent diffusion within the vortex that causes removal of entrained contaminants. Therefore settle plates, strategically placed, are reported to provide a superior method of predicting potential product contamination by mimicking the deposition of microbe-carrying particles (MCPs) into or onto the product. They are inexpensive, may be used to continuously monitor the entire production interval, are less invasive of aseptic operations, and may usually be placed closer to exposed products than volumetric air samplers.

Settle plates cannot be used for quantitative measurement of airborne microorganisms because the sample volume of sedimentation air samples cannot be measured. Air turbulence around an open plate may also effect collection results, and smaller particles may not settle at all. In addition, extended exposure times may result in some desiccation of the nutrient agar, resulting in poor microbial growth.

Volumetric air samplers

As an active sampling method, the volumetric air sampler aspirates a known volume of process air, capturing microorganisms into or onto a nutrient agar medium, a liquid, or a filter. Microorganisms are developed and quantified as an estimate of CFUs present in the sampled environment per cubic foot of air (or other volumetric measurement). The quantitative principles of volumetric (active) air sampling may be expressed by

$$S\,(R_t)\,C = R_f \quad \text{...(2)}$$

where S is source intensity, R_t is transport rate, C is correction factor, and R_f is failure rate.

Volumetric air sampling is accomplished by a number of different methodologies, including impingement, impaction through single or multiple orifices, centrifugal impaction, and filtration. Each method has inherent advantages and disadvantages that affect the value of the data collected relative to the specific application.

Impingement

In an impinger, a known volume of air is drawn through fluid in a glass vessel. Particles separate from the airstream by impinging at the flask bottom, where they are stopped and retained by the liquid as the air continues to flow out through the pump system. High air velocities passing through the impinger effectively break up bacterial/particulate aggregates, resulting in microbial counts, which more closely reflect the actual number of microorganisms, leading to recommendations that impingers be used as the standard reference method for monitoring aerobiologic contamination. However, impingers may require the addition of antifoam agents and replacement of fluid, due to agitation and evaporation loss during longer sampling procedures.

These additional steps increase the possibility of adventitious contamination. It has been demonstrated that the sampling efficiency of an impinger is dependent upon both system design and the particle sizes being sampled. Accuracy and reproducibility of results have been reported to be difficult, and particles of $<5.0\ \mu m$ have been demonstrated to pass through the impingers tested.

Impaction

In slit-to-agar (STA) or sieve impactors, a known volume of air is aspirated through a single orifice (STA), or multiple orifices (sieve), and viable particles, due to their inertia, are forced out of inlet airflow streamlines and impacted onto perpendicular, target nutrient agars as the streamlines abruptly change direction to bypass the target stage. In the centrifugal impaction sampler, high centrifugal forces created by "spinning" air through an impeller turbine at sufficient velocities to cause separation of microorganisms from sample air streamlines result in their impaction onto a nutrient agar strip placed at the inner periphery of the sampling chamber, parallel to the inlet airflow axis.

Sieve impactors are available in single-stage or multistage designs that facilitate both enumeration and sizing of aerobiological contaminants. As the sample air transits the device, sample velocities increase at each stage, resulting in gradient deposition and accurate sizing of microorganisms of smaller diameters and lower mass. Microorganisms aspirated by sieve samplers through a matrix of multiple-inlet orifices impact directly onto an agar medium for development from a single agar plate for each vertically stacked stage, with no further subculture steps required for enumeration. Advantages of sieve samplers are generally high particle deposition rates, the ability to size particles and vary sampling time and volume, and superior collection efficiencies when compared to other methods of aerobiological testing. Single- and six-stage configurations have been reported to be two of the three sampling methods of choice.

Use of STA samplers in isolators and critical process zones should be accomplished using a sterile sampling hose and probe, facilitating remote location of the sampler in a non-critical area. In monitoring a unidirectional slipstream, this hose/probe configuration should be both isoaxially oriented, and isokinetic, in order to minimize disruption of the slipstream. Advantages of the STA include the ability to revolve the plate at varying rates so that the samples may demonstrate changes in aerobiological concentrations directly over time, and the ability to obtain multiple samples with a single petri dish. STA samplers have historically been the standard against which other air samplers are assessed. Agar plates are easily removed from the sampler for development, with contamination enumerated as CFUs per unit of air sampled.

The STA is reported to be both unsuitable for use in the presence of high concentrations of organisms and cumbersome to use. In addition, it has been demonstrated that a significantly higher percentage of particles sized 0.5–0.8 μm, and a significantly lower percentage of particles sized 3.0–25.0 μm, were present in sample air, which had passed through the slit of an STA, than were found in ambient air. This was attributed to fragmentation of larger particles following passage through the slit of the STA.

Due to dehydration of the agar reported to occur over long sampling periods, continuous sampling exceeding 30 min using an impaction sampler is not recommended. Areas of loss have been reported for sieve samplers, including *inlet loss* (the effect of cross-wind at the sample inlet point), *interstage loss* (deposition of particles on internal surfaces other than the impaction agar), and *particle re-entrainment* (particles reintroduced into the airstream due to particle "bounce," resulting from dehydration of the impaction agar)

Advantages of the centrifugal sampler are the capability of sampling large amounts of air (40 L/min) in a short time; it is quiet, lightweight, self-contained, and does not require cumbersome air pumps or external power for operation. Centrifugal samplers provide a good indication of environmental isolates.

Centrifugal sampling cannot be carried out isokinetically, and the accuracy of results is dependent upon the sizes of the particles being sampled. Since particulate sizes in the air volume being sampled are not routinely determined, the validity of the centrifugal sampler as a quantitative device has been called into question, especially for quantification of small particles. Another recent study indicates that centrifugal sampling causes air to move in a turbulent, mixing manner, introducing heavily disturbed airflow patterns around the sampler which may, in turn, impart disturbances to any unidirectional airflow patterns being sampled. Reaspiration of sampled air is also a problem with earlier designs, creating difficulty in discriminating between incoming and outgoing airstreams, which is necessary to quantify microorganisms. Proprietary agar medium strips are specially designed and unique to this system, and require careful technique to insert and remove aseptically.

Membrane filtration

Membrane filtration (MF) sampling is accomplished by capturing aerobiological contamination as it passes through a cellulose membrane filter (CMF) or gelatin membrane filter (GMF). The mechanisms of MF particle removal are inertial impaction, diffusional interception, and direct interception. Following collection, the GMF may be plated aseptically onto an agar petri dish to dissolve, allowing microorganisms to grow directly on the nutrient medium. Dissolution of the membrane into a sterile solution is also possible.

While MF sampling has been demonstrated to be the most effective means of retaining aerobiological contamination, CMF sampling exhibits a lower recovery rate than an impinger when tested against stress-sensitive microorganisms, such as *Serratia marcescens* or *Escherichia coli* due to desiccation on the CMF surface. Studies have indicated that gelatin foam filters incorporated into GMF gave significantly higher recovery rates than CMF over the same sampling period. Recent comparisons of sampling systems indicate that GMF is equally as effective as the STA sampler, irrespective of particle size, and is significantly more effective than centrifugal sampling in the collection of microorganisms with sizes $<5.0\ \mu m$. A recent study comparing the GMF system with centrifugal, sieve, and STA systems in sampling the unidirectional airflow slipstream in the presence of visual tracers indicates the GMF sampler to be the only sampling method capable of isokinetic and isoaxial samplng with novisual disturbance to the laminar airflow pattern. However, in this study, the STA was tested without the remote hose-isokinetic probe device.

Limitations of the GMF are an additional aseptic subculture step, which increases the probability of adventitious contamination, and a proprietary membrane filter, which results in a per-sample cost currently exceeding 12 times that of the one-stage sieve, SAS, STA, SMA, and glass impinger systems, and four times that of the centrifugal sampler.

Growth Media

Growth and collection media used in microbiologic monitoring should be selected on the basis of the target organisms, areas and surfaces sampled, and inhibitory residues that may remain on the sampled surfaces. Under certain circumstances (e.g., when obligate anaerobes are recovered from the product), additional, specific media and methods should be selected by a qualified microbiologist.

Comparison of Aerobiologic Samplers

The different characteristics and operating principles of aerobiological samplers do not facilitate direct and simple comparisons. The user should, therefore, carefully evaluate the numerous advantages and disadvantages of each method in selecting a sampler for the intended application. Two studies that provide basic comparisons of aerobiological sampling systems may offer useful information: A study comparing eight bioaerosol samplers was carried out by Jensen et al. in 1992. Results indicated that the Andersen 6-STG, I-STG, and Ace Glass AGI 30 samplers were the samplers of choice for recovering aerosols of free bacteria (i.e., mostly single cells of *E. coli* and *B. subtilis*, $d_{ae} \geq 2$ μm) under the controlled conditions of the study. Another study, comparing seven samplers commonly used in controlled environments, was conducted by Ljungqvist and Reinmiiller in 1998. This study indicated widely varying results for the impaction samplers tested. The limited number of parallel tests performed prevented an evaluation of comparative collection efficiencies based upon statistical considerations. The salient recommendations of this study are that results should be seen more "... as an indication of a [contamination] level and not be taken as a true absolute value," and that aerobiological samplers be selected carefully, based on practicalities of using different types for different locations or situations. Furthermore, this study recommends the simultaneous use of a discrete particle counter (DPC) to measure the total number of airborne particles present in the area sampled.

Analysis and Interpretation of Monitoring Results

Effective interpretation of data from microbiologic monitoring of the environment can be the most difficult aspect of the monitoring process. Several factors complicate this process, including the inherently nonrandom distribution of most microbial contamination events, errors in sample handling, variation of sampling technique from one monitoring event to the next, and seasonal shifts in the type and level of contaminants likely to be present in the general environment. The purpose of statistical evaluation of sample data is to extrapolate from a collection of individual events to the entire population of events (e.g., 8-h shift). Because microbial monitoring data usually measure the impact of human activity, which is not reproducible exactly from one event to the next, results usually do not fit standard statistical models for normal distributions. In spite of this limitation, it is necessary to summarize the data for comparison to limits. The best statistical methods of evaluation are determined by the nature of the data. Wilson suggests that microbial monitoring data histograms generally resemble Poisson or negative exponential distributions, whereas Akers points out that Poisson distributions may only be appropriate for systems with minimal human intervention. The formula for the Poisson distribution is given by

$$P(C) = \frac{(np_0)^c}{C!} e^{-}np_0 \qquad \ldots(3)$$

where C is individual sample count, np_0 is average count, and $e = 2.718281$.

Trend analysis of results at individual sample locations may be more useful than statistical analysis of data summaries because each sampling location probably reflects a unique situation. Non-traditional groupings of data may also be valuable. For example, grouping all locations where a specific activity was noted on the sample collection form, grouping all data collected during a specific time frame (i.e., just after lunch, or near the end of a production cycle), or grouping all data for each operator may reveal specific problem areas. The example demonstrate four major types of out-of-control patterns. A fifth pattern is due to mistakes, which will usually show up as isolated, out-of-control points. All apply equally to production and sampling operations. All patterns may be observed on both range (R) charts and standard process average charts but are usually more common to charts. Likely causes for each type of pattern can be identified, and a checklist of assignable causes applicable to the particular process should be developed through cause and effect (C&E) analysis. Examples of likely causes for these patterns are:

1. A change or jump in pattern caused by an inexperienced operator, a change in raw materials, or a failure of an equipment part;
2. A trend or steady change in level due to a gradual change in the production environment, a gradual change in equipment performance (e.g. HEPA filter loading), or a gradual tendency toward lax observation of SOPs;
3. Two populations may be due to more than one process line or piece of critical equipment on the same chart, more than one operator on the same chart, or different samplers or sampling techniques; and
4. Recurring cycles may be caused by periodic operator rotation, operator fatigue and rejuvenation cycles, sanitizing and cleaning cycles, and seasonal shifts.

Recurring cycles may be missed if sampling intervals happen to coincide with the cycle frequency, in which case only the low or high range of the cycle may be detected. Out-of-limit trends near the lower limits of the R chart represent superior performance and should be analyzed to identify methods of maintaining these process levels Whatever statistical methods are employed for summarizing data, graphic representations, such as histograms and process control charts can be extremely useful for detecting trends or cyclic patterns in test results.

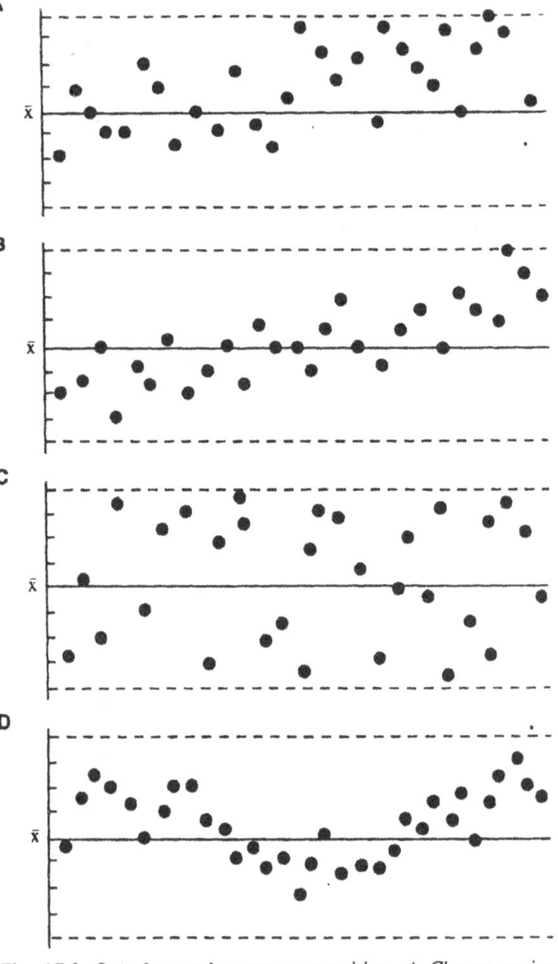

Fig. 17.2. Out-of-control pattern recognition. A-Change or jump in level; B-Trend or steady change in level; C-Two populations; D-Recurring cycles.

There are two types of over-limit results: *Random* results are due to chance (unassignable) causes, whereas *non-random* results are due to assignable causes. For a controlled process and facility, the objective is to differentiate between individual data points that are assignable and those that are not. If the individual over-limit event is not repeated during subsequent, multiple retests, it is not assignable and does not represent a deteriorating trend. All statistical evaluation methods include mechanisms for "discarding" spurious data. There is, however, a cause for any unassignable result, and efforts should be made to identify and understand it. All data have meaning, and may be useful for improving the process or testing procedures.

Speciation

Speciation of microorganisms is indicated when product testing results detect the presence of a specific organism, when evaluating the efficacy of sanitizing compounds and routines, and when monitoring results trigger the corrective action plan. Speciation should be carried out and analyzed by a qualified microbiologist familiar with the sampling equipment, sampling methods employed, and the origins of organisms commonly found in cleanrooms. Speciation should also be conducted periodically to identify isolates normally recovered when the process is operating within limits, and may be useful in identifying the probable cause(s) of any out-of-limit condition. During the initial phase of the corrective action plan, an analysis of probable contamination sources and routes should be made for all organisms identified. Information obtained by speciation may immediately indicate the most likely source. This information may also indicate less common contamination sources, such as perverted cleaning solutions.

Periodic re-evaluation of the monitoring plan should be carried out, and seasonal effects considered in trend analysis. Many sampling methods do not col-lect all organisms with equal efficiency, and organisms likely to be present may vary seasonally. Any seasonal shift (up or down) should be investigated by speciation, and sampler correction factors for the predominant organisms applied.

Corrective Action Plan

The CAP should clearly define and document

1. The method of data analysis;
2. Alert, action, and fail limits;
3. Corrective actions to be employed in the event of detection of a deteriorating trend or an over-limit condition; and
4. A means of confirming the effectiveness of corrective action(s).

A verified trend above the action or fail limit should immediately trigger implementation of the CAP. Because human activity is the most likely source of process control failure, the investigative process normally begins with personnel, and proceeds through the various possible causes from most to least likely. An exception to this general plan is verification of room pressurization, which is a primary indication of engineering control equipment efficiency. Although routine monitoring of pressurization should detect any out-of-limit results, the simplicity of verifying proper pressurization suggests this as a first step. In general, the cause of any deterioration in process or environmental control can be traced to one of three principle systems: (a) personnel controls; (b) process controls; or (c) facility (engineering) controls. Increases in detected airborne microbiologic contamination levels may result from any of several conditions, and a simple set of logical challenges can be applied to the data to determine the most likely cause.

Challenge 1, Is the increase real and reproducible? If it is not reproducible, it may be due to sampling error, or NACs. If it is reproducible, it may be due to an actual increase in levels, or due to enhanced collection efficiency, due to changes in methods, materials, or seasonal or other shifts in the kinds of contaminants present (different organisms have different sampling efficiencies); Challenge 2, If the increase is real, is it due to an increase in source intensity, or to a decrease in the ability of engineering controls to maintain a clean air supply? The easiest way to differentiate between these possibilities is to examine particle count data. There are several possible combinations of test results, each indicating a different cause for increased airborne contamination: (a) If particle counts taken under operational conditions have not risen, but airborne microbiologic contamination has, it is most likely due to a breakdown in personnel discipline and/or gowning procedures; (b) If operational particle counts have risen, but at-rest counts have not, it is again likely that the cause of elevated microbial contamination is personnel activity and that it represents an increase in source intensity (when human activity is eliminated, engineering controls are able to produce the same conditions that were present during the OQ validation phase); and (c) If at-rest particle counts have risen, the increase is probably due to a decrease in the efficiency of the engineering controls. Similar logical tests can be applied to increases in surface contamination levels, which may be due to increases in source intensity, or decreases in the efficiency of barrier controls or cleaning and sanitizing procedures. Flow charts illustrating the logical evaluation of data, and investigation of out-of-limit results are useful as starting points in the development of corrective action plans.

18

PRODUCT DEVELOPMENT

The development of a new chemical entity (NCE) usually undergoes various stages. Our knowledge of the physicochemical and biopharmaceutical properties of the molecule generally improves as it progresses through the development stages. Although many in vivo tests are carried out in drug discovery stage, main focus at this stage is the efficacy of the molecule rather than its development potential. Due to large number of molecules and limited physicochemical information, in-silico simulation based on structure or high-throughput experimental data is often used. However, the developability concept has become ever more important over the last decade, while biopharmaceutical properties are among the most important components. From preclinical development until proof of concept (PoC) initiation, pharmacokinetic (PK) testing is often carried out. PK of different physical forms, salts, and particle sizes of drug molecule can be evaluated in a preclinical animal model. This provides the first opportunity to correlate the in vitro measurement (i.e., dissolution of the molecule) to its in vivo performance, such as C_{max}, area under the concentration time curve (AUC) or deconvoluted, in vivo dissolution profiles. In vivo animal PK data of different physical forms, salts, and particle sizes or formulations also provide the first opportunity for the development of a biorelevant dissolution method. In a recent review published by Li et al., a decision tree for dissolution testing design based on biopharmaceutics classification system (BCS) and physicochemical properties of the molecule has been proposed. This

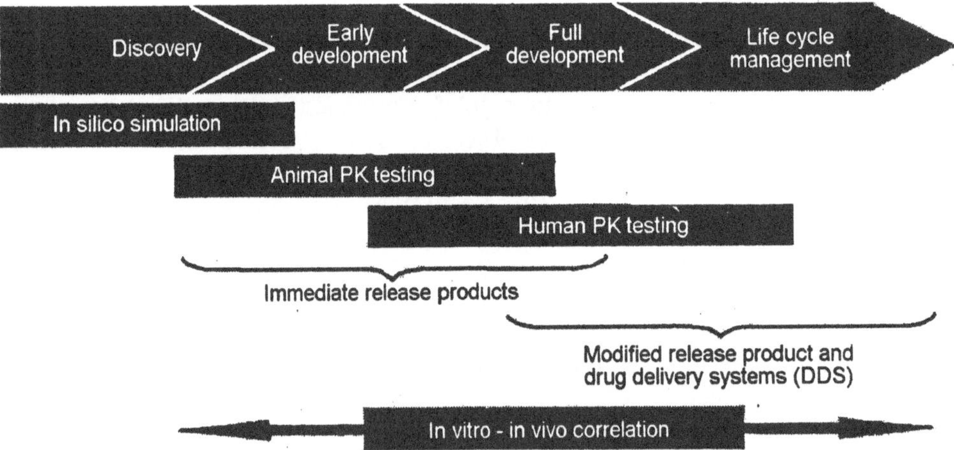

Fig. 18.1. Discovery and development phases of new chemical entity and application of in vitro - in vivo correlation in drug development process.

provides guidance on dissolution method setting, which can be further validated in full development once human PK data are available.

Since formulation development and optimization at a later stage rely on the dissolution method established early on, it is essential the selection of the dissolution method is as meaningful and relevant as possible. When clinical data on different formulations or different particle sizes of the drug substance are available, additional investigations can be performed to verify whether the dissolution test method need be modified or challenged. There is a tremendous scientific and practical value when an in vitro–in vivo correlation (IVIVC) can be established using human PK data, but this often involves a cross-functional team of scientists from formulation, dissolution, and clinical PK development. A significant amount of information is already available in the literature, and successful IVIVCs have been demonstrated for modified release (MR) formulations, on the basis of the 1997 Food and Drug Administration guidelines in which the procedure and acceptance criteria for a successful IVIVC has been clearly defined. In the life-cycle management (LCM) stage of drug development, IVIVC is even more important and has to be considered as part of the development strategy for MR or alternative delivery systems including parental depot, transdermal patch, and so on. Several such successful cases have been reported by Young in this area.

In the authors' opinion, application of IVIVC in new drug development process can be achieved in a four-tier approach. In silico simulation based on compound structure and limited physicochemical information can be performed in drug discovery stage to rank order the absorption potential of a molecule (Tier 1), followed by correlating in vitro dissolution with its in vivo performance in preclinical setting (Tier 2), the dissolution method developed at this stage can be further validated using human PK data (Tier 3), and finally, human PK data from various sources can be systematically utilized to establish a valid IVIVC model to further support future formulation development during life cycle management (Tier 4). The four-tier approach is proposed based on stages of NCE product development. As discussed earlier, IVIVC development is an evolving process, which should be perfected through product development and it is important that such a concept be applied to product development as early as possible.

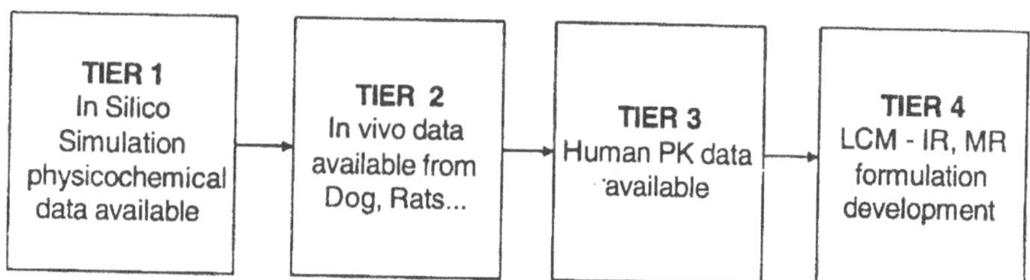

Fig. 18.2. Four-tier approach for in vitro - in vivo correlation development. Abbreviations: PK, pharmacokinetic; LCM, life cycle management; IR, immediate release; MR, modified release.

BACKGROUND

Categories of In Vitro–In Vivo Correlation

Levels A, B, and C IVIVCs are clearly defined in regulatory guidances with the Level A correlation, as point-to-point correlation, which considers complete in vivo and in vitro profiles being the preferred correlation. In the Level A correlation, there is no omission of information from either in vivo or in vitro data. A convoluted plasma concentration profile can be calculated from an in vitro dissolution profile. The benefit of such a correlation includes, amongst other things, the possibility to replace a bioequivalence study with comparative in vitro dissolution data. To develop a valid Level A correlation that can be accepted by the agency for so-called biowaivers, an IVIVC model needs to be developed for at least two formulations, with three or more formulations being preferred. The formulations should have significant differences in their in vitro and in vivo behavior. Validation (i.e., internal and external predictability of the model) also needs to be demonstrated.

The United States Pharmacopeia (USP) also refers to the above-mentioned categories, but does not mention internal and external predictability. Some references describe Level A correlation that consider only one formulation, which do not allow the model to be applied to other formulations or more batches of the same formulations. In this respect, many IVIVC categorized as Level A are not recognized by the regulatory agency. Such correlations, nevertheless, help to assist in the dissolution method development and have the potential to be developed into a true Level A correlation which can be recognized by the agency.

In the case of Level B correlations, the entire course of in vitro and in vivo profiles are also considered, with the information in the profiles reduced to a single parameter. Level B correlation is carried out where the mean in vitro dissolution time is compared with the mean in vivo dissolution time or mean in vivo residence time. However, since the entire plasma concentration profile cannot be predicted based on in vitro dissolution data, the benefit of Level B correlation is therefore limited and is not accepted by authorities for biowaivers.

In the last category, Level C correlation, only one point is taken from the profiles. A typical example of a Level C correlation is the correlation of a percentage of drug released at a certain time point with C_{max}. Immediate release (IR) formulations of good water-soluble substances are usually characterized by this manner. For MR formulations and IR products with less water-soluble drug substance, correlation of partial AUC with drug release at certain time point is rational, since in this case, the dissolution process is usually longer than the gastrointestinal (GI) transit time of the pharmaceutical form, and AUC can be reduced because the drug is not being fully released. In early formulation development stage, a Level C correlation can provide valuable information. In the later phase of development and after process transfer to production, its usefulness becomes limited because the entire plasma concentration profile cannot be predicted, unless a multiple Level C correlation can be established, under which scenario a Level A correlation also becomes very likely.

DEVELOPMENT OF IN VITRO-IN VIVO CORRELATIONS

Deconvolution

In the early days of IVIVC, it was suggested that a correlation should be implemented only for comparable data, where comparison was made between actual data measured in vitro, simulated in vivo data, and vice versa. Correlations are obtained when the in vivo plasma concentration profile is converted via mathematical modeling using model-dependent or model-independent deconvolution into the in vivo absorption profile. The in vivo absorption profile, which is often identical to the in vivo dissolution profile, is then used to establish an IVIVC.

Due to the intrinsic difference between dissolution conditions in vitro and in vivo, the in vitro dissolution profiles can be scaled by mathematical means, represented by Equation 1

$$X_{vivo}(t) = a_1 + a_2 \times X_{vitro}(b_1 + b_2 \times t) \quad \text{if } t > T \text{ then } t = T$$
$$\text{if } b_1 < b_2 \times \text{t then } b_1 + b_2 \times t = 0 \qquad \ldots(1)$$

whereby $X_{vivo}(t)$ represents the absorption profile as a function of time and $X_{vitro}(t)$ represents the dissolution profile. The modifications to the in vitro profile as a function of time t is achieved by introduction of a time scale factor b_2, if the in vitro dissolution process occurs faster or slower than the corresponding in vivo dissolution; or through a lag time b_1 to allow an initial lag time in the in vivo absorption because of necessary preabsorption transit through the stomach; and of a cut-off factor T to accommodate dissolution slower than the GI transit times. The actual correlation is obtained via comparison of the in vivo profile with the scaled in vitro dissolution profile by a linear regression, which provides the slope a_2 and the intercept a_1 as a link function between both profiles.

The aforementioned calculation from the in vivo profile to the in vivo absorption/dissolution profile is known as deconvolution (output to input). The classical methods of deconvolution of plasma profiles include Wagner–Nelson, Loo–Riegelman and numerical deconvolution. The Wagner–Nelson method is a model-dependent method based on one-compartment model, it has a great advantage of not requiring additional in vivo data except oral plasma profile. The Loo–Riegelman method is based on two-compartment model, which requires intravenous dosing data. Model-independent numerical deconvolution requires in vivo plasma data from an oral solution or intravenous as impulse function for the application. All three methods have their limitations, but the requirement of additional data in addition to oral plasma data from a tablet or capsule significantly limit the application of the later two methods. There are numerous literature examples that use model-independent methods, Wagner–Nelson, or Loo–Riegelman methods. Convolution and deconvolution by means of excel sheets are also described by Langenbucher.

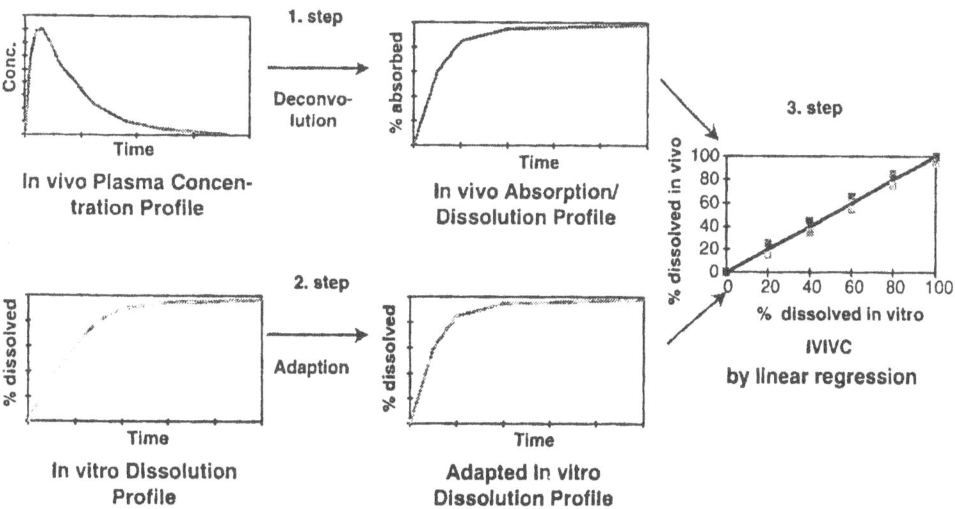

Fig. 18.3. The classical three steps of deconvolution.

Convolution

Conversion of the in vitro dissolution profile to a plasma concentration profile can take place via convolution (input to output). Recently, convolution methods have been established, which convolutes the in vitro dissolution profiles without implementing the correlation of the in vivo absorption/dissolution profile with the in vitro dissolution profile (i.e., physiology based model and simulation software). The model uses multiple differential equations representing various physiological events and convolution-based methods.

A major advantage of convolution-based methods for IVIVC is that no additional in vivo data such as intravenous injections or oral solutions are required. However, these methods can only mathematically fit the data by minimizing the squared error; even though the results obtained are mathematically correct it may not be meaningful PK or physiological models. A critical assessment of the calculated parameters is absolutely necessary. Further, the fitting procedure should be performed several times with different starting values, in order to avoid reaching a local minimum. Last but not the least, these methods should be optimized to as few variables as possible, as the fitting procedure becomes more complex and error-prone with more variables.

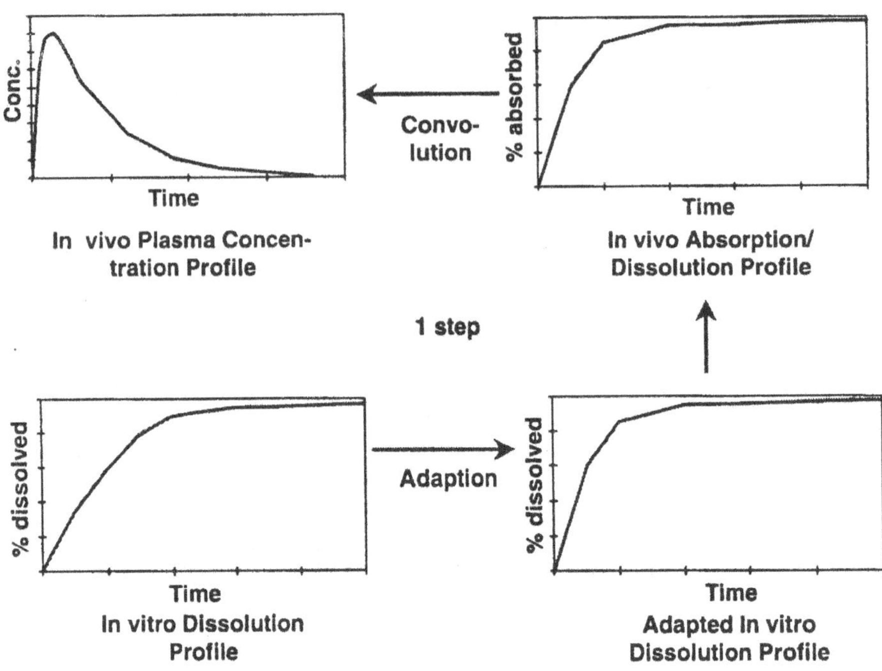

Fig. 18.4. The one-step procedure of a convolution.

Basic Principles of In Vitro–In Vivo Correlation

The in vitro dissolution and in vivo absorption/dissolution profiles play a key role in the development of an IVIVC. Characterization of these profiles warrants a detailed discussion. The cumulative dissolution curves can be well represented by parameters that describe extent of dissolution, time delays, and shape of the profile. The Weibull function depicted in Equation 2 is one of the models that is suitable for such purpose:

$$F(t) = F^{\infty} \cdot \left(1 - e^{((t+t_0)/\alpha)^{\beta}}\right)$$

where α represents the time at which 63.2% of the drug is dissolved, β is a shape factor that, at values below 1, yields a curve with an initially steep slope followed by a flat course; at a value equal to 1, it describes an exponential curve; and at values greater than 1, yields a curve with a sigmoidal shape. Various shape factors can also be interpreted as different release mechanisms. F^{∞} is the dissolved fraction of the dose after an infinite time. t_0 is lag time that considers the delayed start of dissolution process. A perfect correlation can be achieved if all parameters of the Weibull function of in vivo and in vitro profiles are identical.

For example, an in vitro dissolution profile has the following characteristics: $F^{\infty} = 100$, $t_0 = 0$, $\alpha = 1$, and $\beta = 0.5$; whereas the same formulation, when tested in vivo, its in vivo dissolution profile is characterized by the following Weibull parameters: $F^{\infty} = 100$, $t_0 = 0$, $\alpha = 1$, and $\beta = 1.5$. F^{∞}, t_0, and α have identical values, but β (shape factor) is distinctly different. When percentage dissolved in vivo is plotted against percentage dissolved in vitro, a nonlinear relationship deviating greatly from ideal linear curve is obtained. An IVIVC with linear correlation cannot be established.

Whenever appropriate, polynomial functions can be used to obtain nonlinear IVIVC. If there are factors other than in vivo dissolution contributing to the absorption, the usefulness of the IVIVC obtained by nonlinear regression can be very limited. The validity of the correlation has to be verified using

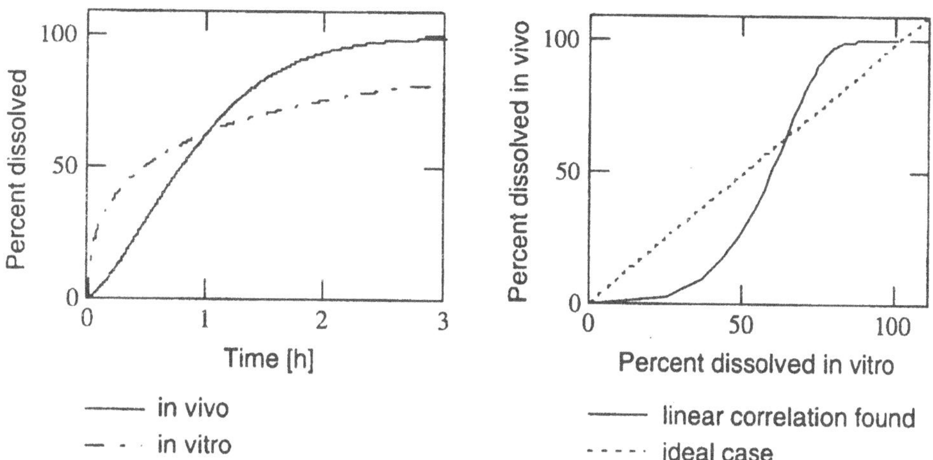

Fig. 18.5. In vitro and in vivo dissolution profiles with different shapes and their linear regression.

the internal and external prediction errors. One could also choose to modify the in vitro dissolution test condition to obtain improved, that is, linear IVIVC.

Similarity between in vitro and in vivo profiles in addition to time factor α is necessary for a successful IVIVC. In the example given earlier, the in vivo and in vitro profiles have the same time factor α. In most cases, however, the in vitro profile may be faster or slower than the in vivo profile. For instance, an in vivo profile ($F^{\infty} = 100$, $t_0 = 0$, $\alpha = 1$, and $\beta = 1.5$) is compared with an in vitro profile ($F^{\infty} = 100$, $t_0 = 0$, $\alpha = 0.2$, and $\beta = 1.5$). F^{∞}, t_0, and β have identical values, but the time factor α is distinctly different. When a time scale factor b_2 is used, which stretches the x-axis by a factor of 5, the in vitro profile can be scaled and fitted very well with the in vivo profile. Equation 3, which is a simplification of Equation 1 with $b_1 = 0$, $a_2 = 1$, and $a_1 = 0$, describes the mathematical relationship with $b_2 = 0.2$:

$$X_{vivo}(t) = X_{vitro}(b_2 \times t) \qquad \ldots(3)$$

The introduction of a time scale factor is acceptable as long as it is used for all formulations and for all further applications of the IVIVC model. The time scale factor can be determined by plotting the time needed for in vivo dissolution versus the time needed for in vitro dissolution of a particular

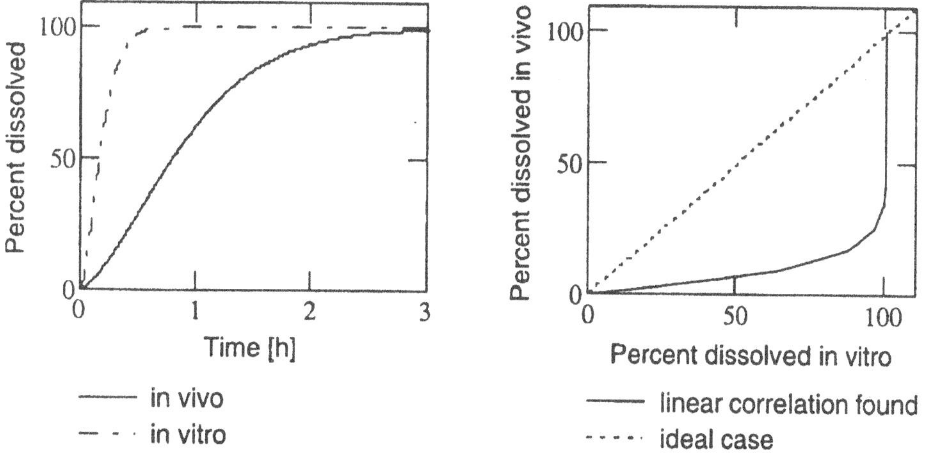

Fig. 18.6. Time scaled in vitro and in vivo dissolution profiles with different time factors and their linear regression.

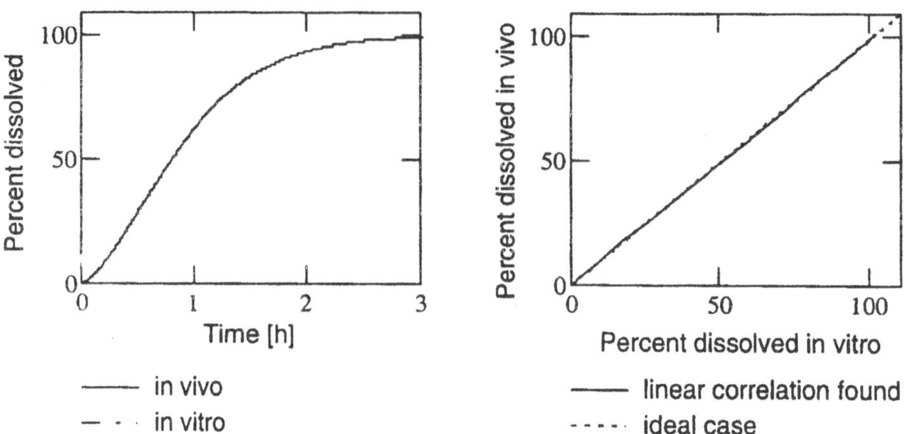

Fig. 18.7. Time-scaled in vitro and in vivo dissolution profiles with different time factors and their linear regression.

amount of drug from the dosage form (Levy plot). After linear regression forced through zero, the reciprocal of the slope of the regression line is the time factor one should use for IVIVC development.

Alternatively, the time scale factor can be calculated as the ratio of the time factors α of in vitro and in vivo Weibull fitted profiles, provided both profiles have an infinite dissolution F^{∞} of 100%.

$$b_2 = \frac{\alpha_{\text{in vitro}}}{\alpha_{\text{in vivo}}} \qquad \ldots(4)$$

Application of the time scale factor can be demonstrated by the following example. Various dissolution conditions were evaluated for an in vivo relevant method, where pH, the agitation speed, and ionic strength of the dissolution medium were varied. The dependence of dissolution on these variables is clearly demonstrated. The similar β values of all in vitro profiles with distinctly different time factors is evident. If a time scaling, based on Equation 4, is implemented for each individual in vitro profile, the time-scaled profiles shown in Figure 18.9 are obtained, where the profiles are almost matching with each other. All profiles obtained under these conditions are suitable in order to achieve an IVIVC, except time scale factors used are different.

Another example in determining the time factor using a Levy plot is shown in Figure 18.10, where the line

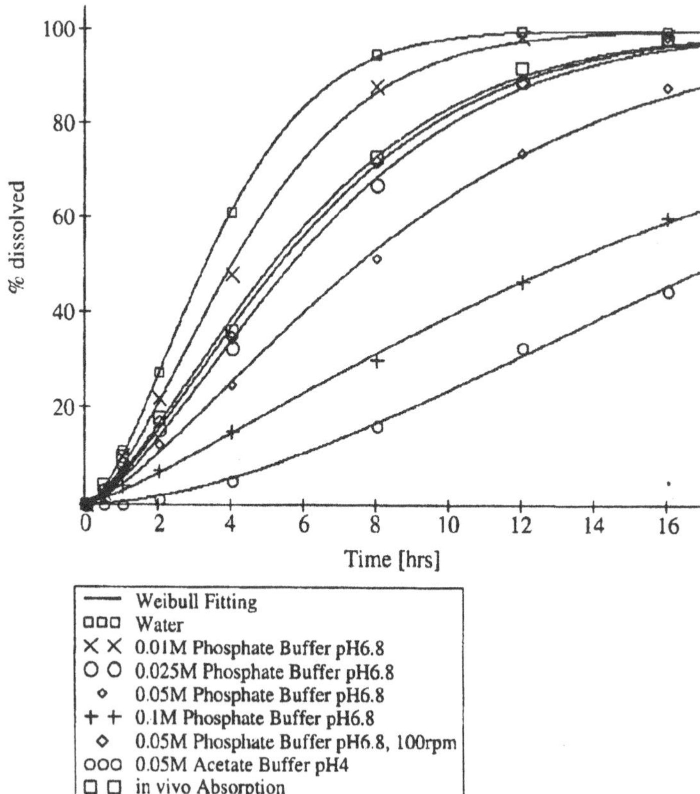

Fig. 18.8. Dissolution profiles depending on pH value, agitation speed, and ionic strength of the medium.

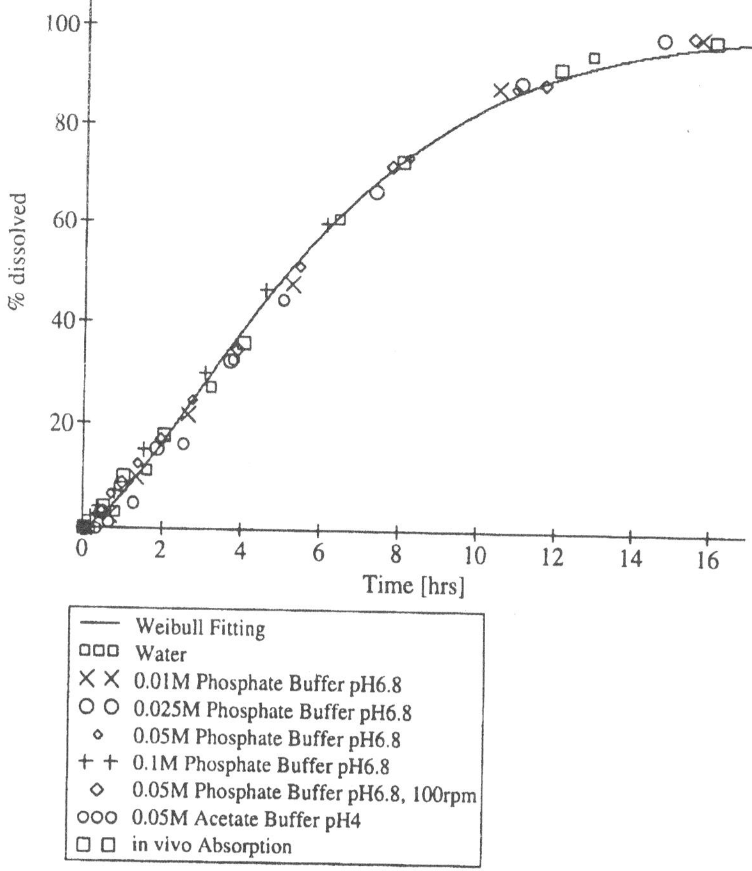

Fig. 18.9. Time scaled dissolution profiles.

deviates upwards after a specific time. Such phenomenon can be explained by the permeability or dissolution change on transit of formulation from the stomach to the intestine and into the colon.

Table 18.1. Weibull parameters and time scale factors

Operating conditions	α	β	*Time scale factor* b_2
Water, 50 rpm	4.11	1.58	0.62
0.01M Phosphate buffer pH 6.8, 50 rpm	5.06	1.54	0.77
0.025M Phosphate buffer pH 6.8, 50 rpm	7.23	1.47	1.10
0.05M Phosphate buffer pH 6.8, 50 rpm	9.73	1.37	1.47
0.1M Phosphate buffer pH 6.8, 50 rpm	17.39	1.25	2.64
0.05M Phosphate buffer pH 6.8, 100 rpm	6.83	1.44	1.04
0.05M Acetate buffer pH 4, 50 rpm	21.21	1.72	3.22
In vivo absorption	6.60	1.42	—

Cut-Off Factor and Function

If the in vivo dissolution is too slow compared to GI transit time, it can result in reduced absorption. If there are regional absorption windows, only partial absorption is possible, despite complete in vivo dissolution. In such cases, the in vivo dissolution profile is not directly related to the in vivo absorption profile; therefore, the in vivo dissolution profile must be further adapted to match the absorption profile, which can be achieved by introducing a cut-off factor.

The cut-off factor Tcan be included as an if-then condition in the IVIVC, as a modification of Equation 5. Alternatively, incorporation of a truncating function in Equation 5 is also possible, which causes a rather gentler subsidence in absorption and can also be used for the numerical solution of differential equations.

$$\varphi(x) = \frac{e^{-\tau(t-T)}}{1+e^{-\tau(t-T)}} \qquad \ldots(5)$$

where $\varphi(x)$ is the truncating function, τ is a measure for the steepness of the function, and T is the cut-off time point.

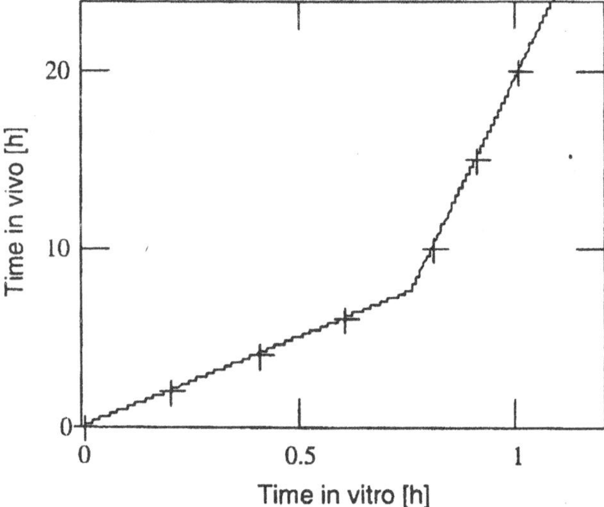

Fig. 18.10. Levy plot with upward curvature indicating change in release mechanism in gastrointestinal tract.

Lag Time

Introduction of a lag time t_0 in Equation 1 is required when there is a delay of in vivo release compared with the in vitro release.

For initial data points, when t is smaller than t_0, the resulting value can be negative. This can be overcome by an if-then condition as shown in Equation 1, or bypassed by the following expression in Equation 6:

$$pos(x) = \frac{1}{2} \times (x + |x|) \quad \text{with pos}(x + t_0) \qquad \ldots(6)$$

This form of expression can be helpful for lag time, particularly with differential equation based IVIVCs, when the mathematical program used does not accept negative expressions or if-then conditions.

Correlation of In Vitro and In Vivo Profiles

Correlation of profiles by means of linear regression is the classical IVIVC method. Altering in vitro test conditions systematically by statistical experimental design is also a very effective tool to match the dissolution characteristics of the in vivo dissolution of the formulations. This approach enabled Qiu et al. to achieve a good linear correlation between percentage absorbed and percentage dissolved of three controlled release formulations.

An alternative method is described by Polli et al., where it represents an extension of linear correlation. For IR formulations in which absorption may be partially permeability limited or regional dependent, a nonlinear correlation may provide certain advantages. Further correlation of in vivo dissolved dosages with in vitro dissolved dosages is described by Dunne et al. by the use of odds, hazard, or reversed hazards functions.

Role of In Silico Simulation in Early Development

In the early research and development stages, one of the frequently asked questions is "What is the oral absorbability of a molecule?" Medicinal chemists who synthesize potential pharmaceutical structures like to know the likelihood of oral absorption even before a molecule is synthesized. Formulation experts, when approached by others to enhance absorption, like to ask what the extent of oral absorption is in order to assess if formulation is really the problem and something they should work on. However, proper in vivo assessment of oral absorption usually requires a radio-labeled molecule, is relatively labor intensive and expensive, and usually takes place much later in the research and development scheme. Additionally, such in vivo experiments involving both intravenous and oral administration are typically done in animal species and are rarely performed in humans for orally administered drugs, for the purpose of assessing the oral bioavailability of a molecule. Therefore, it is desirable to explore in silico approaches to allow for an earlier assessment of absorbability, to extrapolate to situations where experimental data are not available, and to help identify and focus on limiting factors of absorption.

Currently there are two in silico approaches for the predicting absorption: statistical models and mechanism-based models. Statistical models are based on a statistical relationship between inputs, typically molecular descriptors derived from a molecular structure, and outputs, in this case oral absorption percentages. Mechanism-based models rely on a good understanding of absorption processes including physiology, GI dissolution, transit, and permeation.

In Silico Simulation Based on Structure of a Compound

Chemical structure-based statistical models strive to establish a structure-absorption relationship. Lipinski was the first to point out that poor oral absorption is more likely to occur for a molecule when there are more than 10 hydrogen bond acceptors, 5 hydrogen bond donors, and when the molecular weight is greater than 500, and calculated log P is greater than 5. This set of empirical rules was later on frequently referred to as "the rule of 5." More quantitative approaches relate absorption to calculated molecular descriptors and/or parameters such as dynamic surface area, topological structural features, and a composite set of parameters or force fields.

The method by Bai et al. was incorporated into a software called OraSpotter and was evaluated by the author and others using sets of proprietary chemical structures and experimental data. This model used 899 compounds in the training set to relate 28 computed structural descriptors to actual human oral absorption values, reported in the literatures. The input and output of the model are chemical structures and absorption fraction in human, respectively. The absorption fraction, zero to one, was divided into six categories in 0.16 increments. With two test sets of unpublished proprietary compounds, a successful prediction of 79% to 86% was achieved when the predicted values fell within ± one class. This level of prediction is reasonable enough to be useful in rank ordering and prioritization even prior to chemical synthesis of candidate molecules. Calculation using OraSpotter is fast and may be appropriate for high throughput purposes. Since the human absorption data used in the training set represent situations where the dose is relatively low (solubility is probably a less frequent problem) and the formulation may be improved or optimized, the model projection is perhaps biased towards the highest achievable fraction absorbed. This statistical model does not describe the mechanistic aspects of drug absorption, nor does it account for formulation differences and dose levels. Therefore, it may serve as a first filter in improving the odds of success very early on in the discovery stages. Subsequent experimental measurement on solubility and in vitro permeability may help further screen and rank order drug candidates.

In Silico Simulation Based on Experimentally Measured Physico-chemical and Biopharmaceutical Data

As drug candidates progress through research and development, in vitro physico-chemical and biopharmaceutical data gradually become available, which can be fed into mechanistic absorption models. Mechanistic models simulate and model the GI absorption process based on "Advanced Compartmental Absorption and Transit" model in which the small intestine is divided into seven compartments with equal transit time, and the stomach and the colon are treated each as a separate compartment. Drug release, dissolution, precipitation, absorption, and transit across the compartments are explicitly described in the form of specific integrated or differential mathematical equations. Such complex models, together with human and animal physiological parameters, are built into commercial softwares such as GastroPlus. Input to GastroPlus includes some or all of the following:

1. Oral dose,
2. Solubility-pH profile, and human intestinal permeability, which can be estimated from in vitro Caco-2 or artificial membrane assays,
3. Species, GI transit time, GI pH, food status,
4. Formulation release profile, particle size,
5. PK parameters species, GI transit time, GI pH, food status, and
6. PK parameters such as volume of distribution (V_d), clearance (CL), microscopic kinetic rate constants, and so on.

The current version 4.0 of the software contains default physiological GI parameters for human, rat, mouse, dog, monkey, rabbit, and cat. Nearly all parameters in the software are under users' control and can be modified as necessary.

Typical output of the simulation includes

1. Fraction of dose absorbed in each and combined GI compartments,
2. Sensitivity of parameters in affecting absorption, and
3. Plasma concentration-time profile when PK parameters are provided.

In terms of predicting the total fraction of drug absorbed, a correct classification rate was also reported to be approximately 70%, by Parrot and Lave, using a test set of 28 drugs, and eight out 10 correct classification by the author using a test set of 10 proprietary compounds.

The GastroPlus program is a quite transparent system that allows user to grasp an overall picture of the transit and absorption process, the ability to optimize certain parameters, and to run hypothesis testing on IVIVC-related questions. One could simulate the impact of dose, solubility, particle size, release profile, stomach pH, etc., on the extent and time-course of GI absorption. In one example, a question was asked whether or not the particle size of a drug candidate can be relaxed from a current 35 μm to approximately 100 μm without affecting its oral bioavailability. A simulation was therefore carried out, which suggested that the extent of absorption is essentially not sensitive to changes in particle size at least in the range between 35 and 400 μm. This facilitated decision making without having to conduct time and labor consuming experiments. This kind of in silico approach was also used by the author and collaborators for formulation prescreening in which in vitro release profile of candidate formulations were used to simulate the absorption outcome and subsequently narrow down the choices prior to in vivo testing. The author and collaborators also had examples of reasonable outcome in using this approach in the design and selection of a particular in vitro release profile to achieve the desired human plasma concentration-time profile. However, more data including in vivo PK parameters were needed in that case.

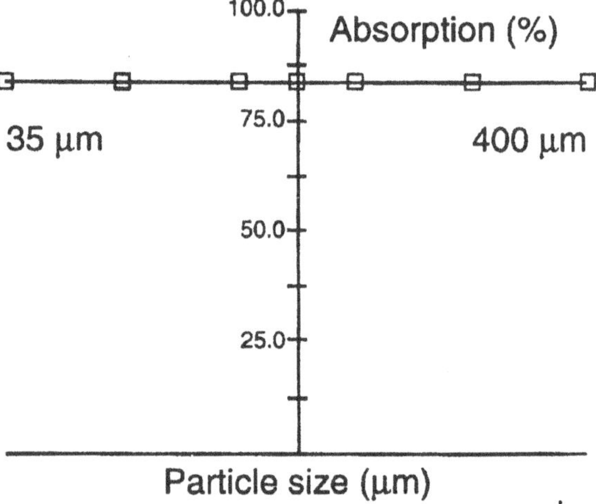

Fig. 18.11. Simulation on the impact of particle size on oral absorption of a drug candidate using GastroPlus.

On the whole, the mechanism-based in silico simulation using physicochemical and biopharmaceutical data appeared to be educational and practically useful in addressing some of the IVIVC-related questions. This approach could potentially save money and time, and spare resources to focus on more critical issues in pharmaceutical research and development.

In Vitro-In Vivo Correlation in Preclinical Settings

As the development phase moves forward, typically during the proof of concept or Phase I stage, the lead candidate is being characterized more thoroughly for its physicochemical properties and its ability to develop. A preclinical PK study is usually performed prior to the Phase I clinical trial. A well-designed preclinical PK study, with the input from the formulation and clinical experts, may provide an opportunity to define the scope for drug substance properties, such as particle size, salt forms, and formulations. Combined with simulations, it would also provide an opportunity to identify the rate-limiting factor(s) for absorption. Further, in vivo data obtained at this stage may be used to better justify the dissolution method development. Among the factors that determine the rate and extent of drug absorption following oral administration, dissolution of the solid drug into solution is of primary importance in the drug release/absorption process.

Polymorphism, surfactant, complexation, pKa, and GI pH profile are among factors that could influence solubility; while particle size and wetting play major roles in drug dissolution. Drug dissolution can be modeled by Noyes–Whitney equation:

$$\frac{dX}{dt} = \frac{A \times D}{\delta} \times (C_s - X_d/V) \qquad \ldots(7)$$

where A is the effective surface area of the solid drug, D is the diffusion coefficient of the drug, δ is the effective diffusion boundary layer thickness adjacent to the dissolving surface, C_s is the saturation solubility of the drug under lumenal conditions, X_d is the amount of drug already in solution, and V is the volume of the dissolution medium.

The most common factors influencing dissolution and its in vivo performance include particle sizes, physical form (i.e., polymorphs and/or hydrates), salt forms, and different formulations. The impact of these factors on in vivo performance of the drug product and several case studies will be discussed in the following sections.

In Vivo Performance of Pharmaceutical Salts

A common approach to improve dissolution of a compound is by forming salts. The dissolution of a pH-dependent drug is usually a function of both bulk pH and the surface pH of the solids. Solubility and pK_a of the compound often determines its surface pH.

The processes for systematic screening and selection of the optimal salts with desirable physicochemical and biopharmaceutical properties have been hindered by lack of prediction of their in vivo behavior. Morris et al., Anderson and Flora, and Gould have published extensively in this field, intending to provide guidance in selecting an optimal salt form from chemical and biopharmaceutical point of view. Selection of salt forms of weak acids and weak bases based on their in vitro dissolution and in vivo PK properties will be discussed in the subsequent chapter with the emphasis on establishing potential in vitro and in vivo correlation. Earlier work on pharmaceutical salts, their dissolution rate, and its impact on bioavailability have been nicely reviewed by Berge et al.

The relationship between diffusion layer pH and dissolution was first demonstrated by Nelson, whereas Mooney et al. discussed the relationship with pH of the unbuffered bulk medium. A direct correlation has also been established between dissolution rates versus diffusion layer pH for various acidic and basic drugs. A self-buffering effect to maintain the steady-state micro-environmental pH may vary from compound to compound, depending on its solubility and/or pK_a values. Despite similar pK_a and pH-dependent solubility of all three compounds studied, pH of dissolution medium (bulk pH) had minimal effect on the dissolution of benzoic acid and 2-naphthoic acid, whereas a more pronounced effect was noticed in the dissolution of indomethacin. Indomethacin has much lower solubility values at different pH than that of other two acids and, as a result, its self-buffering effect in the diffusion layers is limited. The buffer capacity of a dissolution medium also plays a critical role in modulating micro-environmental pH of a drug substance and, therefore, its dissolution rate.

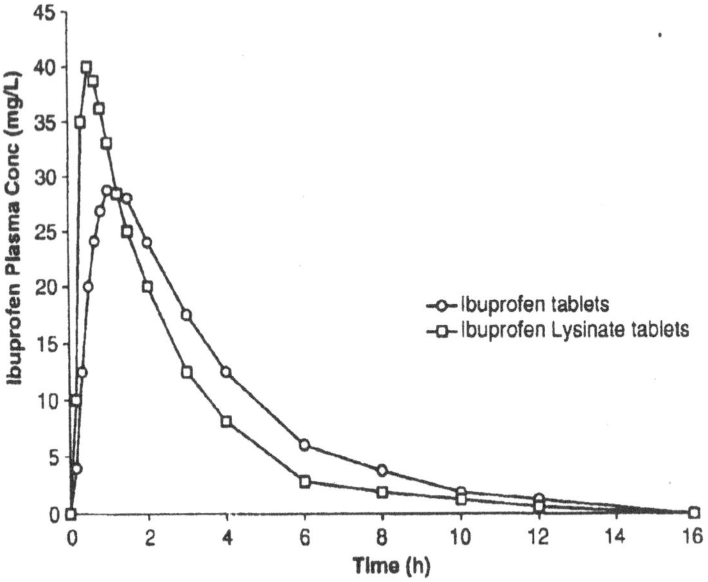

Fig. 18.12. Mean plasma ibuprofen concentration-time profiles in 26 healthy volunteers following administration of 2 × 200 mg of ibuprofen as ibuprofen lysinate tablets or sugar-coated tablets.

Salts of weak acids

The literature reports on human PK profiles of several weak acids and their salts have been reviewed. An example of the salts of weak acids is described herewith. When the PK profiles of ibuprofen and its lysinate salt are compared, the lysinate salt demonstrates a shorter T_{max} and higher C_{max}, whereas the overall AUC was not altered significantly. Similarly, absorption of naproxen and its sodium salt resembles that of ibuprofen. Interestingly, when commercial tablets of naproxen (Naprosyn) and naproxen sodium (Anaprox) were compared for its in vitro release at different pHs in the authors' lab, comparable dissolution profiles were obtained at pH 2.0 and 6.5. Dissolution at acidic pH (pH 2.0) of both forms is low due to their limited intrinsic solubility, whereas dissolution at neutral pH (pH 6.5) is controlled by both the dissolution and disintegration of the dosage form. However, when a dissolution test using a pH switch method to simulate in vivo pH gradient is used, the advantage of rapid dissolution rate of the naproxen sodium versus that of naproxen is evident.

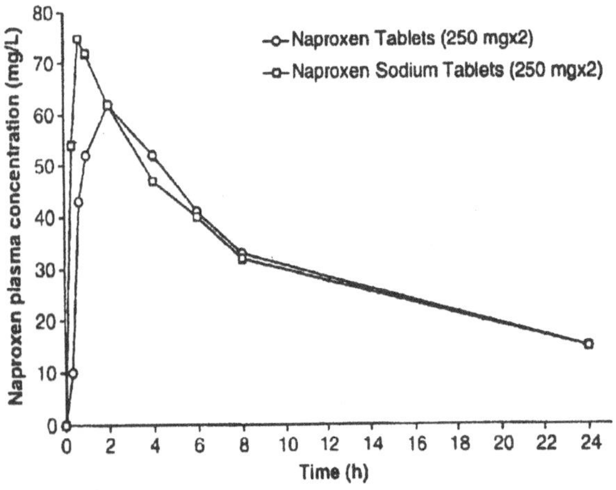

Fig. 18.13. Comparative absorption of naproxen and naproxen sodium.

The dissolution test is performed at pH 2 for 30 minutes followed by pH ramp to 6.5 for 30 minutes by addition of concentrated sodium phosphate, then the pH is ramped up to 7.4. A rank order IVIVC can be established in this case for a weak acid (naproxen) and its salt (naproxen sodium). When salt of the weak acid is dissolved at acidic pH, conversion to free acid may occur, however, the acid coated particle or fine precipitates of acid/salt mixture dissolve rather rapidly when the pH is switched to intestinal pH. The pH gradient dissolution method may be a useful tool at early stage of development when comparing performance of different salt forms.

Salts of weak bases

Prediction of the in vivo performance of weak bases and their salts could be more challenging due to the kinetic nature of the dissolution/precipitation process. In another example, a weak basic drug NVS-1 containing different salt forms of the weak base were intravenous (IV) tested in a dog bioavailability study. The formulations tested are intraveneous formulation containing 3 mg/mL diHCl salt in 20% HP-β-CD and oral formulations, including free base in 0.5% carboxy-methylcellulose (CMC) suspension at 2 mg/mL as well as diHCl and tartrate salts, which are in a dry blend capsule form using generic IR excipients.

The in vivo PK profiles of the three NVS-1 oral variants were tested in three dogs. Absolute bioavailability of the diHCl salt has a mean value of 84%, indicating close to complete absorption. Percentage bioavailability of the salt forms and free base suspension are in the order of diHCl (84%) > tartrate (48%) > free base (12%). Two salt forms of NVS-1 clearly demonstrate their in vivo advantages over that of the free base.

When in vitro dissolution profiles of the three per oral (p.o.) variants (i.e., free base suspension, diHCl salt, and tartrate salt IR capsules) were performed at pH 2, comparable release profiles are obtained for diHCl and tartrate salt of NVS-1, whereas release of the free base suspension was low (<20%) due the limited solubility of free base and its ability to modulate microenvironment pH of the diffusion layer to a higher value.

Given the in vivo difference observed between the diHCl, tartrate, and free base suspension formulation, it warrants an in vitro method that could reflect the potential in vivo performance (i.e., a biorelevant method). When the dissolution of these formulations is tested at different pH levels, distinct different dissolution profiles are evident between the free base suspension, diHCl, and tartrate salt at pH 4. When the percent dissolved at pH 2 and pH 4 were compared with Cmax and AUC of these formulations, it was evident that pH 4 provides a close to linear correlation between the in vitro percent release at 60 minutes and in vivo AUC or C_{max}. Therefore, pH 4 should be used as an in vivo performance indicating method. The above data indicating Level C correlation can be established for NVS-1 using dissolution at pH 4. No further optimization was performed, since NVS-1 is only at preclinical stage. The dissolution method can be further optimized based on deconvoluted profiles, from human PK study.

Effect of Particle Size

The effect of particle size on in vivo drug absorption has been discussed by Johnson and Swindell, in which the effect of particle size on absorption over a range of important variables, including dose, solubility, and absorption rate constant was simulated. With a fixed absorption rate constant of 0.001 min^{-1}, the relationship between dose and solubility as a function of particle size change could be simulated. In general, the relative effect of particle size on the percentage of dose absorbed decrease with increase solubility, with particle size becoming practically irrelevant for drugs at a solubility of 1 mg/ mL with a dose of 1 mg.

Similar simulation can be performed using commercially available software GastroPlus. As discussed earlier in this chapter, physicochemical properties of a compound can be used as input function, animal or human physiology can be selected. Simulation is not meant to be a replacement for scientific experiments, rather, it provides valuable insight on what one would expect to obtain in vivo based on the physicochemical properties of a compound. For instance, when a compound with intrinsic solubility of 1 μg/mL at neutral pH and high effective permeability (3.0×10^{-4} cm/sec) is being tested, a simulation at different dose and different particle size could provide valuable information on the best possible scenario one could expect from such a compound. At a dose of 500 mg, absorption of the compound is practically negligible over the particle size range of 500 nm to 100 pm, indicating that solubility limits the absorption of the compound; particle size reduction would not be helpful in such case to improve absorption. However, at dose of 1 mg, a dramatic shift in absorption dependency from solubility to particle size is evident from the simulation. Here, the use of micronization or nanoparticle system may provide great advantage.

Although one may not be able to obtain an accurate estimate of dose of a new chemical entity until very late in development, formulation scientists could utilize this type of information in a number of ways. At a relatively low dose range, relying on the particle size reduction and improving the wetting properties of a molecule may be quite effective. However, if the molecule is ionizable, such as a weak base, one may want to choose an alternative salt form, which could provide much higher solubility and dissolution rates compared with that of a free base. This would mitigate some of the risk of a potential dose increase at a later stage and, in addition, in vivo variability associated with variability coming from dissolution of the free form can also be minimized.

One key task during the drug development phase is to set a particle size specification. Such a specification is often set based on the impact of change in particle size on processibility or bioavailability. Using the example given earlier in the chapter, a change in particle size from submicron to micron range does not appear to have any significant impact on the percentage of absorption of the molecule. This provides an invaluable tool to assist one to focus the research efforts on the impact of particle size on processibility rather than bioavailability.

Effect of Different Formulations

Physical properties of drug substance will often change during the development process as the chemists optimize their process chemistry, this could result in change in particle size, morphology, and surface properties of the drug substance. A drug product strategy, when greatly impacted by the properties of the drug substance, often needs to be adjusted to ensure a robust formulation that can be produced. A question that may arise is whether the change in formulation will result in bioinequivalence between the formulations. IVIVC can be a very powerful tool in such a case.

One of the questions that is often asked is whether different in vitro release properties will result in different in vivo absorption. It is not uncommon that different formulation approaches such as dry blend/direct compression, dry granulation (roller compaction), or wet granulation may result in formulations with different in vitro release characteristics. NVS-2 has different in vitro release profiles when dry blend and wet granulation formulations are tested in vitro. In early time points, the difference can be as large as 30%. However, when these formulations are tested in vivo in dog, comparable PK profiles are achieved, indicating that the difference in the in vitro dissolution will not have any significant impact on the in vivo performance of the drug product. This would save an enormous amount of time and effort by avoiding the development of a process to match the dissolution profile of the original formulation.

In Vitro-In Vivo Correlations in Full Development and Life Cycle Management

IVIVC can be even more useful at the later development stages or during life cycle management, where a number of human PK study have been performed at different doses and, sometimes, on different formulations. Dedicated discussion will be given to IR products in the following section, since IVIVC on MR formulations will be discussed by others.

The first group of IR products can be described by dissolution of not less than 85% within 30 minutes, and the dose of less than 250 mL of dissolution medium times lowest solubility in vivo relevant pH value range of one to eight. Since it can be assumed that these forms are already completely dissolved under in vivo conditions, all doses are available as a solution for absorption. Such rapid release forms are no longer different from a solution form, in terms of its PK behavior. In addition, if the compound has high permeability, then one could seek a biowaiver according to regulatory guidelines, since it is a BCS class I compound.

The second group consists of conventional IR products that display dissolution-limited absorption. IVIVC are possible with this group, so long as the absorption is dissolution-rate limited rather than permeation-rate limited. Substances from this group, which are mostly classified as class II by the BCS, are suitable candidates for IVIVC, and will be discussed in the following case study.

Immediate Release Product with Solubility-Limited Absorption

This case study refers to a proprietary compound characterized by solubility-limited absorption. To demonstrate the procedure of developing an IVIVC and for a better understanding, a few adjustments were made to the data, which serve to simplify and clarify the presentation of the IVIVC. The method presented in the previous sections for developing an IVIVC will be utilized; the IVIVC will be obtained based on conventional deconvolution using Wagner–Nelson method.

For NVS-3, dissolution tests during the formulation development were performed at 37°C with the USP apparatus 2 (paddle) in 900 mL of water and with the addition of 0.7% sodium lauryl sulfate using a rotational speed of 75 rpm. Since the NVS-3 drug substance showed solubility-limited absorption, USP apparatus 4 (flow through cell) was alternatively used as dissolution test method. The medium in the first hour was 0.1 N hydrochloric acid followed by 0.05 M phosphate buffer pH 6.8 with a flow rate of 16 mL/min and a flow cell volume of 20 mL.

Formulation screening resulted in formulation B, which was produced by roller compaction. Alternatively, a formulation A, which was produced by wet granulation, was also produced. The latter formulation shows a slower dissolution rate and the question is whether similar or different in vivo result would be obtained for these formulations. The formulations (A vs. B) were tested in a single dose, crossover bioavailability study with 12 volunteers under fasting conditions. Blood samples were taken up to 72 hours after the dose was administered. The plasma concentration-time curves are distinctly different with lower C_{max} and AUC values for formulation A compared to B. The in vivo absorption profiles of the tablets

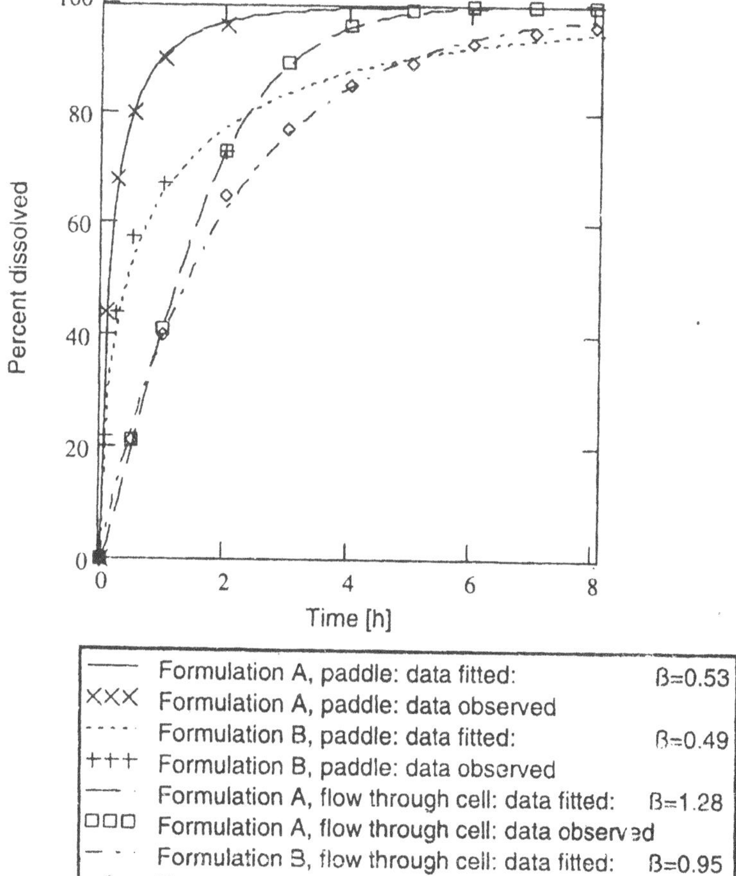

Fig. 18.14. Dissolution profiles of immediate release formulations A and B with related β-values.

are calculated by the Wagner–Nelson method. The in vitro dissolution of both formulations was evaluated using both the paddle apparatus and the flow through cell apparatus.

In order to determine the shape factor β, the in vivo and in vitro curves of formulation B were fit to a Weibull function utilizing least squares minimization. As mentioned earlier, only the curves having the same shape and, therefore, having the same β can be brought to a congruence, which will result in a successful IVIVC. As a consequence, the in vitro dissolution profile of formulation B should show a similar β compared with the β value of 0.38 of the in vivo dissolution profile.

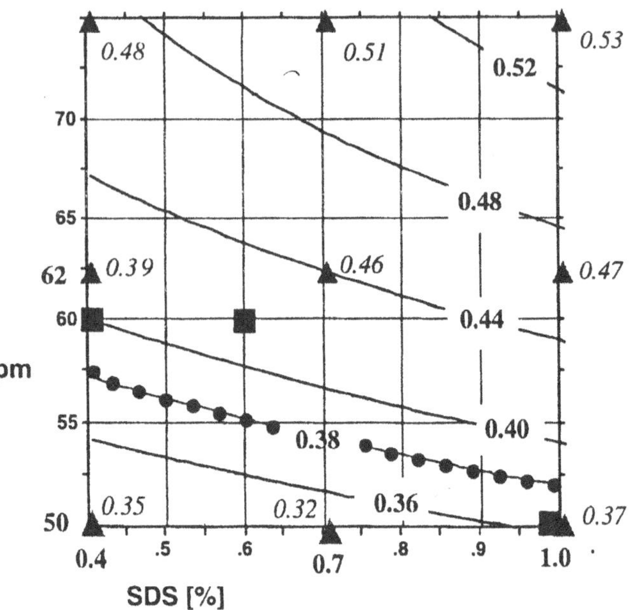

Fig. 18.15. Contour plot of the modeling analysis for the dependence of β from sodium dodecyl sulfate concentration and rotation speed.

The paddle method provides a shape factor of 0.53 that is distinctly closer to the in vivo factor than the shape factor of 1.28 obtained with the flow through cell method, and was therefore considered to be a more appropriate method. The operating conditions of the paddle method were then optimized using formulation B in order to find an in vitro profile for formulation B whose β is most similar to the β of the in vivo profile of this formulation. A 3-level full factorial design was chosen varying the rotation speed (50, 62, 75 rpm) and the concentration of sodium dodecyl sulfate (SDS) (0.4, 0.7, 1.0%). The plot illustrates the dependence of β from SDS-concentration and rotation speed. Each connected black line represents operating conditions that provide the same shape factor. The triangles symbolize the nine operating conditions of the study, the italic values represent the β-values determined in the study. The bold dotted line shows the target value of 0.38, the squares represent the best three operating conditions. The goodness of fit, expressed as r^2, is 0.98. In order to verify the modeling analysis a dissolution test using 60 rpm/0.6% SDS was performed. The predicted value of β according to the model was 0.42 and the observed value was 0.44, which demonstrated the predictive power of the model.

The analysis shows that β increases with increasing rotation speed and with increasing concentration of SDS. The conditions using 50 rpm/1.0% SDS and 60 rpm/0.4% SDS provide the best shape factors of 0.36 and 0.40, compared to the in vivo target factor of 0.38; but the first causes great tablet-to-tablet variability and the latter uses a medium, which is too close to the saturation solubility of the drug substance at room temperature, which caused recrystallization problems during assay of the dissolution test samples. Dissolution conditions using 60 rpm/0.6% SDS overcame the problems of variability and solubility and provide a satisfactory β of 0.42. Therefore, the testing conditions of 60 rpm/ 0.6% SDS were chosen as operating conditions of the final dissolution test method.

In order to bring the in vivo and in vitro profile in an optimum congruence, the in vitro profiles were scaled by a time scaling factor. The time scaling factor of 0.14 was determined by means of Equation 4 with an $\alpha_{in\ vivo}$ and $\alpha_{in\ vitro}$ of 1.44 and 0.21, respectively. This time factor was applied to the dissolution profiles of both formulations. In the initial phase up to 20 hours the curves are in good congruence, but thereafter the simulated profiles lie significantly above the observed profiles. In order to overcome this overestimation of absorption a cut-off factor was introduced, which keeps the profiles at the same plateau after 20 hours. By doing so there is a good congruence between the simulated and observed in vivo profiles. The time-scaled and cut-off factor truncated dissolution profiles as well as the in vivo absorption profiles were used for linear regression.

The relationship between the in vitro dissolution profile and the in vivo absorption profile in accordance with Equation 1, where the lag time t_0 with a value of 0 is not given in the parameters of the Equation, is as follows:

$$X_{vivo}(t) = 7.02 + 0.88 \times X_{vitro}(0.14 \times t) \text{ if } t > 20 \text{ then } t = 20 \quad \ldots(8)$$

In order to validate the IVIVC model, the internal predictability was calculated according to regulatory guidelines. The internal prediction errors for AUC are –4.0% for formulation A and 1.5% for formulation B and for C_{max} 3.2% and 3.1%, respectively.

The initial issue raised in connection with the in vivo relevance of the difference in the dissolution profiles of both formulations can therefore be answered: a slower in vitro dissolution results in a slower in vivo dissolution with a resulting decrease in AUC. IVIVC can be a very useful tool through the various product development stages. In a broad sense, IVIVC can be initiated by in silico simulation at the drug discovery stage. A more experimental based IVIVC with preclinical PK data and physicochemical data of the molecule is also possible. In the preclinical stage salt forms, particle sizes, and different formulations may also be evaluated. Further, human PK testing is an indispensable part of IVIVC development for the purpose of validating the IVIVC model. Last but not the least, IVIVC can be a very useful tool for projects at the life cycle management stage.

19

Technology Transfer Keys

There can be few pharmaceutical companies over the last 15 years that have not undergone the maelstrom of takeovers, mergers, downsizing, centers of excellence or product rationalization. All these events can, and frequently do, result in product or products transfer between manufacturing sites. At best it will be a product or product type that the receiving site is familiar with, or at worst, one with which they are totally unfamiliar. The challenges to effect technology transfer in a timely fashion, within budget and to achieve savings that have probably been precommitted, at the requisite quality, are approximately the same for each aspect. This chapter provides a "ready reckoner" of the issues to consider to achieve these objectives, ensuring that the regulatory issues from both a licensing and inspection perspective are addressed, and maintaining the organization's integrity for its products and with its shareholders. In considering the technology transfer process reference is made to the situation within the EU in the main; however, where useful guides or proposals are available from other regulatory authorities, notably the U.S. Food and Drug Administration, these have been included for completeness.

The purpose of this chapter is to present both an overview of the technology transfer process and to offer specific guidance concerning the key aspects of product transfer management, and how to document outcomes to completely satisfy both internal requirements and regulatory expectations. We provide suggestions on the personnel to be involved in the process, and a checklist to serve as an *aide memoire* to ensure that key steps have been covered. This chapter discusses the principles behind the technology transfer process that can be applied in full or in part, dependent on the nature and complexity of the products involved in the transfer. The requirement to perform a formal technology transfer is prescribed directly and indirectly by the regulatory authorities within the EU For those markets regulated by the U.S. FDA, there are very specific requirements for transfer. While this guideline is focused on the EU, the principles, if applied in full, would also be expected to meet FDA requirements.

Technology Transfer Team

The decision to transfer products between manufacturing sites is frequently driven by economics. This may be the result of a global product or site rationalization program, or it may be driven by attempts to consolidate similar product types at a single site. It may result from a merger or takeover, which generates excess capacity in the supply chain leading to consolidation. Whichever the key driver for transfer, it is likely that due to the sensitive nature of the proposals, both in terms of affected sites and shareholders' confidence, this intention cannot be shared with the affected sites until timescales are already tight. It is against this background that the team responsible for the transfer process is required to operate. It must be accepted that although not ideal, this is an understandable consequence of operating in a highly competitive global business. The structure of the validation team will depend on the degree of fit of the transferred product with the local site capabilities. For example, if the recipient site has a known expertise in solid dose formulations and the transferred product is a straightforward tablet formulation then the team members will be drawn from quality control (QC); quality assurance (QA) and production (or process support where this facility exists). If, however, the product represents a change in complexity (e.g., sustained release formulation) or a change in product type (e.g., capsule formulation where the site has previously only made tablets), then the core team may need to be enhanced for example, by the inclusion of engineering personnel.

Other disciplines, for example, the training function, also need to be considered. If there is a major impact on site quality systems or personnel knowledge base, then extensive training of site personnel throughout all disciplines, but particularly of operations personnel, needs to be considered. It is unlikely that the training can ever supplant the collective knowledge of the donor plant, but it should seek to identify key gaps in the process between donor and recipient plants and deliver a training program to close such gaps. In many situations the timescales will preclude involving all team members full time on the process, unless an organization is specifically resourced to provide this service. However, it is essential that at least one member is full time and has specific responsibility for the project. His role may be project management, co-ordinatory, or "hands on" in the process environment, but he must be focused and not distracted by the pressures of a "day job."

Table 19.1. Proposed team members and responsibilities

Team member	*Responsibilities*
Process technologist	• Central focus for transfer activities. • Collates documentation from donor site. • Performs initial assessment of transferred project for - Feasibility. - Compatibility with site capabilities. - Establishes resource requirements.
QA representative	• Reviews documentation to determine compliance with marketing authorization (MA). • Reviews analytical methods with QC to determine capability, equipment training requirements. • Initiates conversion of donor site documentation into local systems or format. • Initiates or confirms regulatory requirements, e.g., change to manufacturing license; variations to MA if process changes needed.
Production representative	• Reviews process instructions (with process technologist) to confirm capacity and capability. • Considers any safety implications, e.g., solvents; toxic; sanitizing materials. • Considers impact on local standard operating procedures (SOPs). • Considers training requirements of supervisors or operators.
Engineering representative	• Reviews (with production representative) equipment requirement. • Initiates required engineering modifications, change or part purchase. • Reviews preventative maintenance and calibration impact, e.g., use of more aggressive ingredients; more temperature sensitive process, and modifies accordingly.

A regulatory interface is also essential. Despite a supposedly uniform regulatory environment in the EU, the reality for most companies is that even for a single product there may be divergent regulatory requirements; indeed the product registration may not be common to all markets and therefore the impact of change will also be variable. The responsibilities for each team member need to be defined at the outset, so that all the bases are covered and all members understand what is expected of them.

TECHNOLOGY TRANSFER: KEY ACTIVITIES

Timelines

As previously indicated, the timelines for the transfer may well have been preordained by financial or marketing considerations. The first key activity of the team is therefore to do a "*sanity check*" to determine at the macro level whether those expectations can be met. If not, then senior management must be informed to ensure that the implications on the donor site (which may be closing), the recipient site (whose budget may have assumed the transferred volume) market supply, stock market confidence and so on, can be considered. The other time driver may well be the regulatory aspects.

Initially the team will have to make a number of assumptions. For example, it will be assumed that process validation, analytical validation, and cleaning validation are trouble-free. It will also be assumed that actives, excipients, and packaging components are available on standard lead times. A complete time and event schedule at the macro level should be constructed on these assumptions, working backwards from the proposed transfer deadline. Key stages of the process such as:

1. Data collection
2. Data review
3. Regulatory impact with particular emphasis on any change approvals
4. Analytical validation
5. Pilot or full-scale process batch
6. Stability set down (if required)

should be mapped to determine whether the predetermined transfer timelines can be met.

Regulatory Issues

Changes to the approved MA can represent the greatest challenge to the transfer timelines. Most manufacturing units no longer supply a single market, and particularly where centers of excellence have been created, a single unit may supply on a global basis. For even a simple activity, such as registering a site change, the regulatory process can vary from 30 days to 12–14 months. This is why an initial regulatory assessment is so important in determining whether the overall timelines can be met. Fundamental to the transfer process is the decision to implement little (if any) change in the transferred product or process. As the level of change increases, so does the regulatory complexity and the associated timelines. Guidance is available in assessing change in both of the major regulated markets, i.e., the U.S. FDA and the EU. The FDA has published a series of proposals under the simplification process, for example SUPAC (scale up and post approval change) Guidance for Industry for Solid Dose Forms. These provide guidance covering advice on so called "like for like" changes, i.e., the substitution of one granulator for another. A brief resume of some changes considered is given at the end of this section. By using this guidance it is possible to minimize the regulatory impact in those markets governed by the FDA.

Similarly, within the EU, at least for nationally registered products, guidance notes are provided for not only the type of change and its regulatory approval time, but also for the information required to support the change. Changes are divided into 30+ so-called Type 1 variations covering diverse changes ranging from change of site to changes in analytical methods, and other more complex variations, so- called Type 2 changes. In theory a Type 1 variation is approvable within 30 days and a Type 2 variation within 90 days. In practice only some member states of the EU achieve these approval timelines.

Table 19.2. EU guideline on variations to marketing authorization

Nature of change	*Documentation required*
1 Change of manufacturing site	• No change in process, specifications, or test methods. • Proof that proposed site is authorized for the dose form production ("manufacturing licence"). • Declaration in writing of no changes in previously approved specification. • Batch analysis comparison; at least one full size batch, and two pilot batches compared with three full-scale from previous site.
4 Replacement of excipient with comparable excipient	• No change in dissolution profile for a solid dose form. • Justification for change including stability impact. • Commitment to provide ongoing stability and three months' data available up front. • Comparative dissolution profiles of "old" versus "new" product. • Declaration of no change in release or shelf life specifications.
8 Qualitative change in composition of packaging material	• Justification for change including comparative data, e.g., permeability. • For semisolids and liquids proof of no interaction between container and product. • Validation of any analytical methods used to control packaging material. • Ongoing stability and three months data available up front. • Declaration of no change in release or shelf life specifications.
11 Change in manufacturer of active substance	• The specifications, controls, and synthetic route should be the same as already approved (or minor changes justified). • Batch analysis of at least two lots from new source. • Declaration by the MA holder that there are no changes in finished product specifications.
15 Minor change in manufacturing process of product	• Product specifications not affected. • Dissolution profile for one "new" batch compared with three "old" batches (solid dose). • Justification for not submitting a new bioequivalence study.
25 Change in test procedures for product	• Appropriate validation data for analytical method and comparative data between "old" and "new" method.

	• Declaration that release and shelf life specifications remain unchanged.
30 Change in pack size for the product	• Declaration that specifications are unaffected. • Justification that new size is consistent with dose regime. • Declaration that container properties are unchanged. • Declaration that stability studies will be conducted.

FDA Guidance for Industry: Changes to an Approved New Drug Application (NDA) or Abridged New Drug Application (ANDA)

Changes requiring prior approval:

1. Move to a different manufacturing site when the new site has not been inspected by the FDA for the types of operation proposed.
2. Move to a different manufacturing site when the new site does not have a satisfactory good manufacturing practice (GMP) inspection for the operation proposed.
3. Changes that may affect the controlled release of the dose delivered to the patient.
4. Changes in sterilization method for a sterile product.
5. Changes in a viral removal step.
6. Changes from dry to wet granulation or vice versa.
7. Changes in synthetic route for drug substance.
8. Addition of an ink code imprint to a solid dose form.
9. Relaxing an acceptance criteria.
10. Deleting a specification.
11. Establishing a new analytical procedure.
12. Changes in the immediate packaging material.

Changes which can be implemented in 30 days if no adverse comment:

1. Moves other that those requiring prior approval.
2. Moves of testing to another site.
3. Changes in manufacturing process other than those requiring prior approval.
4. Changes to aseptic filtration parameters.
5. Changes from one sterilization autoclave or oven to another.
6. Relaxing an acceptance criteria or deleting a test for a raw material.
7. Change in an analytical method for a raw material.
8. Change in size of a primary container.
9. Addition or deletion of a desiccant.
10. Reduction of an expiration date to provide increased assurance of identity, strength, or purity.

Changes which can be filed in annual report:

1. Move to a different site for secondary packaging.
2. Move to a different site for labeling.
3. Changes to equipment of the same design (see SUPAC guidelines).
4. Change in the order of addition of ingredients for a solution.
5. Changes in specification to comply with *United States Pharmacopoeia* (*USP*).
6. Tightening of specification.

7. Change in container closure system for a solid dose form, e.g., adding a child-resistant closure; change from one plastic container to another of same type.

SUPAC (Scale Up and Post Approval Changes) Guidance for Industry for Immediate and Modified Release Solid Oral Forms (FDA)

Operation	*Equipment type*	*Examples considered essentially similar*
Milling	Fluid mill	Tangential jet
		Loop
		Opposed jet
		Fluidized bed
Operation	Equipment type	Examples considered essentially similar
	Impact mill	Hammer air swept
		Hammer conventional pin or disk
Blending/mixing	Diffusion mixers	"V" blender
		Double cone blender
		Slant cone blender
		Cube blender
		Bin blender
	Convection mixers	Ribbon blenders
		Orbiting screw blenders
		Planetary blenders
		Vertical high intensity mixers
Granulation	Wet high-shear	Horizontal
	Granulator	Vertical
	Wet low-shear	Planetary
	Granulator	Kneading
		Screw
	Extension granulator	Radical
		Axial
		Ram
		Roller or gear
	Fluid bed	All types
Drying	Direct heat, solid bed	Tray and truck
		Belt
Dosing	Tablet press	Gravity
		Power assisted
		Centrifugal
		Compression coating
	Encapsulator	Auger
		Vacuum
		Vibratory
		Dosing disk
		Dosator

Determining the Process Scope

As previously stated, the ideal situation is to simply transfer the total process without change from the donor to recipient site. In practice this is seldom straightforward. During the initial feasibility assessment the comparability achievable is evaluated. Careful comparisons of processing equipment including the sophistication of the control mechanisms available, analytical capability, impact on other site processes, e.g., cleaning validation complexity, training and documentation requirements, all need to be factored into the process scope. Excipients may not be available from the same source or the receiving site may have different preferred suppliers. Actives are normally sacrosanct, although in some cases even this change may have to be made because of other legislation, e.g., restrictions on crossborder trade in controlled drugs. When all unavoidable changes have been identified then the scope of the transfer must be carefully formalized so that all involved parties are aware of the work involved.

Managing change

Following the scope determination, the work needed to support any of the identified changes must be formalized. A single example will provide an illustration. Say, for example, it has been necessary to change the source of an excipient. The following list of questions, although not exhaustive, should be posed.

1. Is the source of the excipient declared in the marketing authorization? If so, regulatory action may be required.
2. Do the routine quality control tests provide sufficient control to characterize the practical use of the excipient? For example, is the particle size, shape, or distribution important?
3. Are there any known interactions of the excipient in the formulation which may be enhanced with the proposed source?
4. Are there any known interactions of the excipient with the container or closure system?
5. Have any lots of donor site excipient been rejected and, if so, did this have any impact on the specification?
6. Do both sources have European Certificates of Suitability, which would indicate that they are equally well characterized by the pharmacopoeial tests?
7. Is the manufacturing process for the proposed excipient significantly different such that it may pose different problems (e.g., presence of solvents where previously none were used, aqueous based extraction which may lead to higher bacterial or fungal counts)?
8. Is the proposed excipient available in manageable quantities (e.g., lifting restrictions may require availability in no more than 25 kg quantities)?
9. Can it be assured that the proposed excipient will not interfere in the finished product analysis (particularly HPLC)? (A minor related substance may co-elute with the active product.)

As can be seen from the previous list, even what on the face of it may be a simple change, can, and does, involve complex issues.

Documentation

In order to maximize the chances of transfer success, as soon as dialog between donor and recipient site can take place, then the team should start to assemble available documentation. It is difficult to provide a definitive list of requirements as this will vary from product to product, process to process and site capability to site capability. However, as a guide the following should be assembled.

1. *Production master formula*: This should be compared to the formula actually dispensed and to that in the MA. It is not unheard of for differences to be seen.

2. *Manufacturing instructions*: These should be compared to those in the MA. In our experience, for older products the detail is likely to be minimal (e.g., granulate the ingredients and tray dry to a predetermined moisture) and differences between actual and licensed can usually be accommodated. For recent products the detail may be substantial (e.g., granulate in a high-shear mixer using both granulator and chopper blades operating a high speed for 30 minutes) and changes require regulatory activity.
3. *Process validation studies or process development studies*: These will provide valuable insight into process robustness, impact of variables on finished product quality, critical control points, etc.
4. *Rejects and deviations*: Again these will indicate process robustness; determine whether manufacturing instructions contain the correct level of detail and whether the donor reacted appropriately to the failures.
5. *Analytical methods and validation*: These should be compared against the MA with particular emphasis on the finished product specification. It is worth remembering at this point that the MA may vary in this and all other respects from market to market.
6. *Raw material specifications with particular emphasis on the active and key excipients*: The latter may be of particular importance in modified release formulations. Care must be taken with any animal delivered products in the current climate of enhanced concern with transmissible spongiform encephalopathy (TSE). Certainly within Europe or where product is likely to be exported outside of the EU, most regulatory authorities will look for the absence of potentially compromising material. If it is recognized that product still contains material of bovine, ovine, or caprine origin (e.g., magnesium stearate), it would be as well during the transfer to substitute a vegetable equivalent. This is one case where like-for-like transfer should be avoided.
7. *Packaging components specifications*: Again these should be compared against those in the MA and the specification should be as comprehensive as possible, particularly as the materials of construction of bottles, plastic tubes, laminates, etc., may well be commercial preparations for which equivalency is potentially difficult to establish.
8. *Safety data*: Particularly where a material has specific safety issues (e.g., irritant or potent sensitizer, solvents, etc.) then all relevant data on handling requirements, disposal, environmental impact, safety data sheets, etc., should be collated.
9. *Other data which may provide a valuable insight into the robustness of the product and the production process*: These include analytical deviation reports and customer complaints.
10. *Where a number of products are to be transferred*: The collation of this repository of information may assist in the prioritization of the transferred products. Choices can be made on degree of difficulty, regulatory issues and the timelines involved, purchasing timelines or sourcing difficulties, and so on.
11. It should be remembered that, where transfer results from the donor site closure, particular sensitivity is needed when dealing with the collation and evaluation of the information. Now is not a good time to be critical of the donor site practices and procedures!

Validation

This is one of the most critical issues in the technology transfer process because it frequently determines the complexity of the process and it is a focus for the regulatory agencies; not only from the licensing side but also during inspections. The approach to validation for any transferred product must always be documented and science based. A number of regulatory guidelines are available: however, they are just that — guidelines. Of necessity they must deal in generalities. It is up to the receiving site team to evaluate each product and the information portfolio, and to determine the level of validation required. In the context of the transfer process we are usually referring to process qualification (PQ), unless of course equipment changes are also involved, in which case installation qualification (IQ) and operational qualification (OQ) may also be needed. Pragmatism also has a place in the decision making process. For example:

1. If the product transferred is a simple liquid in which actives and excipients are dissolved by simple agitation
2. If the equipment in donor and recipient plant is the same or essentially similar
3. If no changes in source or type have been made to excipients and actives
4. If the analytical methods are direct from a major pharmacopoeia

then it may be decided that no prospective validation is required and the transfer success will be measured by ongoing product monitoring.

There are usually three separate validation activities — namely process, cleaning, and analytical validation. Serious consideration should be given to the merits of running a pilot scale (say 10% normal lot size) or even placebo product, if the evidence gathered during the transfer process suggests that the product may be complex or difficult to transfer or validate. This has three advantages. First, it allows all personnel involved to gain some familiarity with the production methods. Second, it may help to avoid costly "write- offs" and third, by working outside of the formal validation protocol, it provides an opportunity to address the issues without compromising the validation protocol or invoking a complex formalized investigation, in the event that something goes wrong.

Process validation

Process validation has probably consumed almost as much time, energy, and money in the pharmaceutical industry over the last 10-15 years as manufacturing commercial products! Many companies also appear to have lost sight of the purpose of validation. In some circumstances, validation *appears* to be performed for the benefit of the validation department or, worse still, the regulatory agencies. There is only one reason to validate a process. That is to *secure* the manufacture of a product, so that it can be *guaranteed*, with a high degree of probability, that the *patient* receives product of the requisite safety, quality, and efficacy each and every time. It also makes good business sense to be able to quickly and reproducibly release good quality products. The approach to process validation will vary with product type and complexity. We will concentrate on the most common dosage forms, as discussion of the transfer of technologically sophisticated products such as inhalation aerosols, steriles, transdermal patches, etc., is best dealt with in a special treatise. As with most validation, three successive and successful repetitions of any of the validation processes given below are the norm.

Solutions

The key to validating solutions is to ensure that:

1. Raw materials specifications for actives and excipients exercise control over critical parameters such as particle size and particle shape, partical size distribution and solubility.
2. The manufacturing process parameters, be they temperature, order of addition, or agitation, are controlled and monitored to effect consistent dissolution of the ingredients.

Once such controls have been established then process validation can usually be effected by monitoring the active content of the individually filled containers produced throughout the filling period.

Creams

Creams may involve solubilization of the actives in either the water or oil phase, or dispersion without solubilization of the active in the water or oil phase. Where the actives are dissolved or dispersed during the cream formation, the energy involved to effect the formation of the oil and water micelle is such that homogenous distribution is almost assured. If the active is dissolved or dispersed after cream formation, this is likely to be a lower energy process and homogenous distribution through the viscous substrate may be more difficult.

In the former case, validation can be affected as for liquids by careful control of the physical attributes of the actives, in particular particle size distribution, and by careful control and monitoring of the homogenization conditions. The active distribution can then be monitored during the filling process by assay of individual filled units. In the latter case, where distribution is effected after cream formation, then active ingredient distribution will normally be monitored at the bulk stage, taking samples throughout the blender as well as the filled units. The purpose of the blender samples is to determine whether the blending plateau is achieved under the prescribed conditions, i.e., the active has been evenly mixed. Sampling of bulks can be technically very difficult: even the introduction of the sampling device may disrupt distribution of the active, although this is less likely in a viscous substrate than in a free-flowing powder (see section 2.5.1.4 on solid dose forms). The sampling regime is to some extent dependent on the blender type, but commonly a matrix of samples is taken by dividing the bulk into top, middle and bottom layers vertically and side — middle — side horizontally.

Ointments

Ointments pose similar, if potentially more challenging, problems than creams. Normally the active is distributed, not dissolved, unless it is reasonably heat stable when it can be dissolved at the molten "fats" stage. Ointments are generally relatively viscous, but due to the lack of water can be blended aggressively without fear of "cracking," i.e., separating phases, then the actives are usually incorporated using some form of high shear mixer. The degree of difficulty in doing this is to some extent dependent on whether the active can be incorporated either when the fats are molten or when they are cool. For the former, distribution should be relatively straightforward; for the latter, the viscosity may demand vigorous or prolonged mixing. Validation sampling is as for creams, i.e., bulk and filled units.

Solids

Validating solid dose forms after transfer has generated significant debate with the industry and its regulators as to the complexity of the validation process. There are probably several reasons for this.

1. The multistage nature of the typical solid dose process, e.g., sieving, mixing, granulating, milling, drying, compression, and coating.
2. The low level of active in the typical tablet.
3. The impact changes or variations in the manufacturing process have on disintegration or dissolution and hence possibly bioavailability.
4. As in most cases the active is not dissolved in the substrate, distribution is accomplished by physical dispersion only.

The U.S. FDA has insisted on blend uniformity studies, even to the extent of requiring them as routine. Within the EU the regulators do not have a declared policy and are driven by good science; normally this requires blend uniformity studies on validation only. A number of companies have taken such studies to extremes and have performed blend studies at every stage of the solid dose process.

This is probably reasonable at the development stage of a product to demonstrate exactly when and under what conditions the mixing plateau, i.e., the point at which the active is homogenously distributed occurs, and to ensure that subsequent demixing does not happen. However, for a previously manufactured product, particularly one for which a large number of lots have been manufactured, consistency of the finished product results should provide a reasonable indication that the process is under control; hence blend homogeneity and finished product homogeneity studies only are required. Sampling at the final blend stage poses particular problems when powder sampling; the introduction of a so-called sample "thief" has been shown to disrupt mixing. Multipoint sampling throughout a blender is normally used, sampling wherever possible a sample size equivalent to the final dose form weight. The regulatory authorities (predominantly the FDA) will accept sample sizes up to three times the dose weight, but even this size is difficult to sample consistently.

Most granulates consist of granules or powders of different flow indices, which upon the introduction of a multipoint sampling device can differentially flow into the sample cavity, leading to apparently heterogenous samples. Even the angle of introduction of the "thief" can impact on the sample characteristics. Final product sampling is usually performed by taking compressed tablets throughout the compression run. Variables that need to be considered are:

1. Interchangeability of compression machines to provide production flexibility.
2. The impact of the change of overhead feed drums and whether segregation occurs as the drum or hopper empties.
3. The impact of compression machine speed on dose reproducibility.
4. The impact of vacuum transfer parameters such as velocity, fluidization air volumes.

Direct compression formulations can be more problematic than wet granulation formulations as the incorporation of active in the former is physical only. Each formulation transferred should be considered on a case-by-case basis to determine the most appropriate validation approach. It may be appropriate, if time and economics permit, to manufacture a 10% scale pilot batch with additional sampling to gain an understanding of the manufacturing dynamics before resource is committed to a full-scale batch.

Acceptance criteria

It is difficult to set general acceptance criteria for each dose form as it is dependent on so many different factors. However, as a guide the following criteria have gained acceptance within the industry and with the regulatory authorities. For a *tablet product* the criteria outlined in the *USP* for uniformity of dose should be applied, but the relative standard deviation (RSD) should not be greater than 5.0%. If it is wished to control content uniformity by weight during routine manufacture, it will be necessary to demonstrate a closer relationship of weight to content. It is unlikely that this may be assured with an RSD greater than 3.0%. For *liquids, creams, ointments and gels* it is normal to take samples at several stages during the production process. The sampling points are dependent on the complexity of the manufacturing process and the mechanics of incorporation of the active. For example, if there are several aggressive mixing stages in the process it may be possible to only sample at the end of the process: for a more gentle process it may be necessary to demonstrate homogeneity at several steps.

For *intermediate* stages acceptance criteria using a 95% two-sided confidence interval about the mean could be used which would ensure that the true batch mean is contained within the data with 95% confidence.

The calculation:

$$X \pm t_{df,0.025} S \sqrt{n},$$

where

X = mean of n values

S = standard deviation of n values

n = number of unit samples

df = n–1

$t_{0.025}$ = 97.5 percentile of the t distribution with df degrees of freedom.

For *final* product it is normal to expect all finished product samples taken throughout the filling run to meet in full the finished product specification.

Cleaning validation

This is another area in which careful risk assessment is required when transferring products. As a practical example, the receiving site is used to dealing with fairly innocuous solid dose forms and then has to manufacture a tablet containing highly potent active. It is quite possible that local cleaning methods will prove inadequate based on the normal criteria used to assess cleaning efficacy (less than 0.1% of the standard daily dose of the "contaminant" present in the daily dose of the recipient product).

Consideration would need to be given to either:

1. Reevaluating the cleaning methods, which might be an onerous task requiring extensive revalidation.
2. Assessing whether a change in detergent might be sufficient to effect removal.
3. Or whether a facility would need to be dedicated to the new product.

Similarly, if the receiving site was used to handling creams and then had to deal with a fatty ointment, once again current cleaning methods may prove inadequate. Depending on the status of the donor plant, analytical methods may be available which are sufficiently sensitive to detect around the parts per million rate, and this method development will need to be factored into the timelines. Finally, a new product may bring with it additional microbiological demands, e.g., products containing natural ingredients, high sugar concentrations, poorly preserved, and so on. This will probably need the services of a competent microbiologist to assist in the risk assessment.

Analytical validation

The technology transfer of analytical methods can almost be considered as a project within a project, in that the ideas and thinking behind the overall product transfer apply equally to the analytical area. All relevant documentation, method validation reports, out-of-specification reports, laboratory investigations and typical analytical results, should be reviewed by a transfer team. This transfer team should consist of all parties who will be using the methodology, and should include a minimum representation from all those involved in routine testing, stability, and process validation support, plus at least one knowledgeable individual from the donor site, when possible. Each test should be reviewed against its history in the hands of trained analysts, the skill set of the receiving site, and the sophistication of the methodology.

In addition, emphasis should be placed on site-specific operating procedures, to highlight ways in which differences could impact the way the test is implemented at the respective sites. A record of the rationale used to decide on the level of technology transfer necessary for each test should be made at this stage. The preparation of a validation master plan (VMP) may prove a useful vehicle in which to record these decisions. Guidance on the level of technology transfer necessary for specific test procedures is given in the IPSE guidance on technology transfer. However, recommendations on some of the more common test requirements as applied to common pharmaceutical formulations are detailed below.

Assay

Assays should always be transferred although matrixing can be used on similar formulations. Typically this will be carried out by two analysts at each site, in triplicate, on three batches, on three different days. The analysis should consist of independent preparation of reagents, standards, etc., and should use different batches of analytical columns if appropriate. During the analysis any standard system suitability tests must be met and the acceptance criteria are usually based on the mean assay and variability obtained together with a visual comparison of the chromatography. Typically limits of plus or minus 5% of the mean assay between donor and receiving site are considered acceptable.

Impurities and degradants

These should always be transferred. The samples analyzed and the analysts used are the same as for the assay. Transfer should also include confirmation of the limit of quantitation and response factors for those substances where quantitation is calculated from the relative response to that of the drug peak. Old samples are often useful in these transfers, especially for products that typically have low levels of impurities. Acceptance criteria are usually based on mean and variation values (variation may be expressed in absolute rather than relative terms) and a visual comparison of the chromatography.

Dissolution

Typically transferred but often limited to one analyst, one batch and a dissolution profile on 12 units at each site. Acceptance criteria are typically mean meets specification with an absolute difference of not greater than plus or minus 5% and profiles are comparable.

Identity

Identity varies widely in techniques and complexity but is typically carried out on one batch only with acceptance criteria based on showing equivalence.

Microbiological testing (including sterility and LAL)

Transfers are not normally carried out on these test procedures as these are usually subjected to "in house" validation before use. Validation is usually completed in triplicate on three different batches.

Compendial methods

Transfers are not normally considered necessary. However, care should be taken. These methods are not always described in sufficient detail to ensure comparable results are obtained (e.g., column packing details, extraction times, etc.). If the receiving site has had no experience of the formulation, a limited transfer may be prudent. As with all such guidance different approaches are equally valid, and provided a sound rationale is recorded then this should be acceptable to the regulators. The conclusions reached should be acceptable to all parties involved but, in general, and in the experience of the authors, this is not always the case. There are a number of pressures present at this time: some subconscious, others more direct. The vast majority are to reduce the workload and speed up the whole process, but it is our experience that more time has been lost through foreshortening of the process, than in carrying out unnecessary additional work. It is important to remember: this is a *knowledge transfer* process as much as a *technology transfer* process.

Protocol

For those methods where a formal technology transfer has been deemed necessary, it is important for the whole process to be recorded in a protocol, prior to any completion of testing. This protocol should ideally be generated by the donor site, since it is considered expert in the methodology. However, alternative arrangements can be made if necessary, but it is preferable that any such protocol be generated by individuals who will not participate in the subsequent analysis.

This protocol should include the following sections:

1. *Objective* — a clear statement of the objective of the transfer, from which laboratory the method is transferred and which of the receiving sites' laboratories are included in the transfer.
2. *Scope* — a clear statement of the methods transferred and what is involved in the transfer.
3. *Definition of responsibilities* — who is responsible for what and when, e.g., who writes the report, who signs the report, when does responsibility for the method transfer from the donor site to the receiving site.
4. *Definition of terminology* — do not make assumptions that everyone has the same understanding of terms used (this is especially important in transfers between different countries).
5. *Materials, methods, equipment to be used* — should include details on how the transfer analysis will be transferred, define the samples to be used, the number of replicate sample preparations,

different analysts, days on which the analysis is to be completed, replicate injections of samples and standards and how they should be treated (individually, meaned, etc.).

6. *Prequalification activities* — what training, if any, is required to be carried out by staff at the receiving site before the main part of the protocol is executed. What if any trial runs will be completed and what will happen to the results.
7. *Experimental design used* — if a number of similar formulations are transferred at the same time it may be prudent to investigate the potential for reducing the workload by the use of experimental design. If this course is followed the design and the rationale for its use should be included.
8. *Acceptance criteria* — detail what acceptance criteria will be applied to which results, include any statistical assessments to be made.
9. *Remediation process* — if all goes well this section should not be needed, but including it at this stage enables subsequent actions to be more easily justified. It should include details of those involved in any investigations undertaken and any additional training requirements.
10. *Documentation* — should make reference as to whether the transfer will be completed using the donor site's documentation or whether this is to be converted to the receiving site's format ahead of the transfer work. It should also include how documentation generated during the transfer is identified, handled, reviewed, and stored.
11. *Raw data* — how the raw data is to be identified, handled, reviewed, and stored.
12. *References* — references to any external documentation used during the assessment prior to generating the protocol and any site SOPs used during the transfer.
13. *Approval signatures* — who will approve the protocol and subsequent report. Should include name, job function, date and where working across time zones, the time and time zone.

For older products, where validation data to modern standards is not necessarily available, consideration should also be given to revalidating the methodology to International Committee for Harmonization (ICH) requirements as the movement of the product may open up discussions with the regulators on these aspects of the license. Only when this protocol has been agreed should analytical work commence. When the analytical work is complete there are, in common with other qualification-type work, a number of possible outcomes. Hopefully these and the necessary remediation were included in the original protocols. However for those that were not, the normal processes of investigation and further work should be followed. Do not forget that the underlying reason for the transfer is to ensure that the method is robust, compliant, and can be used reliably at the new site. The outcome of the protocol should be recorded in a formal report, any deviations discussed and justified and the report duly approved by the same signatories. Depending on the sophistication of the test and the general skill set of the receiving site, consideration should be given to how additional staff will be trained in these new methodologies.

Packaging Issues

This section will concentrate on primary, i.e., product contact packaging, although the regulatory issues involved in declaring a change of site on label, leaflet, or carton can be considerable!

Issues to be considered are availability and comparability. Most sites will have a purchasing strategy of preferred suppliers to secure economies of scale. Major items will be purchased from a single supplier, bottles and laminates often fall into this category. Wherever possible, supply chains will also be kept short, purchasing from as close to the manufacturing unit as possible.

Where product is transferred across countries or continents this may cause conflict between the needs of purchasing and the regulatory position in a product transfer. Significant changes in primary packaging are likely to require at least 3 months upfront stability and for sensitive products possibly 6 months at 25°C and 60% relative humidity (RH) and 3 months at 30°C and 75%RH.

Compatibility may also be an issue on a number of fronts. First, as the plastic compounds used in both bottles and blister pack laminates are often commercially sensitive, it is sometimes difficult to directly compare them except by resorting to IR trace comparison. While this may provide a chemical compatibility, the bottles or laminates may still have different barrier properties and it may be necessary to compare minimum vapor transmission rates (MVTR) as well. Second, although not normally considered a problem with solid dose forms, liquids, creams or ointments may need data generated on extractables and there is a potential for migration of the printing inks into the product. Similarly, some products may interact with the container causing discolouration or even cracking.

Stability Requirements

In the previous sections the need to consider stability for transferred products has been mentioned several times. As before, the best avoidance tactic is to make no changes in either process or packaging components. Practically this can be a difficult position to sustain, and in most cases sufficient changes will need to be made which precipitate a stability requirement. By the time a 10% pilot scale batch has been produced, samples taken (and presuming stability indicating assays are available and validated), 3 months may have elapsed until the first stability time point; a further 1 month for results generation and reporting; then a total of at least 6 months can elapse. Clearly, this has an important impact on the transfer timelines.

If changes appear unavoidable then an early dialogue with the regulatory authority is recommended, to ascertain whether upfront or concurrent stability is required. Provision of previous data coupled with MVTR data, product compatibility studies or declarations from the container manufacturer of its suitability (conformance to FDA or DIN standards) for pharmaceutical use may be sufficient to allow stability data to be produced post-commercialization.

If there are a number of different strengths of the same formulation, it may be possible to use matrixing, i.e., provide data on the lowest and highest strength to negate the need for data on products in between. For older products another complication may be the stability conditions themselves. Older products may only have had stability data generated at room temperature (18–25°C) and ambient humidity. Upon transfer, stability data meeting ICH conditions will be expected, i.e., 25°C and 60%RH. This may be too severe a challenge for either the formulation or the packaging system. The latter may be correctable by increasing the barrier properties of the bottle or blister film (although not forgetting that this may have an economic impact) while the former may stop the transfer at worst, or require a reduction in the shelf life. Depending on the market competition, even this option may be unpalatable to the sales and marketing group.

Training

Regulatory agencies are paying increasing attention to training of operational staff, as do most companies. This assumes even more importance during technology transfer for a variety of reasons. First, time constraints are normal and cutting training may be considered a soft option to save time. Second, the formulation, its manufacturing process, and the handling characteristics of the ingredients, may all be unfamiliar to operational staff. Third, the transfers will be under scrutiny, both inside and outside the operational unit, thereby increasing pressure on the staff. Spending time on involving all relevant personnel in the process, providing appropriate and timely training, and encouraging staff to contribute to the process itself, will all help to minimize the likelihood of failure at what can be a stressful time for the organization. It perhaps goes without saying that all training must be documented and increasingly "validated."

Technology Transfer Report

Regulatory inspectors and sometimes assessors will ask for evidence of successful transfer. This is more likely when the technology transferred, be it the process or analytical method, is new to the site or poses particular challenges, e.g., the introduction of bioassays. The report should also serve a similar function to the original development pharmaceutics report in that it provides a "ready reckoner" of key aspects of the product and a reference point in the future if problems are encountered.

Contents

Generally the process consists of two stages:

1. The generation of a protocol (a proposed structure for which is given below).
2. A final technology transfer report, which includes all the raw data, or reference to where it can be found, together with a critical evaluation of the results.

Protocol structure

1. *Scope* a clear statement of the transferred product and of what is involved in its transfer, i.e., process validation, analytical validation, cleaning validation, etc.
2. *Change management* a statement of any changes being made as a result of the transfer, e.g., changes in source of actives, excipients, components, analytical methods and equipment, together with justification.
3. *References* — cross-references to the original donor site documentation, e.g., manufacturing formula, manufacturing and analytical methods, specifications for actives, excipients and components. Copies of these documents may usefully be attached to the report as appendices.
4. *Acceptance criteria* — a statement as to how the success of the transfer will be measured (see the Acceptance Criteria section) for each of the processes involved.
5. *Sampling regime* — a statement of the number, size, and source of all samples and at what stage they will be taken.
6. *Recipient site documentation* — reference to any source documents used in determining the transfer approach, e.g., pharmaceutical development reports, analytical validation or process validation reports from the donor site.
7. *Additional requirements* — for example, if it has been determined that stability is needed then a copy of the protocol or reference to where the report may be found.

It may also be worth considering adding a section regarding the level of training considered necessary if the production, cleaning, or analytical methods are complex or new to the site. The completed protocol will be supplemented with all the raw data (or references to workbooks, data files, etc.), to form the final report and a clear critical evaluation of the data and conclusion. If all acceptance criteria have not been met then a number of options need to be explored.

The transfer team, together with regulatory support, need to consider the nature of the failure and its impact on the robustness of the transfer. For example, if the cleaning validation fails, it can be considered that the manufacturing process is uncompromised, but a report addendum will have to be prepared clearly stating what corrective action has been taken and what results were achieved after implementation of the action.

Failure of the analytical validation clearly disrupts the program as process validation cannot be initiated with a flawed analytical technique; or indeed any stability testing initiated.

Failure of the process validation is clearly very significant and it may be very difficult to pinpoint what actions are required to correct the process. The normal causes of failure are inadequate distribution of the active and change in the dissolution profile.

Causes for the former may be:

1. Inadequate mixing, over mixing (leading to demixing).
2. Disparate particle sizes of active and excipients.
3. Physical segregation caused by vacuum transfer systems.
4. Different bulk density leading to higher or lower loading in the granulator and subsequent changes in swept volume.

For the latter, over-mixing leading to "slicking" of the lubricant is a common source of failure. Normally an extensive sampling regime is required to determine the root cause, taking samples potentially at every stage of the process. This additional testing should be defined by a new protocol which once more sets out the purpose of the additional work, the acceptance criteria, etc., and the work carried out. It may be helpful to include the corrective action report as an addendum to the original report. It may be wise to maintain an increased sampling regime following any corrective action, to provide additional confidence that the source of variability has indeed been identified. It should be noted that the technology transfer report may be requested by the licensing authority in approving the site transfer, or by the inspectorate, as part of a preapproval or normal GMP inspection.

Approval Process

The normal signatories of the technology transfer protocol are the team involved, regulatory affairs personnel, with a final approval to start from quality assurance. If the process involved is technically very complex it may be worthwhile, at the protocol initiation stage, to seek sign-off from experts at the donor site to ensure that (based on their better understanding of the process) all key criteria have been covered. Once the work required to enact the protocol has been completed, and where timescales are very tight, it may be worth considering if commercial production can be effected against a review of the raw data, rather than waiting for the completion and signoff on the finally completed report. This decision should be formalized prior to the initiation of the transfer process, not subsequent to it.

Post-Transfer Evaluation

During the period of the transfer, close scrutiny of the process involved is maintained by the transfer team and hence it can be considered that the validations are somewhat "artificial." It is therefore worth considering putting in place a post-transfer evaluation process where, say, the first 6 or 10 lots produced under standard production conditions are reviewed. Additional final product samples may be analyzed and the results plotted using Shewarts charts or similar to establish process robustness. Dissolution profiles rather than simply drug availability after a set time period may be considered. These results can be collated and added as an addendum to the original technology transfer report to provide powerful evidence of the success of the transfer validation. In those countries where annual product reviews are mandated, then any recently transferred product should be given priority review status.

Technology Transfer Checklist

Below is a checklist that summarizes the details that should be collated during the process, the majority of which have already been referenced.

1. Copy of Part 2 of marketing authorization.
2. Production master formula.
3. Manufacturing instructions.
4. Dispensing instructions.
5. Analytical methods.
6. Previous process validation.

7. Previous analytical validation.
8. Cleaning instructions and previous cleaning validation.
9. Stability reports.
10. Excipient specifications and source.
11. Active specifications and source.
12. Primary packaging material specifications and source.
13. Packaging instructions.
14. Customer complaints.
15. Process deviations file.
16. Analytical deviations file.
17. Reject and rework file.
18. Specimen manufacturing batch record.
19. Specimen cartons, labels, leaflets.

20

Animals in Drug Development

The use of animals in scientific investigation has been traced back to several centuries BC. For instance, the writings of Aristotle (384–322 BC) and Erasitratus (304–258 BC) indicate that they had studied the anatomy of various animals. Early investigations such as these were the beginning of the basic sciences that today form the foundations for new drug development.

History of Animals Use in Drug Research

Until the end of the last century, experiments using living animals were carried out on domestic or easily captured wild species. The choice was usually limited and based on availability. By the end of the nineteenth century, the concept of the laboratory animal had begun to emerge as an animal deliberately chosen for its inherent suitability for the purpose; it was especially bred in captivity or obtained from its environment not merely on grounds of convenience but rather for its usefulness for the particular investigation at hand.

Need and Rationale for Animal Use

Tests in intact animals are necessary to understand how a drug will work in the context of the myriad metabolic and homeostatic mechanisms that are active in vivo. Screening tests are commonly conducted with in vitro systems and isolated tissues or organs to identify and, in some cases, to act as a bioassay to help purify pharmacologically active agents. However, the variable processes of absorption, distribution within the organism, metabolism to either inactive or more active products, and excretion will modulate the expression of pharmacologic activity in vivo. The only way this modulation can be estimated is by studying the new drug in intact animals.

Aside from studies of pharmacologic activity, side effects of new drugs must be identified and an initial assessment made of their risk-to-benefit ratio. Again, mechanisms of action and effects on specific organs can be studied by using in vitro techniques. However, to identify unexpected adverse effects and to estimate the dosages that may be pharmacologically active without producing unwanted effects, in vivo studies must be conducted.

Extrapolation from Animal to Human

For most substances, the mechanism of action will be the same in humans and other mammals. Therefore, quantitative rather than qualitative differences in response are most common. Humans may be more sensitive to some drugs than certain laboratory animals are, but in many cases some animal species are more sensitive than humans are. For example, the mouse is most sensitive to atropine, the cat is less sensitive, and the dog and the rabbit tolerate atropine at doses 100 times higher than does the human.

Species differences in sensitivity can often be explained by differences in metabolism, including quantitative and qualitative differences in the ability to detoxify drugs and also differences in the rates of absorption, transport, distribution, and elimination of chemicals. After oral administration, absorption in laboratory animals is generally considered to be similar to that in humans, although there are quantitative differences for some compounds. For example, species differences in the absorption and action of some compounds are related to differences in the bacterial flora of the gastrointestinal tract. The distribution and storage of drugs are reasonably consistent among mammalian species, including humans, although plasma binding tends to be more extensive in humans than in small mammals. Urinary excretion in different animal species depends to some extent on their different diets, because diet influences urinary pH and thus the extent of ionization of compounds. Biliary excretion is quite variable from species to species and is apparently more extensive in mice and rabbits than in rats and humans. Species differences in response to drugs appear to be related mainly to rates of biotransformation, which are generally more rapid in small laboratory animals than in humans.

Animal Models in Drug Discovery

Twenty years ago, the initial screening of new compounds for pharmacologic activity was conducted using whole animals or tissues and organs isolated from animals. Today most of the initial screening for new drugs is done in vitro using the techniques of biochemistry and molecular biology. Only after a new drug candidate has been identified and studied in vitro are studies in animals initiated. The purpose of the animal studies is to verify the pharmacologic activity of the new drug, identify any unexpected pharmacologic activity, and develop an initial data base on the action of the drug in vivo.

An ideal approach would be to have an in vivo screening program designed to allow for the detection of unique profiles of activity or combinations of activities. Therefore, in addition to a set of initial screening models, relevant secondary tests would be conducted to generate additional information on specificity, mechanism of action, and possible side effects.

The following sections describe some representative models currently in use in screening for new pharmacological compounds. Descriptions of most of these models were derived with permission from standard operating procedures of the former Pharmakon Laboratories, Waverly, PA 18471. Many other models, as well as variations on the models to be described, are available.

CNS

A convenient test for initial screening of compounds for CNS activity would be the *neuropharmacologic profile* or open field behavior test in mice or rats. In this test, animals are dosed with the compound and placed individually in an open area consisting of a square box about 2–4 feet on each side with an open top. The animals are then observed continuously for alertness, depression, spontaneous motor activity, defecation, urination, grooming behavior, ataxia, and convulsions. The animals are systematically observed to measure time of onset, peak effect, duration, and character of drug action. This kind of test can provide an initial pharmacological appraisal of chemical compounds and an estimate of acute toxicity. CNS depressants, tranquilizers, antidepressants, central and peripheral skeletal muscle relaxants, psychostimulants, analgesics, anticonvulsants, and diuretics may be detected by this test. Other classes of drugs, however, will generally not be detected. The Randall–Selitto assay is a specific test for analgesia. In this test, a suspension of 20% brewer's yeast in water is injected into one hind foot of a rat. This causes an edematous condition that increases the rat's sensitivity to pain. The test compound is administered 2 h after the yeast injection, and after an additional hour, the pain thresholds of the inflamed and non-inflamed paws are measured. This is done with a device, the Analgesy Meter, which exerts a force that increases at a constant rate. The rat paw is positioned on a teflon platform, and the force is applied to the volar surface with a blunt teflon cone.

Table 20.1. Major therapeutic classes

CNS	Sedative–hypnotic
	Anticonvulsant
	Muscle relaxant
	Anesthetic
	Analgesic (narcotic and non-narcotic)
	Anxiolytic
	Dementia/cognition
	Antidepressant
	Neuroleptic/antipsychotic
Cardiovascular	Antihypertensive
	Anti-arrhythmic
	Cardiotonic
	Antithrombic
	Anti-anginal
	Cerebrovasodilator
Metabolic	Hypolipidemic
	Hypoglycemic
	Diuretic
Immunopharmacologic	Anti-inflammatory
	Anti-edema
	Anti-allergenic
	Anti-asthmatic
	Bronchodilator
	Immunostimulant
Gastrointestinal	Anti-ulcer
	Gastrokinesis
	Antisecretory
Antimicrobial	Antibacterial (Gram positive and negative)
	Antiviral
	Antifungal
	Antitrichomal

The *phenylquinone writhing* assay is also a test for analgesic activity. In this test, mice are given an intraperitoneal injection of 0.25 ml of 0.02% phenylquinone in 5% ethanol. This will cause 100% of the mice to writhe within 10 min. Characteristic patterns of writhing consist of torsion of the abdomen and thorax, drawing the hind legs close to the body, and raising the heels off the floor. Complete blocking of the writhing syndrome for 10 min after the phenylquinone injection is considered a positive response. The ability of a test compound to cause reversal of tetrabenazine-induced ptosis in mice is an indication of CNS stimulant effect. Mice are dosed with test compound and then given an intraperitoneal injection of 32 mg/kg of tetrabenazine methane sulfonate. Thirty minutes after the tetrabenazine injection, the mice are graded for the degree of ptosis. Lack or partial reversal of ptosis is considered a positive response.

Inhibition of pentylenetetrazol-induced seizures is used as an indication of hypnotic, tranquilizer, or anticonvulsive activity. Mice or rats are given the test drug, and after 30 min a dose of pentylenetetrazol, which will cause 50% of the animals to convulse (CD50), is administered intramuscularly. A drug that increases the CD50 may have activity of the type mentioned above.

Cardiovascular

Spontaneously hypertensive rats can be used to screen compounds for antihypertensive effects and for effects on heart rate. The animals are dosed for one or a few days. Blood pressure and heart rate are measured by means of an inflatable cuff around the tail. Most classes of antihypertensives will be detected. Agents such as beta-adrenergic antagonists will be detected by decreased heart rate. Other rat models include deoxycorticosterone acetate (DOCA)-induced hypertensive, renal hypertensive (one or both renal arteries clamped), and stroke-prone spontaneously hypertensive rats. Hypertensive dogs produced by clamping one or both renal arteries may also be used to test or verify antihypertensive activity in a second species. Because of the ease of introducing intravenous and intra-arterial catheters and measuring blood flow and blood pressure, dogs are commonly used to conduct hemodynamic studies. These studies evaluate the effect of the test compound on systolic and diastolic blood pressure, heart rate, cardiac output, *dp/dt*, respiration, ECG, and ventricular pressure. From these data, effects desirable for treating angina pectoris, congestive heart failure, coronary vasospasm, and myocardial infarction can be detected.

Anti-inflammatory

Two commonly used models to detect anti-inflammatory activity are carrageenan-induced paw edema and adjuvant-induced polyarthritis in rats. The former represents an acute and the latter a chronic inflammatory process. Non-steroidal anti-inflammatory agents inhibit the formation of carrageenan-induced paw edema. However, to detect activity in the developing and established phases of chronic inflammation, the polyarthritis model is well accepted. In both tests the measured endpoint is volume of the hind paw. This is done by immersing the hind paw in the well of a mercury displacement plethysmograph. In the carrageenan test, 0.1 ml of a 1% suspension of carrageenan is injected into the plantar surface of one hind paw of a rat. After 1 h the test compound is administered, and after a further 3 h the volumes of both the carrageenan-treated and non-treated hind paws are measured. The net difference between the two measurements is an indication of the amount of edema remaining after test compound treatment. The smaller the net difference, the greater the anti-inflammatory activity of the test compound. In the polyarthritis model, 0.1 ml of a sterile 0.75% suspension of finely ground *Mycobacterium tuberculosis* or *Mycobacterium butyricum* (Freund's adjuvant) in paraffin oil is injected into the hind paw as done for carrageenan. The polyarthritis disease state takes about 20 days to develop. Therefore, to test a compound for activity in the developing stages of chronic inflammation, the test compound is administered during the first 20 days after the single injection of Freund's adjuvant. To test a compound for activity against fully developed chronic inflammation, the test compound is administered for 4–10 days, starting about 20 days after the Freund's adjuvant injection. In both the carrageenan and polyarthritis models, drug effects are expressed as the percentage inhibition of paw edema in drug-treated animals compared to non-drug-treated controls. In the *croton oil topical inflammation* test in mice, 20 μl of a 3% solution of croton oil is applied topically to the anterior and posterior surfaces of one ear and 20 μl of the test drug is applied to the same ear 30 min later. Inhibition of ear swelling by more than 50% relative to vehicle-treated controls measured 2 h after croton oil application indicates acute topical anti-inflammatory activity.

Immunomodulation

Inhibition of oxazolone-induced delayed-type hypersensitivity is used as an in vivo test for inhibition of the cellular immune response. The shaved abdominal surfaces of groups of mice are sensitized by topical application of 0.1 ml of 5% oxazolone. The test drug is given intraperitoneally an hour later and then daily for five consecutive doses. After an additional 4 days, the animals are challenged by application of 0.5 ml oxazolone to one ear. Ear thickness is measured 24 h later. A decrease in ear thickness relative to untreated controls is an indication of immunosuppresion.

Inhibition of sheep red blood cell lysis by serum from sensitized mice is an indication of suppression of the humoral immune response. Groups of mice are sensitized by the intravenous injection of 0.2 ml of a 2% sheep red blood cell suspension. The test drug or vehicle is administered intraperitoneally to groups of mice for 3 consecutive days beginning 2 h after sensitization to sheep red blood cells. Nine days after sensitization, blood samples are collected, complement- inactivated serum prepared, and serial dilutions made. Sheep red blood cells and complement are added to aliquots of the serum dilutions. The serum titer is then expressed as the reciprocal of the dilution causing complete hemolysis. A lower than normal titer may indicate immunosuppression, and a higher than normal titer may indicate immunostimulation.

Antitussive

Dogs are surgically prepared by implantation of a small iron slug in the lumen of the trachea. After a 2-week recovery period, the cough response of the dogs is determined in response to electromagnetic stimulation of the implanted tracheal slug. The stimulus is imposed for 3- to 5-s periods, and the total number of coughs elicited during and 30 s after stimulation is recorded. After establishing each dog's control cough response, test substances can be administered at weekly intervals and compared with the effects observed after administration of a standard antitussive agent.

Endocrine

A simple assay for antidiabetic activity is the determination of changes that occur in blood glucose levels in rats after oral administration of a test compound followed by a subcutaneous injection of glucose. Rats are fasted overnight, administered the test compound, usually by gavage, and then immediately given a subcutaneous injection of 125 mg glucose. Two hours after test compound administration, the rats are anesthetized and blood drawn for plasma glucose determination. Decreased plasma glucose relative to controls not treated with test compound is an indication of antidiabetic activity.

Antimicrobial

Many animal models use infections artificially introduced into the animal either systemically or into specific organs or tissues. The behavior of infections and the efficacy of antibiotics in eliminating those infections differ, depending on the organ or tissue involved. The type of local pathology, the penetration and pharmacokinetics of antibiotics, the local host defense system, and the clearance rates for the bacterial inocula differ among the various organs and tissues of an animal. Therefore, to get a reliable prediction of how effective an antibiotic will be clinically it is mandatory to test new antibiotics in vivo. There are a great variety of such models. For descriptions of many of these, the reader is referred to a three-volume series.

Anticancer

New drugs suspected of having anticancer activity are tested in standard animal models in which tumors are transplanted from one generation of animals, generally mice, to the next and are thus perpetuated in vivo. In vitro tumor cell culture systems are commonly used to determine if a new drug has cytotoxic or growth- inhibiting activity. However, the in vivo test is considered to be a better predictor of activity in humans.

The L1210 lymphoid leukemia model is commonly used. This tumor is carried as an ascites tumor in BDF1 or CDF1 mice. Ascites fluid from carrier mice containing 100,000 cells is implanted in the test mice. Twenty-four hours later, treatment with the test drug is started. After 6 or 7 days of treatment, the numbers of survivors are determined and the animals weighed. The results are evaluated by comparing drug-treated groups to untreated ones. Drugs resulting in a greater proportion of surviving mice compared with non-drug-treated controls may have anticancer activity. Many other similar models are available.

Animals in Drug Safety Testing

Before a new drug can be given to people, it must be tested in animals to determine its side effects and at what dosage those side effects will appear. This testing must be done in vivo because the effects of the processes of absorption, distribution, metabolism, excretion, the interactions among these processes, and the interactions among the various organs and neuroendocrine systems within the whole animal cannot be duplicated in vitro. To characterize the nature of the side effects to be expected from a new drug, it is usually necessary to give much higher dosages than would be given clinically and sometimes to give the drug over prolonged periods of time. This is because the dosages of drugs needed to elicit pharmacological or toxicological effects are often higher in laboratory animals than in humans, and because the side effects of drugs suitable for clinical use are usually provoked only by exaggerated dosages. In some cases the drug may accumulate within the body or within particular organs or tissues and thus give rise to toxic manifestations. Some side effects appear only after long periods of repeated administration.

In addition to the requirement to test new drugs in animals, it is also necessary to test in more than one species of animal, because extrapolation of the results of testing in animals to humans is less than perfect. Certain species may be more sensitive or predictive than others. To ensure that the safety of a new drug has not been overpredicted and that any potential side effects have not been overlooked, it is routine practice to test new drugs for safety in at least two species. In most cases, these will be a rodent and a non-rodent species.

The variety of animal tests and the length of the studies required for a new drug depend on the nature of the drug (pharmacological or chemical class), the intended clinical use of the drug (for example, length of the usual course of treatment), and, to some extent, on the requirements of the countries in which the new drug will be registered for marketing. These factors will be discussed further in the following sections.

Acute Toxicology

In acute toxicology testing, animals are given single doses of a drug. The most common study design is to give groups of rats or mice (such as 5 per sex) single treatments over a wide range of dosages and then observe them over a period of 7-14 days for survival and for physical or behavioral signs of toxicity. In most cases a LD_{50} (the dosage at which 50% of the animals die) will be determined; however, this is not always feasible or necessary. The acute toxicity test may be conducted for several reasons. This is the first toxicity test that will be done for a new drug, and it provides the basis for choosing dosages that will be used in subsequent toxicity studies involving repeat dosing. This test provides information regarding the effects of single large doses of a new drug. This information may be used to predict the effects of overdosing (either accidental or purposeful) in humans. The acute toxicity test is a convenient safety check on new batches of drug. Even though extensive chemical analyses are conducted on new batches of any drug, a quick test in live animals to assure that there have been no dramatic changes in acute toxicity provides a desirable level of comfort before making the new drug batch available for human use. The acute toxicity test is also a convenient method to determine any interaction between two drugs that would cause unexpected toxicity in clinical use. Thus, if a new drug will be commonly used clinically in combination with other drugs or in patients who commonly receive certain medications, it might be prudent to test the new drug in combination with these other drugs in an acute toxicity test in order to predict such an interaction before using the new drug clinically. Apositive finding in such a combination study would likely be followed up by longer-term, repeat-dosing studies.

Acute toxicity studies may be conducted by administering the drug by any of several routes (oral, intravenous, intramuscular, intraperitoneal, subcutaneous, or dermal). The route chosen usually is that intended to be used clinically. Rats and mice are generally used for acute toxicity work; however, rabbits are commonly used when the route of administration is dermal.

If a drug is to be given parenterally, acute vein and muscle irritation studies are commonly conducted in rabbits. These studies help assure that a new parenteral formulation will not cause unnecessary pain or tissue damage in people. They are also useful in developing new formulations for parenteral use with minimal potential for such effects. In a vein irritation study, groups of drug-treated and vehicle-treated rabbits are given injections via the lateral ear veins. The reason rabbits are used for this test is because the lateral ear veins are large enough, long enough, and easily visible, so as to facilitate making the injections and identifying the injected portion for subsequent sampling for histological examination. The animals are observed during the injection and at intervals (such as 2–4 h) afterward for indications of discomfort during the injection and of swelling, erythema, or tenderness of the injection site. Twenty-four hours after injection, the animals are killed, and the injection site veins are examined histologically for evidence of tissue damage or inflammation.

In a typical muscle irritation study, groups of male rabbits are given intramuscular injections of 1.0 ml of drug formulation or vehicle with a 23-gauge needle inserted vertically to a depth of about 15–20 mm into the sacrospinalis muscle. The injection site is marked by drawing a circle of ink around the site. The animals are observed during the injection and daily thereafter for 7 days for discomfort during injection and for signs of swelling, erythema, or tenderness at the injection site. On 1, 3, and 7 days after injections, blood samples are taken for measurement of creatine phosphokinase activity. Elevation of this enzyme in blood is an indication of muscle damage. Also, 1 and 7 days after injection, rabbits from each group are sacrificed and the muscle tissue surrounding the injection site taken for histological examination for evidence of tissue damage or inflammation.

Subchronic and Chronic Toxicology

Repeat-dosing toxicity studies are conducted to determine what side effects will arise from repeated administration of a drug at lower dosages than those used in acute toxicity studies and to determine safe dosages to be used in the initial human clinical trials. These studies range in duration from 1 to 2 weeks to 1 to 2 years. The length of studies required for a drug depends mainly upon the duration of treatment and the intended clinical dosing regimen. These studies are conducted in stages so that the results of one study can be used to design the subsequent study of longer duration. The first are usually 2 weeks in length followed by 1-month, 3-month, 6-month, and then 1-year studies. Parallel subchronic and chronic studies are almost always conducted in two species, usually the rat and dog, because there is a large historical data base for these species and they are easy to work with, relatively economical to house, and readily available from commercial vendors. However, special circumstances may dictate that other species be used. For instance, if a drug causes excessive vomiting in dogs, which are known to be particularly sensitive to such effects, then some other non-rodent species such as the monkey may have to be used. Also, if the absorption or metabolic handling of a drug in the rat or dog is found to be markedly different from that in humans such that one of these species would not be a reasonable predictor of toxicity in humans, then another species would be used.

The usual protocol for subchronic and chronic studies includes groups of animals containing equal numbers of both sexes receiving at least three dosage levels of drug plus vehicle or other control groups. These animals are observed daily for clinical signs of toxicity. Their body weights and food consumption are measured frequently. These three parameters—clinical signs, body weight, and food consumption—can be very sensitive indicators of toxicity. Complete hematology and serum chemistry profiles are determined at least at the end of the administration period and in some cases at intervals during the period of administration. Thorough physical examinations by a veterinarian or a trained technician are conducted at regular intervals. Periodic electrocardiograms are commonly recorded in studies with dogs. At the end of the period of drug administration, all the animals are subjected to a complete necropsy under the supervision of a veterinary pathologist. The tissues are then subjected to complete microscopic examination by a veterinary pathologist to detect morphologic alterations in the tissues that may have resulted from drug administration. In some cases it may be desirable to allow some animals from the drug-treated groups to live for a period of time after the end of drug administration to determine if any drug-related changes will disappear upon withdrawal of the drug.

As mentioned, the results of the subchronic and chronic studies are used to help determine the dosage to be used in the initial human clinical trials. To do this, the lowest dosage causing no toxicity (the no-toxic-effect dosage) is determined for each study, and a safety factor is applied depending on the species. For instance, for rats the no-toxic-effect dosage is divided by 10 and for dogs by 6 to arrive at an estimate for the initial human dosage. These factors are derived from the observations that laboratory animals can usually tolerate higher dosages of drugs and other chemicals without exhibiting toxicity than can humans and that the differences in tolerance vary with differences in basal metabolic rate, which in turn varies with body surface area to weight ratio. This ratio varies by a factor of approximately 10 in rats and 6 in dogs relative to humans. The descriptions of toxic effects elicited in the subchronic and chronic studies allow clinicians conducting clinical trials to know which side effects to anticipate so as to protect the patient volunteers.

Reproductive Toxicology

Reproductive toxicology covers the entire process of reproduction from mating to pregnancy, birth, weaning and, sometimes, the reproductive function of subsequent generations. The species most commonly used in these studies are rats and rabbits, although in special circumstances, other species such as mice, dogs, or monkeys may be used. A series of studies is usually conducted so as to cover all the phases reproduction. Within each study, groups of animals corresponding to untreated controls and two or three drug-treated groups are used.

One type of typical study, usually conducted in rats, provides information on fertility and general reproductive performance, particularly on gonadal function, estrous cycles, mating behavior, conception rates, and early stages of gestation. This study is usually referred to as a fertility study. Mature male rats are treated with the drug for 28 days prior to mating. This period is considered to be sufficient to detect effects on male reproductive organs when used in conjunction with thorough histological evaluation of testes. This fertility study in male animals is conducted prior to large-scale (Phase III) clinical trials in men. Female rats are treated for 14 days and then mated to treated males. Daily vaginal inspections are made and the finding of sperm or a copulation plug is considered as Day 0 of pregnancy. The females are sacrificed on Day 13, and the number of live and dead embryos, the number of implantation sites, and the number of copora lutea on the ovaries determined.

Some of the dams may be allowed to deliver normally, and the newborn pups are counted, examined, sexed, and weighed. The pups are again weighed and counted on Days 4 and 21 (weaning). From this test, preimplantation death, derived from the number of implantation sites in the uterine horns compared to the numbers of corpora lutea on the respective ovaries, post-implantation death, derived from the number of resorption sites compared to the number of implantation sites in the uterus, and the survival and growth of the offspring are determined. This study is generally conducted prior to any clinical trials involving women of childbearing potential. However, in the USA and Europe, women of childbearing potential confirmed to be non-pregnant and using effective birth control may be enrolled in Phase I and Phase II (usually small-scale) studies prior to completion of the female fertility study.

The second typical study, commonly called the teratology study, is usually conducted in two species, rats and rabbits. Rabbits are commonly used as a second species in Segment 2 studies because after the thalidomide tragedy in the early 1960s, rabbits were found to be more susceptible than were other commonly used laboratory species to the teratogenic effects of thalidomide, one of the few proven human teratogens. In the Segment 2 test, inseminated females are treated only during the organogenesis period, which for rats and mice are Days 6–15 and for rabbits are Days 6–18 of gestation. One day prior to birth, the dams are sacrificed and the fetuses delivered by cesarean section. The fetuses are weighed, sexed, and examined for gross abnormalities. The fetuses from each treatment are then randomly divided into two groups. One group is preserved in fixative for subsequent soft tissue examination. In the other group, the tissues are cleared and the skeletons stained for skeletal examination. The main endpoints in this study are numbers of live and dead fetuses, sex ratio of the fetuses, fetus weights, grossly observable abnormalities, and soft tissue and skeletal abnormalities. This test procedure was developed based on the well-established principle that the embryo is most susceptible to induction of birth defects during the organogenesis period. Previous exposure of the dam, as in the Segment 1 test, can lead to infertility or elevation of detoxification mechanisms, and thus to underestimation of the potential of a compound to cause birth defects. A separate phase of testing was developed to specifically assess the occurrence of birth defects. This study is usually completed prior to any human studies involving women of childbearing potential (proven non-pregnant and using effective birth control) in Europe and Japan and prior to large-scale Phase III studies involving women in the USA.

In a third type of study, called the perinatal/ postnatal test, pregnant females are treated during the last quarter of pregnancy and through lactation until weaning. The weanlings are necropsied to detect any internal anomalies. The purpose of this study is to determine the effects of the drug on late fetal development, labor, delivery, lactation, neonatal viability, and growth. It also assesses potential effects on neonates due to drug being excreted in the mother's milk. The endpoints for this study are the numbers of live and dead pups, the sex ratio of the pups, the numbers of surviving pups at 4 and 21 days after birth, and the growth and development of the pups. Postnatal testing of pups commonly includes developmental indices such as days on which the following events occur: balanopreputial separation in males, vaginal opening in females, eye opening, pinna unfolding, and incisor eruption. Tests for reflex development and learning and memory are also commonly included. The reproductive competence of the offspring may also be tested. The potential of a compound to induce changes in these endpoints can be masked by infertility in the fertility and general reproductive performance study, which would lead to insufficient numbers of offspring to detect a change. This study must be completed prior to applying for marketing approval.

Mutagenicity

New drugs are routinely screened for their potential to cause gene mutations and/or chromosome aberrations by in vitro tests. An in vivo test is also required by most regulatory agencies. Further mutagenicity tests in whole animals are usually conducted only if the in vitro tests prove inconclusive or questionably positive. A new drug showing a strong positive response in an in vitro mutagenicity test probably would not be developed. In vivo tests serve to determine whether a drug has potential to cause genetic alterations under conditions closer to those that one would obtain under clinical use. The significance of these studies to the safety of a drug is twofold. First, a drug that causes genetic damage could produce such damage in the sperm or ovaries of the patient and thus potentially cause genetic abnormalities in the children of that patient. Second, it is widely accepted that any agent capable of causing genetic damage is also likely to be a carcinogen. The most common in vivo tests for genetic damage are chromosome damage tests and the dominant lethal test in mice or rats. Chromosome damage can be assessed in mice and rats by bone marrow cytogenetic analysis and by bone marrow micronucleus assay. In both methods, bone marrow is examined after animals have been treated with either a single high dose or after several (2–4) daily doses of the drug. After the single dose, bone marrow is collected 6, 24, and 48 h after dosing for cytogenetic analysis or 24, 48, and 72 h after dosing for micronucleus determination. After the repeat dosing schedule, bone marrow is collected 6 h or 24–30 h after the last dose for cytogenetic or micronucleus assay, respectively. For cytogenetic analysis, the animals are treated with colchicine 2–3 h prior to euthanasia to block dividing bone marrow cells in metaphase, femoral bone marrow is collected and fixed, and metaphase spreads are prepared on microscope slides.

After Giemsa staining, the numbers of chromosomes and their normal or abnormal appearance in metaphase spreads are determined. In the micronucleus test, femoral bone marrow smears are stained with Giemsa or a fluorescent dye such as acridine orange, and the numbers of polychromatic erythrocytes containing micronuclei are determined. Normal polychromatic erythrocytes contain no nuclei. In the process of red blood cell maturation, the nucleus is expelled just prior to the polychromatic erythrocyte stage. Micronuclei represent chromosomes or chromosome fragments that are left behind in the cell after expulsion of the nucleus.

The dominant lethal assay is used to detect mutagenic damage to male germ cells. The principle behind this assay is that theoretically there are a large number of chromosomes that, when damaged, could lead to lethality during early gestation if included in a fertilized egg. Hence, the target size relative to the genome is large for dominant lethality, and therefore the test should be a sensitive indicator of genetic damage. In this test, male animals (usually rats or mice) are treated with the drug daily for 5 days. They are then mated with separate groups of females each week for 8 weeks. The 8-week interval covers the entire spermatogenic cycle. The females are killed at mid pregnancy, about 14 days after the midweek of mating. At necropsy the uteri are examined and the numbers of corpora lutea, living implantations. and dead implantations are counted. The endpoints for this assay are (1) the numbers of preimplantation losses, determined by subtracting the numbers of implants from the numbers of corpora lutei, and (2) the numbers of dead implants. Agents that cause increased numbers of preimplantation losses or dead implants compared to vehicle or historical control levels are considered positive in the dominant lethal assay. Because of the serial mating scheme, it is possible to know which stage of spermatogenesis is affected if a positive result is obtained.

Several transgenic animal models are available for mutagenicity testing in vivo. The most widely used are the Big Blue and Muta Mouse models. These animals have portions of the E. coli galactosidase operon inserted into their genome. This bacterial DNA is used as the target for mutagenicity testing when the animals are treated with test chemicals. After chemical treatment, the bacterial DNA is removed from the tissues and packaged into bacterial viral (phage) particles. The phages are used to infect bacteria growing on agar plates. The bacteria multiply to form colonies that can be counted. Because of a color reaction that can be catalyzed by the galactosidase protein, a color reaction formed in the bacterial colonies can be used to assess the presence or absence of mutations formed in the target DNA from virtually any tissue within the treated mice.

Carcinogenicity

Carcinogenicity bioassays are long-term studies in mice and rats conducted according to standard guidelines established by the National Cancer institute and the International Conference on Harmonizationj] In these studies the animals are treated repeatedly for periods of 18–24 months for mice and of 24 months for rats. Treatment is by a route consistent with the intended clinical route. The study design usually includes vehicle control and two or three drug-treated groups. The highest dosage is selected as the maximum dosage that will be tolerated by the animals. This dosage may cause minimal signs of toxicity but should cause no more than a 10% decrement in body weight gain compared with control groups and should not cause toxicity, other than that related to a neoplastic response, that would be predicted to shorten the animal's natural life span. This high dosage is necessary to give a maximum test of the potential of a new drug to cause cancer. The animals are examined frequently for palpable masses. At the end of the treatment period, the animals are necropsied and histologic examinations of the tissues are conducted with particular attention given to the detection and identification of tumors. Recently, transgenic strains of mice that allow detection of a carcinogenic response within 6 months of treatment rather than 2 years have become available. Examples of these are the $P53^{+/-}$ (P53 knockout), TG.AC and the rasH2 mouse models. These animals contain deletions of genes involved in suppressing the formation of tumors. The use of these animal models is justified based upon the fact that these same genes are known to be involved in many human tumors. Thus, the mechanisms leading to enhanced tumorigenic response in these animals is known to be relevant to human tumorigenesis.

Primary Irritation Testing

If a new drug is intended to be applied to the skin or eyes, one of the first tests to be conducted would be to determine if the drug, or the formulation containing the drug, will cause irritation of the skin or eyes. Even if a drug is intended only for dermal application, eye irritation testing may also be required because of the possibility of inadvertent exposure to the eyes. For instance, an antibiotic intended for topical treatment of acne would be applied on the face, and the potential for eye contact would be considerable. These tests are usually conducted in rabbits because of their widely accepted sensitivity to dermal and ocular irritation and because of the scientific literature describing such tests in rabbits. Other species, such as guinea pigs or mice, may be used for dermal irritation studies under special circumstances.

Table 20.2. Dermal irritation scoring system

Skin reaction	*Value*
Erythema and eschar formation	
No erythema	0
Very slight erythema (barely perceptible)	1
Well-defined erythema	2
Moderate to severe erythema	3
Severe erythema (beet redness) to slight eschar formation (injuries in depth)	4
Edema formation	
No edema	0
Very slight edema (barely perceptible)	1
Slight edema (edges of area well defined by definite raising)	2
Moderate edema (raised approximately 1 mm)	3
Severe edema (raised more than 1 mm and extending beyond the area of exposure)	4

A typical dermal irritation assay is conducted as follows. Six male albino rabbits are be clipped free of hair on the back. One area of skin is left intact, whereas another is abraded in a tic-tac-toe pattern with the point of a hypodermic needle so as to incise the superficial epidermis layer without causing bleeding. The test material, 0.5 ml of liquid or 0.5 g of solid or semisolid is applied to each site under a 1 × 1 in. gauze pad. The entire trunk of the animal is wrapped with an impervious material and held in place with tape for 24 h. The patches are then removed and excessive material wiped off.

The mean values of the six rabbits for erythema and eschar formation at 24 and 72 h for both intact and abraded skin (four values) are added. The mean values of the six rabbits for edema at 24 and 72 h (four values) are also added. The total of eight values is divided by 4 to give the primary irritation index. Values of 5 or greater are considered indicative of a positive irritant.

A typical ocular irritation test is conducted as follows. Six albino rabbits of the same sex are given thorough ophthalmological examinations within 24 h before use to ensure absence of preexisting ocular damage. The animals would be firmly but gently restrained. The test formulation is be placed in one eye of each animal by gently pulling the lower lid away from the eyeball (conjunctival cul-de-sac) to form a cup into which the test substance is dropped. The lids are then gently held together for one second and the animal released. The other eye, remaining untreated, serves as a control. For testing liquids, 0.1 ml is used. For solid, paste, or particulate substances, the amount used must have a volume of 0.1 ml weighing not more than 100mg. The eyes of each rabbit would be examined 24, 48, and 72 h after treatment. After the 24-h examination, the treated eyes may be rinsed with tap water or saline. At this time the eyes may also be examined with the aid of fluorescein stain. One drop of fluorescein sodium ophthalmic solution USP is dropped directly on the cornea. After flushing out the excess fluorescein with tap water or saline, injured areas of the cornea appear yellow and are best seen under ultraviolet illumination.

The test may be considered positive if three or more animals exhibit positive reactions at any observation period. Equivocal tests are repeated. For humane reasons, formulations known to be corrosive or to be severely irritating in the dermal irritation test are assumed to be ocular irritants and not tested.

Antigenicity Testing

New drugs may undergo testing for antigenicity depending upon the chemical structure (suspected of being a sensitizer because of similarity to known sensitizers) or because of the intended use of the drug. Formulations intended for topical use are usually tested for delayed contact sensitivity. However, new drugs intended for systemic use are sometimes tested for their potential to induce anaphylaxis. These tests are commonly conducted in guinea pigs, but rats or mice are sometimes used.

Delayed contact hypersensitivity can be evaluated by several standard protocols in guinea pigs. A typical procedure is to sensitize groups of 10 guinea pigs each by injecting 0.1 ml (0.05 ml for the first injection) of a 0.1% suspension or solution of test material intradermally in the upper dorsal area three times per week for a total of 10 injections. Additional groups are similarly treated with a positive control compound such as dinitrochlorobenzene and a negative control (saline). About 2 weeks after the tenth injection, the animals are challenged by intradermal injection of 0.05 ml of the respective test compound, positive control, or saline in the dorsal lumbar area. The animals are shaved at least 18 prior to each injection.

The erythema and edema grades are recorded separately. A dermal irritation score for each sensitizing injection and the challenge injection for each animal are calculated by adding the 24-h and 48-h scores for both erythema and edema (four scores) and dividing by 4. The dermal irritation scores obtained from the initial sensitizing injection and the challenge injection for each animal are used to determine whether sensitization had been produced. When the challenge score exceeds the initial irritation score for a given animal by 1 or more, the animal is considered sensitized.

The potential of a compound to induce anaphylaxis can be evaluated in both active systemic anaphylaxis (ASA) and passive cutaneous anaphylaxis (PCA) tests in guinea pigs or rats. In both tests, the test compounds and positive and negative control substances are injected subcutaneously or intraperitoneally three times per week to groups of 6–10 animals for a total of 6 injections. In the ASA test, the animals are challenged 2 weeks after the final sensitization injection intravenously with the respective test compound or positive or negative control and observed for signs of anaphylaxis. These would be graded as:

Negative: No anaphylactic symptoms

Mild: Restlessness, rubbing of the nose or ears, coughing, espiratory acceleration, or piloerection

Moderate: Urination, defecation. dyspnea, or ataxic gait

Severe: Convulsion followed by recovery

Fatal: Death by a fatal anaphylactic reaction

In the PCA test, serum is collected from the sensitized animals 2 weeks after the final sensitization injection. This serum is diluted with saline to a dilution of 1/8 or more and injected intradermally on the backs of previously untreated guinea pigs. Four hours later, these guinea pigs are given intravenous injections of 1.5–2.0 ml of saline containing 0.5% Evans Blue plus the respective test compound or positive or negative control. Thirty minutes after the intravenous injection, the animals are examined for the presence of blue areas of skin surrounding the earlier intradermal injections. A blue spot having a diameter of 5–10 mm is considered a positive reaction.

Governmental Requirements

Governmental regulatory agencies such as the USFDA have established guidelines describing the kind of safety tests that should be conducted in animals in order to have a new drug approved for use in clinical trials and in order to get approval of a new drug application (NDA) for marketing. The rationale and circumstances for conducting reproductive, mutagenicity, carcinogenicity, irritation, and sensitization studies have already been mentioned. These descriptions are limited to the requirements of the United States, Japan, and Europe because these areas represent the largest pharmaceutical markets in the world today. These requirements have been developed at the International Conference on Harmonization to provide uniformity among the three regions. Phases I, II, and III refer to the different phases of human clinical trials. Phase I refers to the initial trials, limited to one or a few doses to determine absorption, pharmacokinetics, and an initial estimate of safety. Phase II refers to larger-scale studies to establish safety and to get an initial estimate of clinical efficacy. Phase III refers to the final, large-scale, multicenter trials aimed at establishing efficacy.

Care of Laboratory Animals

Proper care of laboratory animals used in research is a basic requirement to assure the validity and reproducibility of the results obtained. Animals used in drug research are subject to the strictest standards of care beginning with the animal supplier. For the most commonly used laboratory animals, these standards of care often apply for the entire life of the animal. Guidelines for proper care of research animals are provided by the Department of Health and Human Services. The American Association for the Accreditation of Laboratory Animal Care provides the service of certifying laboratories complying with those guidelines. All reputable industrial drug development houses strive to achieve and maintain certification by the association.

Sources of Laboratory Animals

Laboratory animals for drug research in industry are virtually always obtained from reputable animal suppliers who observe strict standards of care of the animals they provide. Animals that are not properly cared for often result in lost time—and therefore lost money—in drug development.

The U.S. Department of Health and Human Services publishes the Guide for the Care and Use of Laboratory Animals, Publication No. (NIH) 78-23. This was prepared by the Committee on Care and Use of Laboratory Animals of the Institute of Laboratory Animal Resources of the National Research Council. The "guide" contains recommendations regarding housing, sanitation, husbandry, veterinary care, personnel qualifications, personal hygiene, occupational health, and physical plant. The National Institutes of Health (NIH) requires that grantees and contractors using live, vertebrate animals in projects supported by NIH follow the guidelines prescribed in the guide. The Public Health Service further requires that grant-seeking institutions either be accredited by the American Association for Accreditation of Laboratory Animal Care (see later) or have an institutional committee that reviews its animal facilities and practices for compliance with the guide.

American Association for Accreditation of Laboratory Animal Care (AAALAC)

AAALAC is a non-profit corporation directed by representatives of 24 scientific and professional organizations that are members of the corporation. It was organized in 1965 to conduct a voluntary program for the accreditation of laboratory animal care facilities and programs. AAALAC encourages optimal care for laboratory animals by providing a mechanism for peer evaluation of animal care programs by the scientific community. Humane treatment of laboratory animals, protection of personnel from hazards associated with the use of animals, and control of variables that could affect animal research adversely are among the principal objectives of the accreditation program. Ani-mal care facilities of applicant institutions are visited and a thoroughly evaluated by two experts in laboratory animal science, who submit a detailed report to the Council on Accreditation. Following the standard listed in the Guide for the Care and Use of Laboratory Animals, the Council determines whether AAALAC accreditation should be granted. Accredited facilities submit annual reports on the status of their animal facilities to AAALAC, and site visits to accredited facilities are conducted at least every 3 years. These annual reports and site visits determine whether accreditation will be continued. Full accreditation by AAALAC is accepted by the NIH as assurance that the animal facilities are evaluated in accordance with their policy on laboratory animals.

21

Microbial Control of Pharmaceuticals

Pharmaceutically active products (drug products) are expected to be efficacious, however; the presence of microorganisms in these products may have adverse effects on their efficacy. The severity of the effects that microorganisms may have on any particular drug product is a function of the nature of the product, its intended use, and the nature of the microorganism concerned. At one end of the spectrum, microbial contamination of a sterile parenteral product may, on injection into a debilitated patient, result in fatality; at the other, patients may refuse to begin or continue a course of medication because of aromas, off-flavors, or discolorations of microbial origin. In either situation, or in any related situation, the presence of microorganisms ought to be avoided in drug products.

Microbiological standards for drug products are published in the pharmacopeias and/or are required by regulatory agencies for their registration. Generally, these standards are concerned with the protection of the public from infection by limiting the numbers and types of microorganisms to levels that are unlikely to be harmful. In addition to standards applying to the products themselves, there are also microbiological standards applying to the conditions under which drug products are allowed to be manufactured. These manufacturing standards (Good Manufacturing Practices, or GMPs) are intended to ensure that finished product standards are being attained consistently.

Microbial control of pharmaceuticals is primarily concerned with minimizing the opportunities for drug products to be contaminated by microorganisms. It is secondarily concerned with minimizing the potential for any microorganisms that may have contaminated drug products to increase to levels that may risk the efficacy of the product. The testing of product samples for compliance with microbiological standards is only one small part of this. By and large, microbiological test methods are product-destructive and, as a consequence, it is unusual to find valid statistical sampling and testing being done at batch release. Finished product testing is at best confirmatory and in some cases may be dispensed with when manufacturing controls ensure that products are highly unlikely to become microbiologically contaminated (parametric release in its broadest sense).

Minimizing the risk of microbiological contamination of drug products is assured by the application of microbiological and physical standards and controls to starting materials, product-contact packaging components, manufacturing facilities, manufacturing processes, and equipment. By and large, these assurances are obtained by applying controls that protect materials, equipment, and processes from sources of microbiological contamination. In recognition of the fraility of protective measures in all but the most extreme circumstances, microbiological contaminants are also routinely controlled by removal, inactivation, or destruction. The microbiological standards applying to drug products are expected to be maintained until time of use by the patient (or healthcare professional) and throughout their shelf-lives. This presents two areas of concern relevant to microbiological control: first, that the product should be protected (usually by its packaging) from additional contamination after release to market, and second, that the product should be formulated to prevent proliferation of any microorganisms that may have been present at tolerable levels at the time of release.

Different types and levels of microbial control are applicable to different types of products. The single major division is between sterile and non-sterile products.

Microbial Control of Sterile Products

Sterility is defined as the total absence of all viable life forms. Parenteral products and ophthalmic products are expected to be sterile. Parenteral products must be sterile because their route of administration overrides the body's external physical barriers to infection. Ophthalmic products must be sterile because eye damage is often irreparable. No distinction can be made between microorganisms that are known to be specific causative agents of disease and those that are not. Any microorganism may be opportunistically pathogenic if administered parenterally or if applied to susceptible tissues (the transparent parts of the eye have a particularly poor blood supply and, therefore, a less sensitive immunological response than do other parts of the body) or to debilitated or immunocompromised patients.

Sterility, the Sterility Test, and Sterility Assurance

Sterility has an absolute definition (absence of ALL viable life forms). As with all absolutes, it is difficult, if not impossible, to prove.

Sterility tests

The pharmacopeial standard applying to sterile products is that they must be capable of passing a Test for Sterility. These were "harmonized" along with the Japanese Pharmacopoeia and the requirements of the Australian Therapeutic Goods Administration in 1999, but they still have some minor differences in detail. The Test for Sterility relies on the detection of viable microorganisms within a sample that is directly or indirectly inoculated into broad-spectrum microbiological recovery media. Detectable microbial growth is confirmation of non-sterility, whereas sterility can be assumed from the absence of growth. In other words, the Test assumes sterility unless non-sterility can be demonstrated. The Test for Sterility is really a test for non-sterility, and even within that redefinition of its terms of reference, its indication is limited to those microorganisms capable of producing discernible growth under the specified test conditions. Many microorganisms are not recoverable under these conditions. When the Test for Sterility first appeared in the USP and in the *British Pharmacopoeia* (BP) in the 1930s, it was described in the same terms as any other pharmacopeial test method; that is, as a method whereby a microbiologist could determine whether a single article presented for analysis was sterile.

There was no indication in the pharmacopeias until 1955 in the USP and until 1968 in the BP that the results of the Test should be or could be extended to apply to batches of product required to be certified as sterile. The USP initially required 10 units to be tested from each batch of autoclaved products and 20 units from each batch of other sterile products, the BP required 20 units. In the current pharmacopeias, the sample size for the Test for Sterility is 20 units in all but a few exceptional circumstances. However, with such a small sample size, successful results (no growth inferring with sterility or "passing" the Test for Sterility) provide little assurance that there is not a significant proportion of contaminated units in the batch. This has been recognized and debated for many years, even before the pharmacopeial requirements were first published. In 1949, Knudsen pointed out that when using a sample size of 20 units, batches containing 5% contaminated units would be "passed" as sterile on 35 of every 100 occasions. Brewer elaborated further on the statistical limitations of sterility testing by showing that sample sizes of 20, 50, and even 100 units are hardly better than sample sizes of 10 units for detecting contamination in batches of product containing 0.1% contaminated units. The pharmacopeial sampling requirements for the Test for Sterility are a compromise; they have been known to be, and shown to be, statistically unsound for decades. They are a compromise between the fact that the Test is destructive to the units sampled and the self- evident requirement for a very high level of assurance that batches of supposedly sterile product do not contain non-sterile units.

In practical terms a "pass" in the Test for Sterility should not be perceived to be of any more significance than any other successful measure of compliance with microbiological or physical standards or controls applicable to the manufacture of sterile products. A "pass" in the Test for Sterility must not be allowed to overrule any failure to comply with other environmental or control standard(s) because it is quite possible to "pass" the Test and still have a significant number of non-sterile units in the batch. On the other hand, a "failed" Test for Sterility is likely to be a good indicator of a genuine problem that has not been disclosed by some other microbiological or physical means.

Methods for sterility testing

The Test for Sterility may be performed in one of two ways, by direct inoculation (direct transfer) or by membrane filtration. In direct inoculation, the product samples are put aseptically into the microbiological recovery medium and incubated. Clearly this approach is only suited to products that are not likely to be inhibitory to the growth of microorganisms in the recovery medium. An incubation period of 14 days is specified. In the membrane filtration method, the product samples are put aseptically into a volume of non- inhibitory diluent and then passed through a sterile 0.45 μm membrane filter. The membrane is rinsed through with additional volumes of diluent, then aseptically cut in half. Half is transferred to a container of soybean casein digest medium (SCDM) and the other to fluid thioglycollate medium (FTM).

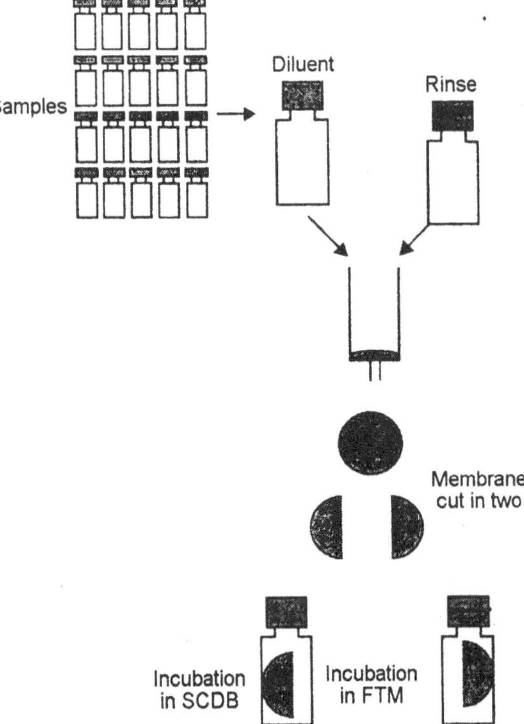

Fig. 21.1. Generalized scheme for the test for sterility by the membrane filtration method.

A variation of membrane filtration is the use of "closed" systems such as the Millipore Steritest system. At the heart of the Steritest system are two presterilized canisters, each with a membrane filter sealed into its base. The product under test is inoculated into its diluent and transferred via a peristaltic pump into the canisters and through the two membranes. During transfer the diluent is automatically split in two parts. After product filtration, the media are transferred into the canisters, SCDM to one canister and FTM to the other, by the same means. No manipulation of the membranes is required. The canisters are incubated at the temperatures specified in the pharmacopeias. Whichever variant of the membrane filtration method is used, SCDM is incubated at 20-25°C and the FTM at 30-35°C for 14 days.

Before 1999, the pharmacopeias allowed incubation for only 7 days. Now the USP allows 7-day incubation only for terminally sterilized products. This extension of the incubation period from 7 to 14 days is a curious situation. The stimulus was an article published by the Australian Regulatory Agency indicating that it was possible for some drug products to be contaminated with microorganisms that would require more than 7 days of incubation to produce demonstrable growth under the conditions of the Test for Sterility. This was not, however, a remarkable new discovery. Brewer and Schmitt observed (albeit with ethylene oxide sterilized medical devices) in 1966 that "slow growing" microorganisms (e.g., micrococci and diphtheroids) might take up to 4 weeks to produce demonstrable growth under the conditions of the USP Test for Sterility. There has been no actual evidence of patients having come to harm as a result of requiring only 7 days of incubation in the Test for Sterility. One can only suggest that some compromise was reached during the "harmonization" discussions, and the benefit must be for exporters to Australia where the "preharmonization" Test for Sterility was far more demanding and restrictive.

Conditions for sterility testing

The Test for Sterility is vulnerable to false-positive and false-negative results. A false-positive means that a genuinely sterile product fails the test because of incidental contamination during the preparation of the sample or during the Test. A false-negative means that a non-sterile product passes the Test because viable contaminants fail to grow.

Both circumstances can have serious consequences, but false-positives are less likely to go unnoticed because high frequencies of false-positives have a commercial impact, at least delaying the release of product and at worst leading to suspension of manufacture.

The avoidance of false-negatives is addressed at length in the pharmacopeias. Each batch of medium used in the Test for Sterility must have been shown to be capable of supporting the growth of low inocula of a specified array of microorganisms. Each Test for Sterility applicable to each specific product must be validated by repeated demonstration that the viabilities of low inocula of a specified array of microorganisms are not inhibited by product traces contained in the medium (direct inoculation) or on the membrane filter.

The pharmacopeial attitude to false-positives changed in 1999, beginning in the 8th Supplement to USP 23 and in the 1999 Supplement of PhEur. An expectation of some level of false-positives had been tolerated in the Test for Sterility since its inception. This was in acknowledgement of there being a finite probability of the Test becoming contaminated as a result of the large number of aseptic manipulations required in its performance. However, times and technologies have changed.

When the Test for Sterility was first published in the 1930s, it was, at best, being done in glove boxes. The pharmacopeias recognized the probability of incidental contamination and permitted, in the event of Test failure, an automatic right to retest without further ado. However, with the advent of HEPA filtration and laminar flow technology in the 1960s, the actual frequency of false-positive diminished, but the automatic right to retest remained. Isolation technology became available for doing the Test for Sterility in the last decade of the 20th century.

The automatic right to retest still remained in the pharmacopeias until in the 1999 revisions, it was recognized that the testing technology was available whereby the probability of incidentally contaminating a Test for Sterility could be less than the probability of the sample actually being non-sterile. The current pharmacopeial situation is therefore that retesting is only permitted when it can be unequivocally demonstrated that the contaminant in the Test arose incidentally during testing. Strictly, this is not a retest but a repeat Test because the first Test is at fault.

The consequence of this approach is that repeat testing is allowed only with a great deal of information about the microbiological conditions pertaining during the Test, and a large element of professional judgment by the functions held responsible for product release. Many companies have balanced the potential for the increased risk of commercial loss as a result of failures in the Test for

Sterility with the potential for regulatory action in the event of disagreement over the judgment involved in repeat testing. They concluded that isolation technology is the only sensible future for the Test for Sterility.

Sterility assurance

Despite the attention, capital and resources given to the Test for Sterility, batches of product cannot be confirmed to be sterile by end-product testing. The Test for Sterility is in fact only a test for a specific broad range of microbial contaminants, and its sampling statistics are not capable of disclosing frequencies of contaminated units that would put patients at risk owing to non-sterility. This has been recognized by the pharmacopeias, notably the PhEur, which for some years has carried a statement:

... a satisfactory result only indicates that no contaminating microorganism has been found in the sample examined in the conditions of the test.... The sterility test is ... the only analytical method available to the authorities who have to examine any product for sterility.

Then, how can sterility of batches of supposedly sterile products be confirmed by those functions within companies that are held responsible for product release? The answer is in the use of validated manufacturing processes based on sound scientific evidence that each product unit is most probably sterile. This raises a second question of how much confidence must one have to claim sterility? The answer to this question, for terminally sterilized products, is that there must be no more than one chance in a million that viable contaminants survive in any one unit. This is called a sterility assurance level (SAL) of 10^{-6}. The answer for aseptically filled products is that the SAL must be as close to 10^{-6} as is technically possible, with the proviso that the degree of protection given to the process must afford no more than one chance in a thousand of any one unit becoming contaminated. This is called a contamination rate of 10^{-3}, and unlike the SAL it relates only to the protection given to the process and not to the potential for contaminants surviving or proliferating in actual products.

The concept of the SAL is founded in academic studies of how microbial populations reduce in numbers in response to inimical treatments. In 1945 McCulloch showed that for steam sterilization, a population of bacteria: "exposed to a lethal degree of heat ... decreases in a fairly orderly manner. Thus if 90% of the viable population is killed during the first minute of exposure, approximately 90% of the survivors will be killed during each subsequent minute, which will continue until nearly all of the population is extinct."

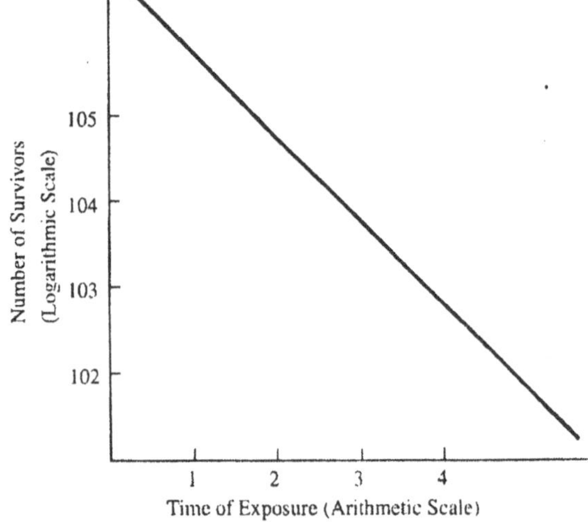

Fig. 21.2. Exponential inactivation of microorganisms.

This exponential order of inactivation of microbial populations has subsequently been demonstrated to be a general characteristic of microorganisms in all processes of sterilization. The logarithmic axis of the exponential survival curve has no zero point. Thus, there can be no time of exposure at any temperature, no dose of radiation no matter how high, that can guarantee 100% inactivation of any microbial population. Exponential inactivation is the basis of the concept of sterility assurance. If the behavior of microbial populations in response to a particular sterilizing procedure is regular and exponential over the region of the survival curve within which their response can be monitored, then the treatments required to achieve SALs of 10^{-6} can be extrapolated. The aseptic filling process is not suited to the calculation of SALs in this way. This is because aseptic filling is not based on exponential inactivation and therefore provides no basis for extrapolation. The principle of aseptic manufacture is that, first of all, the drug product and its product-contact packaging components are sterilized to comply with SALs of 10^{-6}, and then they are brought together in ways that are intended to avoid further contamination (asepsis). Ideally, the finished product would still have an SAL of 10^{-6}. The short-fall from this ideal is primarily a function of the technology used in the aseptic filling process. Where sterile isolation technology is being used—this is a developing rather than an established technology at the time of writing in 2000—it is likely that there is very little shortfall. With standard technology, a level of process protection from microorganisms demonstrable through media fills offering a contamination rate of no more than 10^{-3} is nominally acceptable to regulatory bodies worldwide.

Microbiological GMP in the Manufacture of Sterile Drug Products

As far as manufacture is concerned, there are two broad categories of sterile products: those that are terminally sterilized (filled and hermetically sealed within their final containers before being exposed to a sterilization treatment), and those that are aseptically manufactured (the drug product and its product-contact packaging components are sterilized and then brought together in ways that are intended to avoid further contamination. Serious measures to protect the manufacture from microbiological contamination are necessary for both categories but are clearly most critical in the poststerilization stages of aseptic manufacture. There are several sources of standards and limits that may be applied to the manufacture of sterile products. They can be divided into sector-specific standards which are focused specifically on the manufacture of sterile pharmaceuticals and generic standards that are focused on particular technologies, irrespective of how the technologies are to be applied.

Sector-specific standards applying to manufacture of sterile drug products

There are five significant sources of sector-specific standards applying to the manufacture of sterile products. Two are mandatory, three are voluntary. The two mandatory standards are Annex 1 of the European Union's GMPs and the FDA's 1987 Guideline on Sterile Drug Products Produced by Aseptic Processing. The FDA document is under review at the time of writing this article. The first of the two non-mandatory standards is contained in Section 1116 of the USP. It should be explained that this is a general chapter of the USP and is not therefore mandatory unless referenced in a USP monograph. At time of writing, Section 1116 is not referenced in any monographs. The second of the voluntary standards is IS 13408, applying to both medical devices and to pharmaceuticals according to the International Standards Organization (ISO) definition of "healthcare products." Here, it should be explained that the ISO is a voluntary body whose membership is drawn from national standards organizations. ISO standards have no legal authority in any country or territory unless the national standards body elects to adopt the ISO standard instead of publishing its own standards.

The third voluntary standard is The International Society of Pharmaceutical Engineer's (ISPE) Baseline Pharmaceutical Engineering Guide. This is one of a series of ISPE guidance documents that has limited endorsement by the FDA. It should be understood that only minimal standards are being endorsed and there are many reasons why specific sterile products and applications could be seen by the FDA to require compliance with higher standards.

Working with these five documents is not easy; they use different terminology and definitions and have different emphases that in part, may be a function of the 10-year span that encompasses publication dates. All of them are concerned with controlling microbiological contamination that may arise from the environment, from personnel, and from materials and equipment. Some individual standards within these documents may relate to microbial numbers, others to physical characteristics that relate to contamination control.

All of these documents stress a requirement for room classifications according to the concentration of non-viable airborne particles at 0.5 μm and larger. The EU GMPs subordinate classification of the various areas applicable to sterile manufacture according a broader based grading system. Grades A to D are defined in terms of a range of independent characteristics such as the concentration of non-viable airborne particles at two sizes in operational and nonoperational conditions, the concentration of airborne viable particles in operational conditions, and several other indices of microbial contamination on surfaces and hands, etc. The inclusion of microbiological limits within this grading system is important in that it emphasizes that it is not solely the concentration of non-viable airborne particles in cleanrooms (room classification) that determines their suitability for manufacture of sterile products.

Generic standards for technologies used in the manufacture of sterile drug products

The most important generic standards applying to technologies used in the manufacture of sterile drug products relate to the protection of manufacture from contamination from the air. The air supply to facilities for sterile manufacture must be filtered, in some specific applications, it must be unidirectional, its velocity may have to be controlled within specified limits, and there must be pressure differentials between adjacent areas. In the late 1990s, there had been a great deal of ISO activity in the harmonization of various standards applying to air quality. The first three parts address classification of air cleanliness, methods for testing and monitoring, and metrology. Parts 1 and 2 cover much of the ground but are not identical to FS 209. The significant question emerging as these standards are published has to do with the reaction of the pharmaceutical regulatory agencies. Whereas we can with confidence be sure that the standards applying to the specifications of HEPA filter media and to the in situ HEPA filter integrity test will be accepted, there still are some doubts about the standard for room classification. Both of the two mandatory sector-specific standards currently require room classification according to Federal Standard 209. This is a U.S. government standard; its current revision is FS 209E, and it will not be automatically replaced by IS 14644. Thus, we are dependent on the next revision of Annex 1 of the EU GMPs and of the FDA's Guideline on Sterile Drug Products Produced by Aseptic Processing to determine whether they will be adopted for the manufacture of sterile drug products.

Validation and Control of Sterilization Processes

Although there are many sterilization processes used in association with the manufacture of sterile drug products, the three primary processes are steam sterilization, dry heat sterilization, and sterile filtration. Dry heat sterilization is, in the context of the manufacture of sterile parenteral products, a subset of dry heat depyrogenation.

Steam sterilization

Steam sterilization is widely used as a terminal process for drug products in glass ampules, vials, syringes, and plastic containers. It is also used for sterilizing closures, filters, manufacturing equipment, and cleaning equipment, etc. Steam sterilization in autoclaves has a long and strong scientific basis. The essence of validation of steam sterilization processes is to demonstrate that temperature and time conditions are being achieved uniformly through every item included the autoclave load and that the lethality being achieved in practical situations corresponds to that which would be expected from sterilization theory. Thus, compliance with limits for temperature uniformity throughout empty autoclaves (heat distribution studies) is an index of the way in which the autoclaves are engineered. Compliance with limits for temperature uniformity within items loaded into the autoclaves (heat penetration) is an index of the way in which items are wrapped for sterilization (where applicable) and how they are loaded into the autoclaves in relation to the positions of steam inlets, drains, racks, trays, and thermal sensors.

With modern autoclaves, the major impediment of concern to successful sterilization is air in porous loads. Air may be present as a contaminant of the steam supply such that the temperatures theoretically achievable at particular steam pressures are depressed, or air may be present within the load, insulating it from the contact with the steam required for predictable lethality.

Pure steam generators are designed to deliver steam of satisfactory quality—standards are published in a UK document, Health Technical Memorandum (HTM) 2010 but non-condensable gas like air and nitrogen can accumulate in the steam through poorly insulated and trapped distribution systems and therefore should be tested periodically close to point of use. Autoclaves suited to sterilization of porous loads require some form of air removal, most often by deep pulsed vacuums, before the introduction of steam. The effectiveness of air removal is difficult to monitor by physical means; air entrapment may be a local phenomenon in particular locations in loads, in particular materials (e.g., in cartridge filters), or where items come into contact with one another (e.g., with rubber closures in bulk). Therefore, it is normal to use biological indicators to ensure that there is correspondence between theoretical and practical reality. Biovalidation of steam sterilization, although done extensively, is all very complex and, to an extent, a poorly understood. The basics are that a suitable biological indicator should be resistant to sterilization by steam (but not necessarily the most resistant microorganism known—spores of *Bacillus stearothermophilus*) are approved by the USP, PhEur, and others and are most often used. The biovalidation cycle must be of lower thermal lethality than the lowest thermal lethality allowable within the routine production-cycle specification.

Steam sterilization is not confined to autoclaves. Many items of manufacturing equipment, including some quite massive applications to vessels, pipe-work, filters, etc., are now sterilized in place with steam (SIP). It is essential that the equipment holds pressure, that air is removed, and that condensation does not accumulate in low points of the system. Biological validation is generally unsophisticated and is normally done by ensuring that the process inactivates several biological challenge test pieces, each carrying 10^6 spores of *Bacillus stearothermophilus* (D_{121}-values undefined but presumably meeting the pharmacopeial criteria of equal to or greater than 1.5 min) placed at critical points. Academically, it is problematic to equate this approach with the sterility assurance level concept that applies to the sterilization of groups of items. Steam sterilization processes are monitored for compliance with strict specifications of temperature, pressure, and time. Routine monitoring with biological indicators is not necessary. Indeed, any item of steam sterilizing equipment that is operating so erratically as to merit routine monitoring with biological indicators should be replaced.

Sterilization by filtration

Filtration is a means of sterilizing fluids by removing, rather than inactivating, microorganisms. The sterilization of liquids is used extensively in aseptic manufacture, sterilization of gases is used both in terminal sterilization and in aseptic manufacture. Most applications use cellulose-esters, polyvinylidine fluoride, polytetrafluoroethylene, nylon, and other polymeric materials. The removal of microorganisms from fluids by passage through filters is very complex; sieving, or surface retention, is only one of a series of mechanisms that depend on interactions among the chemistry and surface characteristics of the membrane, the microorganisms, and the suspending fluid.

The FDA defines sterilizing filters as those that have pore-size ratings of 0.22 μm or smaller and relates this to a microbiological particle passage test using *Pseudomonas (Brevundimonas) diminuta*: A sterilizing filter is one which, when challenged with the microorganism Pseudomonas diminuta, at a minimum concentration of 10^7 organisms per cm^2 of filter surface will produce a sterile effluent. It is essential that the microbiological particle passage test is performed as part of the development of new sterile formulations. Because of its very specialized nature, the test is normally performed only by the filter manufacturers, who then provide limits for secondary physical tests (e.g., bubble point, pressure decay, forward flow, etc.), which can be applied to verify the pore size rating and integrity of the membrane filters.

Maintenance of Sterility After Product Release

The sterility of a sterile dosage form can only be guaranteed while it is protected from the surrounding non- sterile environment within a container made from materials impermeable to microbial penetration. Container and closure systems for sterile products must be capable of withstanding process conditions, storage, and transport without compromizing the sterility of the product. This has been recently emphasized by the FDA, which has omitted a former obligation to provide data from the Test for Sterility in stability program for new sterile products in favor of verifying the microbial integrity of the container-closure system.

There are no standard methods for verifying microbiological integrity of container-closure systems. Documents such as that published by the Parenteral Society in 1992 and the PDA in 1998 may be helpful in relating microbiological integrity to secondary physical tests, but they do not specify detailed microbiological test methods. There are two general approaches, wet tests and aerosol challenge tests. Wet tests consider penetration of microorganisms in liquid suspension into sealed containers usually previously filled with sterile medium. The basic assumption is that the most vulnerable route for penetration of liquid filled containers by microorganisms is in the event of a continuous liquid film or "bridge" forming between the outside and the inside of a container. Aerosol challenge tests are less critical than wet tests and should be applied only when total exclusion of moisture from the containment system can be ensured by secondary barriers.

No discussion of maintenance of sterility is complete without addressing multiple-dose ophthalmic presentations. The normal circumstances for sterile parenteral products are that they are unit dose or, if multiple dose, they are penetrated only by sterile transfer devices (syringes, giving sets, etc.) and used on one patient only. This is not the case for ophthalmic ointments and drops: unit-dose presentations are quite unusual and generally used only in hospital practice, for example, after eye surgery.

The multiple-dose presentation is the norm for ophthalmic products. The container is breached at first use and therefore has no further microbiological integrity over subsequent applications by the patient for an undefined period possibly up to the expiration date of the product. Under these circumstances, contamination of the drug products can and must occur; the proliferation of the contaminating microorganisms the products is controlled by use of antimicrobial and preserved formulations. After opening they are, effectively, non-sterile products. Why, therefore, do we go to the trouble to manufacture ophthalmic ointments and drops as sterile products? There is no clear answer to this question; it is an anomaly. It has been a worldwide regulatory requirement "since the beginning of time" for ophthalmic products to be manufactured as sterile, and there is undoubtedly little point in contesting its logic or consistency. Another possible anomaly concerning sterility may be arising from the FDA's 1997 proposal to require all aqueous inhalation products to be sterile. This example is anomalous because only in very exceptional circumstances is the equipment used to administer inhalation products supplied and maintained sterile and, of course, neither are the nasopharyngeal and bronchial passages of the patient.

Pyrogens, Lipopolysaccharides, and Bacterial Endotoxins

Parenteral products are expected to be sterile because of the risk of infection. Another critical biological characteristic is that they should be free from pyrogens. Pyrogens are substances that, when injected in sufficient amounts into the human body, give rise to a variety of extremely unpleasant symptoms of which the most recognizable is a rise in body temperature. In extreme conditions, the rise in body temperature can be so rapid and to such an extent that the patient dies (endotoxic shock).

In the pharmacopeias, pyrogenic products have traditionally been defined in terms of the temperature rise induced in injected rabbits. The causative agent of the pyrogenic response is lipopolysaccharide. This material is of microbiological origin, and although all bacteria appear to be capable of producing lipopolysaccharide, it is found primarily in the cell envelope of Gram-negative species. Naturally occurring lipopolysaccharide is referred to as bacterial endotoxin.

Bacterial endotoxin reacts with a high degree of specificity with a "*clottable protein*" contained in the amoebocyte cells of the horseshoe crab (*Limulus polyphemus*). This has allowed the development of in vitro testing of drug products and other substances for bacterial endotoxins. The pharmacopeias are progressively replacing their former requirements for in vivo rabbit pyrogen testing of parenteral products with the in vitro Limulus Amoebocyte Lysate (LAL) test. There are a variety of test systems now marketed (gel clot, turbidometric, chromogenic, etc.), but the pharmacopeias regard the gel clot method as the reference test. In the gel clot method for the LAL test, a quantity of LAL reagent of defined sensitivity (λ), e.g., 0.03 EU (endotoxin units) per milliliter, is mixed with an equal quantity of the product under test (or a dilution thereof). The mixture is incubated for a defined period and then inverted. The production of a gel is evidence of bacterial endotoxin in the product sample at a concentration equal to or greater than the sensitivity of the LAL reagent.

Product endotoxin limits are based on dosage regimes derived from a formula K/M, where K is the threshold dose for any substance capable of giving a pyrogenic response in humans. With some exceptions K has been given a fixed value of 5 EU/kg body weight of the patient, and adult patient body weight is standardized to 70kg for calcualtion. M is the maximum dose of endotoxin per kilogram of body weight of a patient that is permitted to be given in a single 1-hr period. Endotoxin limits are therefore unique to each dosage form. Because K is fixed, it is usually only necessary to determine M from the maximum human dosage indicated in the product instructions. The validation and performance of the endotoxin test require rather elaborate and detailed attention to use of controls.

Control of bacterial endotoxins

Although bacterial endotoxins are of microbiological origin, they are not lost with loss of viability. Of the sterilization processes commonly used in the manufacture of sterile parenteral dosage forms, only dry heat is capable of destroying bacterial endotoxins in a reasonable time frame. There is therefore no practical way of removing bacterial endotoxins from finished drug products: thus, they must be controlled at source. The most likely source of bacterial endotoxins is water and product-contact packaging components that have been in contact with water. This is because bacterial endotoxins are most frequently found associated with Gram-negative bacteria, and Gram-negative bacteria have evolved to be primarily waterborne. Water used in manufacture of sterile parenteral products must comply with pharmacopeial limits for endotoxin of no more than 0.25 EU/ml (limits in the USP and PhEur for water for injection). In principle water complying with this limit can be produced by distillation, reverse osmosis, and ultrafiltration. PhEur allows only distillation to be used for the manufacture of ingredient water for parenteral products; the USP allows distillation and reverse osmosis. Only the Japanese Pharmacopoeia allows water for injection to be manufactured using ultrafiltration.

Product-contact packaging components, such as glass vials, which are required to be sterile, are usually sterilized and depyrogenated by dry heat in ovens or tunnels. The standard required by the FDA for acceptable depyrogenation processes is that they should be capable of reducing a bacterial endotoxin challenge by a factor of 10^{-3} (3 logs). Unfortunately, inactivation of bacterial endotoxins by dry heat is complex, and satisfactory process specifications are difficult to predict; inactivation of purified lipopolysaccharide may approximate to pseudo-second-order reaction kinetics. It appears that there may be a threshold temperature of approximately 160–170°C, below which a 3-log reduction of bacterial endotoxin cannot be achieved regardless of time of exposure.

Microbial Control of Non-sterile Products

Non-sterile dosage forms are a diverse group of products. The microbiological risks that non-sterile products present to the patient are equally diverse. A single microbiological standard cannot sensibly be applied to all non-sterile products, and this is well reflected by pharmacopeial and regulatory requirements. Similarly, there can be no single standard applied to the microbiological control and prevention of contamination during the manufacture of non-sterile products.

Microbial Limit Test

Microbial limit standards for some, but not all, non-sterile dosage forms are given in USP monographs. PhEur takes a slightly different approach. One of these categories is for products for topical and respiratory use, the other for product's for oral and rectal administration.

In setting appropriate limits for particular non- sterile products, both pharmacopeias take account of the significance of microorganisms to different types of product, to the way in which the product is used, and to the potential hazard to the patient. For instance, 47 of 48 monographs defining microbial limits listed in USP 24 for oral dosage forms restrict microorganisms (*E. coli* and/or *Salmonella*) that are pathogenic by gastrointestinal ingestion. These are, of course, not the only microorganisms that could endanger a patient taking an oral dosage form. They have been selected as indicators of the general type because there are well defined methods for their recovery and they are easily recognizable in culture. Similarly, the USP typically (but not universally) restricts from topical products only those microorganisms (*Staphylococcus aureus*, *Pseudomonas aeruginosa*) that have the potential to cause skin infections. Sixty- seven of 68 monographs in the USP 24 require the absence of at least these two species, and of these 67 only 11 have additional requirements. These limits applying to the absence of specific indicator microorganisms appropriate to the product's usage may be supplemented by general hygiene restrictions on total numbers of microorganisms per gram or milliliter (typically to no more than 100 cfu per gram or milliliter). A very similar overall approach is taken by the PhEur.

Requirements are not specified in the pharmacopeias for sample sizes appropriate to testing batches of non-sterile products for compliance with microbial limits. The test is destructive to the product, and it is extremely unlikely that statistically valid sampling plans are in use anywhere; samples composed of 10 1-g amounts taken from 10 separate 15-g tubes of cream, or of three 3.3-ml amounts taken from three separate 500-ml bottles of syrup, may be typical.

The Microbial Limit Test is, like the Test for Sterility, only confirmatory. It is not generally mandatory to test each batch of every non-sterile product for compliance with microbial limits. The exception is in the United States where it is mandatory to test every batch of non-sterile product. At the time of writing (early 2001), the FDA has proposed a relaxation of this rule for future registrations. However, in the case of tablets there is no requirement to register microbial limits, and therefore testing is not mandatory. The logic behind this is that the water content of tablets is too low to allow proliferation of microbiological contaminants.

It should also be kept in mind that the major regulatory agencies (FDA, MCA) would not want to have the pharmacopeial limits on numbers of microorganisms perceived as tolerance of microorganisms contaminating and proliferating in non-sterile products. The acceptance of these limits is only an acknowledgment of the reality that when products are not manufactured as sterile, some microbiological contamination is inevitable. Well formulated non-sterile products manufactured under microbiologically controlled conditions are extremely unlikely to have bioburdens approaching the pharmacopeial limits (typically 100 cfu per gram or milliliter). Most regulatory bodies now expect companies to set tighter microbial limits on their non-sterile products based on their typical results, these being seen as alert limits indicative of some loss of microbiological control if exceeded.

Microbiological GMP in the Manufacture of Non-Sterile Drug Products

The extent to which the microbiological controls are required to be applied in the manufacture of non- sterile dosage forms is primarily a function of two factors: consequences of infection to the patients and probability of microorganisms proliferating in the product. The seriousness of the risk to patients of infection from non-sterile dosage forms is primarily dictated by the route of administration of the dosage form. The probability of contaminating microorganisms surviving and proliferating in a non-sterile dosage form is generally a function of its water content. The precise allocation of "stars" is a matter of opinion, but at one extreme there is little doubt that aqueous inhalations merit "5-star" microbiological controls in manufacture, and possibly may soon be required to be sterile. Near the other extreme, the FDA, for example, does not require microbial limits to be registered for solid oral dosage forms.

There is little published guidance to microbiological controls for non-sterile manufacture. Equipment and facilities should be designed to minimize the opportunities for contact with air, personnel, and water. Exposure to air is unavoidable, either as local atmospheric (environmental) air or as air from compressors used to operate manufacturing equipment and in fluid bed dryers, etc. Even for "1-star" non- sterile manufacture, the air supplied to areas used for manufacture and filling should be filtered. HEPA filters should be used in "5-star" non-sterile manufacture but are generally not necessary in "1-star," intermediate classifications of manufacture, requiring decisions on air filtration to be made from sensible risk assessments.

Personnel should be restricted from all areas of pharmaceutical manufacture to those who are necessary. Protection from contamination from personnel is by training in hygiene, enforcement of hygiene rules, and provision of protective clothing. Hair is the major source of contamination from personnel, and "street clothes" is the second most significant source. Hair- covers should be provided and worn properly in all areas of sterile manufacture; beards, moustaches, and other excessive facial hair should be covered. Overall sleeves should extend to the wrist and be elasticated or studded to provide a neat fit. Because dogs are still allowed to soil the streets, protective footwear or shoe covers should be provided to all personnel allowed to enter pharmaceutical manufacturing areas.

Water is often the major ingredient in non-sterile products. When it is used as an ingredient, it must meet the pharmacopeial limit for purified water of not more than 100 cfu/ml. Well designed and operated pharmaceutical purified water production and distribution set ups meet far tighter standards than these. Water is also often the principal cleaning fluid for equipment and facilities and is therefore unavoidable. It is a potent source of contamination because it usually contains sufficient nutrients to allow survival of metabolically versatile microorganisms, particularly *Pseudomonas* spp.

When water is left to stand, Pseudomonas spp. do not only survive, but increase in number. Water should not be permitted to stand on equipment (particularly in crannies and crevices), on floors, or in sinks and wash bays. Contamination spreads with water that forms films over surfaces and on the hands and clothing of personnel. Waterborne contaminants may be aerosolized by vibrations or when water falls more than a few centimeters. To restrict the opportunity for contamination from water, there should be air breaks of approximately 5 cm installed between equipment drains and the tun dishes leading to foul drains. The FDA has published guidances on the design and control of water systems.

Maintenance of Microbiological Quality of Non-Sterile Products After Release

It is not desirable for those few microorganisms that may be present in non-sterile products at the time of release to increase to numbers to levels at which they may present a risk of infection to the patient or "spoil" the product. Additional contamination in the period up to the first use by the patient or healthcare professional is provided by the packaging. It is neither necessary nor usual to find that non-sterile product packaging has been specifically designed or tested to be impermeable to microbiological contamination. On the other hand, many products are given good microbiological protection as a secondary consequence of the protection given to the stability of their active ingredients, etc. For instance, tablets packed individually in strips or foils are microbiologically protected until time of use. It is also unlikely for microorganisms to be able to contaminate pressurized metered-dose inhaler containers.

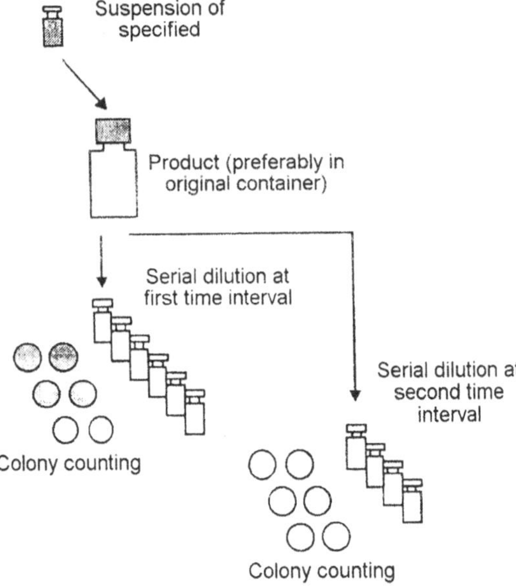

Fig. 21.3. Generalized scheme for preservative efficacy testing.

Microbiological protection of multiple-dose presentations such as liquid inhalations, nasal sprays, oral liquids, creams, and lotions is more complex. Once opened they are susceptible to microbiological contamination. If they are aqueous-based, they are in principle susceptible to proliferation of these "new" contaminants. To avoid this, they are formulated with antimicrobial agents or preservatives and are expected to be able to comply with preservative efficacy standards specified in the pharmacopeias.

22

Research and Development in Pharmaceutical Industry

The structure of discovering and developing new drugs has shifted greatly over the past 20 years. In the early years of this industry, from its rebirth following the Second World War through roughly the end of the 1970s, the major pharmaceutical companies developed "in house" most of their primary products, largely by testing large numbers of available compounds. Scientific knowledge was obtained primarily from freely available sources. There were perhaps 40 highly integrated firms worldwide that contributed to this effort. Since then, the process of drug development and discovery has become increasingly complex. A new technology appeared, termed "biotechnology," which placed this process on a more scientific basis. A new set of firms appeared: smaller and interposed between the scientific community and the major pharmaceutical firms. It is reported that between 25% and 40% of sales by the major pharmaceutical companies currently are from products that originated in the biotech sector.

New Technology for Pharmaceutical Research

Since the mid-1980s the pharmaceutical industry has been shaken by the rapid pace of technological change. Unlike most other industries, however, this change has had little effect on production processes used to produce new or existing products. It has not led to cost-saving innovations that permit lower production costs; indeed, it has had little to do with the manufacturing process. Instead the new technology relates to the process by which new products emerge in this industry. At the same time, the new technology has not had so great an impact on the process by which new drugs are tested and evaluated. The extensive testing of new drugs required by the U.S. Food and Drug Administration (FDA) and similar agencies elsewhere has not been greatly affected by the new research methods.

At the dawn of the modern industry, in the 1950s and 1960s, the process of drug discovery was largely empirical and had little of a theoretical base. This fact was acknowledged in studies written during this era, such as the book by Jewkes, Sawyers, and Stillerman (1958). Those authors emphasized the distinction between systematic and empirical research. In the former, "the new idea has a certain completeness and unity from the outset," while in the latter, "the new idea is a nature of a discovery arising from a search, more or less informed, among many possibilities." The latter approach was characteristic of new discoveries in the chemical industry. Jewkes et al. suggested that "many modern chemical inventions... have risen from the vague intuition that a chemical compound with a given structure might have certain desirable properties, followed by the experimental verification of the hypothesis". This characterization was applied directly to pharmaceutical research during this era. Thus, a former medical director of a division within Pfizer stated in 1960: There can be no question that some very wonderful, exciting, extremely important, and productive research has been and is being done within the pharmaceutical industry. However, we do not think that it would detract in any way from these fine and worthwhile activities to point out that much that is called research in the pharmaceutical industry has little relationship to what most people engaged in academic and research activities would consider to be scientific research.

If this picture applied to the early postwar years, it does not describe the pharmaceutical research process very well at the beginning of the twenty-first century. What was once a largely empirical discovery process has developed into a more theoretical activity. The science of pharmacology has become more advanced so that researchers can develop a greater understanding of how drugs work in the body. This greater understanding has shifted the character and setting for pharmaceutical research.

The shift to a more science-based process, however, is not fully complete. It occurred more rapidly in some therapeutic categories than in others, and in some pharmaceutical companies than in others. These two dimensions are, of course, not independent for companies whose work is more heavily concentrated in areas where science-driven activities have taken hold more fully and have in turn adopted the new approach more quickly. A striking feature about this technological shift has been the considerable heterogeneity in the adoption process. The diffusion of this change has not been rapid or complete. One reason is that firms who want to employ the new technology cannot merely invest in basic research. Cockburn and Henderson (1998) emphasize that "it is also important for the firm to be actively connected to the wider scientific community". They developed the concept of "connectedness," as measured by the extent of collaboration in writing scientific papers across institutional boundaries, and conclude that "firms wishing to public sector research must do more than simply invest in in-house basic research: they must also actively collaborate with their public sector colleagues... . The extent of this collaboration... is positively related to private sector research productivity". The process by which firms acquire this new technology is not simple or direct, nor obtained without cost.

Cockburn, Henderson, and Stern (1999) emphasize the importance of organizational factors and the distribution of power relationships within the firm for the speed at which new research methods are employed. Some firms are more suited to the new technology than others. The authors note that all their informants emphasized "that differences in the historical experience of the firm, in their 'knowledge capital,' were critically important in shaping the adoption decision". To examine the diffusion process empirically, Cockburn et al. explore the relationship between patenting and publishing by the company's scientific staff. When the older, more empirical approaches were employed, these activities were considered substitutes, and the publication of research findings not encouraged. In contrast, research organizations using more science-based methods saw the publication of research findings differently. These activities were encouraged as promoting increased interdependence with the scientific community. For this reason, patenting and publishing were now complements rather than substitutes in the research process. Cockburn, Henderson, and Stern also study the manner by which the new technology was adapted. They find that the new technology was an important factor for pharmaceutical research and yet has been characterized by a relatively low rate of diffusion. The increasing importance of new biological discoveries for the design of pharmaceutical products required new capabilities.

As Gambardella (1995) notes, "Although a public good, science is not a 'free' good. Internal scientific capabilities are critical for taking advantage of the public good". From interviews with research personnel at various companies, he observes the different decisions taken at different companies to develop their scientific capabilities. Some made a major effort in this, while others did not. Where the new technology was employed, research personnel were encouraged to participate in the broader scientific community and publish their findings in the scientific literature. There was also increasing collaboration by industry researchers with nonindustry scientists located at university and government laboratories. As part of these increasing interactions, there have been a greater number of research collaborations and agreements between drug companies and other scientific institutions. Gambardella provides a list of 59 such relationships between large U.S. companies and universities and other research institutions from the 1980s. While research institutions benefit from the infusion of industry funds, the companies gain greater access to scientific discoveries.

To test these observations, Gambardella estimates the relationship between company patents and a lag structure of its scientific publications, together with the level of research expenditures. He reports that "scientific research and drug discovery appear to be intimately connected" and that "in the 1980s, the productivity of applied research increased which is related to significant advances in scientific knowledge and in the technology of experimentation (e.g., computerized drug design)". From his data, there were clear advantages to firms who adopt the new technology. Cockburn and Henderson (1998) examine the importance of public funding for the development of the most important new drugs. Although they find that more than three-fourths of the leading 21 drugs introduced between 1965 and 1992 had at least some input from the public sector, this does not mean that public-sector research was sufficient for their development. Of these products, most relied on enabling discoveries from the public sector. However, for only 2 of the 21 did public-sector research contribute to the synthesis of the relevant compound. Even when creation of new drugs was facilitated by public research efforts, there were still important parts of the discovery process carried out in industry research laboratories. In large measure, industry and nonindustry research efforts are complementary.

To study this matter further, the authors investigate the extent to which scientists in industry research laboratories collaborated with their public- sector counterparts, using coauthorships as a measure. Not only did they find a large number of such collaborations but also that coauthorships are positively related to the number of important patents taken out by the firm. They conclude that "firms wishing to take advantage of public-sector research must do more than simply invest in in-house basic research: they must also actively collaborate with their public-sector colleagues. Further,. . . coauthorships across institutions are correlated with private sector research productivity... [so that there are] substantial differences across firms in their ability to access public knowledge". This is another factor affecting the rates of diffusion of the new science-based technology.

Although the trend in pharmaceutical research activities has been toward a more scientific basis, there remains a substantial empirical component to these activities. Schwartzman and Cognato (1996) argue that "pharmaceutical research remains empirical, notwithstanding the increase in knowledge." Even is cases where drugs were allegedly rationally designed, "it was essentially still a matter of following leads and not hypotheses suggested by general theories". Although acknowledging that pharmaceutical research efforts have become more structured in recent years, these writers suggest that it is still largely an empirical exercise. An important corollary of these changes has been the growing connection between university and industry research activities. Schwartzman and Cognato report that the number of scientific publications authored by researchers at industry laboratories rose sharply in the years between 1973 and 1986. However, they indicate that this result does not apply to all companies.

Biotechnology

The initial scientific discovery by Stanley Cohen and Herbert Boyer, leading to the new technology in 1973, provided the basic technique for recombinant DNA. As this discovery became increasingly understood, its commercial implications became recognized. New firms were created to employ this new technology. Zucker, Darby, and Brewer (1998) observe that "the primary pattern in the development of the industry involved one or more scientist-entrepreneurs who remained on the faculty [of a research university] while establishing a business on the side.... We see the university as bringing about local industrial benefits by permitting its professors to pursue private commercial interests while their faculty appointments tie them to the area". These writers emphasize that the new scientific knowledge is not a "free good" usable by an unlimited number of potential users at little cost. Instead, it is a form of human capital that was held originally by only a small group of discoverers and co-workers who had gained this knowledge by working at the "bench-science level". Strikingly, this new technology was not immediately available to the major pharmaceutical firms. At its outset, the new technology was the province of a host of small companies that typically focused on one or a few potential products. Scriabiane (1999) estimates that there were 1,308 such firms in the United States in 1996. Of these, only 260 were public corporations. Many start-up firms had their roots in university science. Another survey reported that fully 1,100 new biotechnology companies were created between 1980 and 1994 from licenses granted by universities.

Historically the new firms created to pursue this technology saw themselves as representing a different industry, distinct from the broader pharmaceutical industry. Their original goal was not only to discover new drugs but also to manufacture and sell them. But only a few actually reached that goal. An important reason is that the discovery of a new drug is only the first step along the path to launching a new product successfully. The FDA requires extensive clinical testing for new drugs, and the costs of large-scale trials, particularly in Phases 2 and 3, can be substantial. As noted below, the costs of clinical trials and other product development efforts represent more than half of total research and development costs. Since the new start-ups had generally employed most of their resources in the more scientific, discovery phase of this research, they were often not prepared to support the additional testing costs that were required. Furthermore, the marketing of a new drug is often as costly as its total research expenditures. Those outlays are typically concentrated in the first two years following a product's introduction. Marketing costs effectively double the total outlays required for a new product's launch. This level of resources was generally available only from the major pharmaceutical companies.

Increasingly, the large pharmaceutical companies formed partnerships and alliances with smaller biotechnology start-ups. In addition to providing needed capital, they facilitated the clinical trial process and supplied essential managerial support. However, interactions between the two types of firms were often difficult as they developed from different cultures. A solution was the purchase of the more successful biotechnology firms by large pharmaceutical companies. These included the following acquisitions: Genentech by Hoffman- Laroche, Chiron by Ciba-Geigy (Novartis), Genetics Institute by American Home Products, Sphinx Biotechnologies by Lily, and Affymax by Glaxo. While some leading biotechnology firms remained independent, for example, Amgen, most joined the pharmaceutical industry. Prospects for an independent biotechnology industry soon disappeared.

Although the difficulty of raising sufficient capital from private investors was an important reason, there is also a second explanation, which resulted from the distinction between single-project and multi-project firms. As Guedj and Scharfstein (2004) observe, "the problem with single-project firms is that, if they have poor investment opportunities, they may still invest because managers are reluctant to return funds to shareholders.... This conflict is mitigated in an internal capital market to the extent that higher-level managers can retain funds for investment, but have a broader range of projects in which to invest". Small biotechnology start-ups, which often have only a single research project, sometimes continue to invest funds even when prospects are relatively dim.

To test this proposition, Guedj and Scharfstein compare start-up biotechnology firms with major firms that have a larger number of projects. They report that single-project firms were more likely to move their products from Phase 1 to Phase 2 trials within a two-year period than were mature firms. However, their products were also less likely to demonstrate good results in Phase 2 trials, and less likely to move into Phase 3 trials within a three-year period. The authors interpret these findings as suggesting an agency problem between investors and managers for smaller, single-project firms that often leads to over-investment in research. Larger, multiproduct firms were therefore more efficient.

Although the early biotech firms had an advantage in their understanding of the new scientific technology, they faced the economic hurdle of raising sufficient capital to conduct their research, carry out the extensive trials required by FDA, and bring their products to market. As with other start-ups, they originally sought investor funding, although this was soon joined by contracts and grants from leading pharmaceutical companies. In return for providing the necessary funds, the larger companies sought alliances through which they would share in the returns from any new products that resulted.

An important feature of the biotechnology sector is the increasing formation of alliances between small start-up firms and larger pharmaceutical companies. These alliances represent a middle ground between fully independent transactions and the acquisition of the smaller firm by the larger company. By the 1990s, funding by the leading pharmaceutical companies for their alliance partners became a major source of biotechnology financing. In four years -1994, 1995, 1997, and 1998- alliance funding represented more than half of the amounts received by start-up biotechnology firms and exceeded 60% of total financing, although it was somewhat lower in other years. While the new start-up firms received financing, the large pharmaceutical companies came to rely increasingly on these alliances for their new product pipelines. Of the 691 new entities approved by the U.S. Food and Drug Administration between 1963 and 1999, fully 38% were in-licensed rather than developed fully in industry research laboratories. Through this process, the major companies gained access to the new technology, and the new biotech products that resulted became important members of their overall menu of drugs.

These alliances required that smaller biotechnology firms accept diluted property rights in their new products. Not only would the returns be shared but decisions and control over the research process would now be negotiated with an outside partner. An obvious question is why they were willing to do so. One answer is that these steps were needed to raise capital that would not otherwise be available. However, if that were the only factor, other investors than the large pharmaceutical companies would have equal standing and be as likely to respond. This capital is typically provided by pharmaceutical companies, which suggests that other factors are also important. To examine these matters, Danzon, Nicholson, and Pereira (2005) investigate the research performance of biotechnology alliances, paying particular attention to whether this performance varied with the experience of the originating and licensing companies. The issue studied was whether the gains from collaboration, and particularly the expertise that each firm brings to the alliance, exceed any likely disincentive effects following from the dilution of property rights. The latter might result because each firm's efforts were not fully internalized, and each bore only a portion of the research costs associated with bringing a product to market.

Danzon and colleagues collected information on nearly 200 compounds under development in the United States during 1988–2000. Nearly half of the compounds were developed within an alliance, both for large firms as well as for smaller and medium-sized ones. For Phase 1 trials, they report that the size of the originating firm was not related to the percentage developed within an alliance, which confirms the conventional wisdom that small firms generally have the same skills and resources needed for small-scale trials as larger firms. In contrast, they find that small and medium-sized originating firms more frequently had compounds in development through Phase 2 and 3 trials within an alliance than otherwise. The smaller firms seemed to require the resources and expertise of a major firm to pursue these larger and more expensive trials.

The authors also examine the experience and size of the licensing firms. Again, they find that the number of past trials had little relationship with the prospects for success on Phase 1 trials, but the number of past trials did have a substantial positive effect on later phases of research. Having performed more trials in the past was predictive of greater success with the Phase 2 and 3 trials. They report that "large firms have higher success rates on in-licensed compounds than on compounds that they originate in-house". These findings suggest that large pharmaceutical companies have an advantage in carrying out latter-stage clinical trials as compared with new start-ups, but not in discovering new drugs or in performing Phase 1 trials. There appears to be an important division of labor by which biotechnology is employed to discover and develop new drugs. Nicholson, Danzon, and McCullough (2002) examine the relationship between alliance payments and product features as related to the characteristics of the parties. They find that "biotechnology companies signing their first deal receive a 60% discount relative to firms that signed at least two prior deals, controlling for product characteristics and some measure of the rights transferred." Also, "the discount for inexperience declines to 30% on a biotech firm's second deal and is insignificant for subsequent deals".

Learner and Merges (1998) review a sample cf 200 alliances between smaller biotechnology firms and larger pharmaceutical companies, or among biotechnology firms, between 1980 and 1995. They seek to understand the role of control as between the two parties and report "evidence consistent with the hypothesis that the financial condition of R&D firms affects their ability to retain control rights in technology alliances" (p. 146). As expected, smaller biotechnology firms with more revenues prior to the alliance were less likely to negotiate away their control rights. Learner and Tsai (2000) also consider the nature of biotechnology alliances and how they are influenced by whether or not they were formed in periods of sufficient external financing. They report that when external financing was more readily available, control was more frequently maintained by the smaller biotechnology company then when external financing was more limited. This study also finds that when control was maintained by the smaller biotechnology firm, the alliance's performance was better as measured by the probability that their drug would advance to the next stage of testing or be finally approved. On the other hand, performance was "significantly worse" when control was assigned to the large corporation. This issue is important because only when the research entity retains control is the project likely to be managed efficiently. However, when it does not have sufficient financial resources, and must transfer increased ownership to a pharmaceutical company, prospects for the larger project are reduced.

Scale and Scope of Pharmaceutical Research

These issues of scale and scope in regard to pharmaceutical R&D have been studied most extensively. The first concerns the relative productivity of different sized research efforts, and whether R&D dollars are more effective when aggregated together in large-scale enterprises or when divided among a larger number of smaller firms. The critical issue here is the importance of specialized people and equipment. Second is the issue of economics of scope, which refers to the advantages of specialization or diversification within research facilities, whether there are advantages within a given scale of research activities of concentrating on a limited number of research problems or alternatively in spreading the effort more broadly. These findings were disputed by Vernon and Gusen (1974), who instead report for the 1965–1970 period that larger firms were better at innovation than smaller firms. To be sure, as those authors acknowledge, the latter period followed the introduction of the 1962 Drug Amendments that required demonstrations of efficacy as well as safety for the introduction of a new drug, while my earlier study preceded the new law. A possible explanation, therefore, for the reported differences was the new conditions under which pharmaceutical research was then carried out. Jensen (1987) reviewed these earlier studies and provided new estimates. She did not find that marginal product of research expenditures depended on firm size. Her results instead suggest that, except for the smallest firms, there is no particular advantage for new products of either large research scale or large firm size.

The current literature on this subject has advanced beyond these early studies. Much of the progress is attributable to the work of Cockburn and Henderson, who emphasize differences between the discovery and development of new drugs. Discovery includes both the basic science and the application of the science to the selection of candidate drugs. In this effort the research process is particularly risky in that only a few candidate drugs are actually continued into development. Drug development, on the other hand, largely includes the three phases of testing required by the FDA. Although outcomes are more certain than before, it remains a risky process in which many prospective drugs are discarded.

Although the development segment of pharmaceutical research has a lesser scientific component than the discovery phase, it remains a substantial undertaking that absorbs more than half of total industry research budgets. Cockburn and Henderson (2001) report that the relative cost of development efforts has accounted for between 60% and 70% of pharmaceutical research activities since 1970. The costs of this work are largely determined by FDA requirements.

For their original study on this subject, Henderson and Cockburn (1996) gathered project level data from 10 large pharmaceutical companies, which together accounted for approximately one-fourth of total industry research and development. When their data are aggregated to the firm level, they report no evidence of scale economics: "the implied long-run elasticity of important patent output with respect to research spending in every model was between 0.4 and 0.5". However, their analysis of program- level data leads them to different conclusions. Although they report "quite sharply diminishing marginal returns to increasing investment in any single program... programs embedded in larger and more diversified firms appear to be significantly more productive". Therefore, they find both economies of scale and scope at the firm level.

Cockburn and Henderson (2001) acknowledge that their early results pertain only to the discovery phase of pharmaceutical research, and not to development. To correct for this omission, they gathered additional data from the same 10 companies they had examined earlier. This information was for 708 development projects conducted between 1960 and 1990. On average, these firms undertook approximately 16 individual projects simultaneously, with average total spending per project exceeding $18 million. Over the 30-year period, mean expenditures per project roughly doubled. Furthermore, there was a wide range of product duration, running from 1 to 26 years, although 90% of them lasted 10 years or less. As expected, projects that failed to generate a new drug application (NDA) were concluded earlier than those that led to NDAs.

Their primary results were based on log it regression models used to explain the project's probability of success, where success was indicated by a new drug application. Their primary explanatory variables are: Scale - the firm's total development spending, Scope - the number of therapeutic classes in which the firm was active, and Experience - the stock of previously obtained NDAs. When these explanatory variables are included together in the estimating equation, the Scale effect was not statistically significant while the Scope effect has a major impact on the probability of the project's success. The firm's past success in the therapeutic class was also significantly and positively associated with successful outcomes. The authors conclude that "relocating the average project to a firm active in one more area would increase the probability of success by about 0.03". However, they also find that both of these purported effects disappear when firm dummy variables are introduced into the analysis, from which they conclude that "much of the variation in the scope measure is between rather than within firms".

The different ways in which research is organized as between firms in the Henderson-Cockburn sample have striking effects on the probability of success. The authors note the presence of "enduring idiosyncratic differences among firms in the organization and management of the drug development process.... Differences in development strategy - in the pace and timing of development spending, and in the formulation of research strategy that guides clinical development - [can be] important determinants of development productivity". That conclusion raises the question of why less efficient organizations and managements continue and are not replaced by more effective alternatives. Overall, Cockburn and Henderson (1999) emphasize the presence of knowledge spill-overs both within and across firms. The success of a given project is enhanced, they argue, by the success of a related program within the firm as well as in other firms. Even more important, they write:

The most statistically important determinant of a research program's success, however, is its past productivity. The keys to this determinant are the "*knowledge capital*" accumulated by the program as an organizational unit as well as the skills and experience of individual scientists... . The primary advantage of size has [therefore] become the ability to exploit internal returns to Scope - particularly the ability to exploit internal spillovers of knowledge - rather than any economy of Scale per se.... [Furthermore,] the benefits of spillovers can be realized only by incurring the costs of maintaining "*absorptive capacity*" - the ability to capture new spillovers." The firm's scientific base, and the knowledge capital acquired by that base, they contend, dominates any simple economies of either scope or scale in determining the success or outcomes of a firm's research and development process. Scope and scale by them selves are less important than the knowledge capital accumulated by the firm.

The unique contributions of Henderson and Cockburn arise in part from the data set they have been able to acquire. While earlier studies used the firm as the observational unit, they probed within the firm to the level of the research project, and in doing so, provided rich insights that were not available earlier. A dimension of the increasing disintegration of pharmaceutical R&D is the growing use of contract research organizations (CROs) to conduct clinical trials of new drugs. By 1999, 23% of trials were out sourced to CROs. In general, the more data-intensive projects are out sourced, while knowledge-intensive projects are more frequently undertaken within pharmaceutical companies.

Productivity and Costs

There are two ways of approaching the question of the productivity function and the cost function, which of course are duals of one another, and the economic literature deals with both. Except in perverse circumstances, conclusions regarding one have direct implications for the other. This principle applies to research costs and to research productivity. The increasing research cost of new drugs is directly related to the declining productivity of pharmaceutical R&D. An important feature of pharmaceutical research in the past few decades is that despite the substantial scientific achievements that have occurred, and that are reflected in the increasing application of biotechnology to new drug development, the rate of new product generation has been fairly steady. As Cockburn acknowledges, however, "counts of new molecular entities (NMEs) are a noisy measure. On average, over the long term, these numbers have been remarkably steady, but they fluctuate sharply from year to year, so that peak-to-trough changes over shorter time periods can be highly misleading".

To be sure, simple counts of new products introduced do not encompass either their medical or their economic importance. Some introductions are invariably more important than others. Indeed, as Grabowski and Vernon (1990, 1994) point out, there are major differences in sales among products so that the relevant distributions are highly skewed. Furthermore, pharmaceuticals have various indications, and the medical and/or economic importance of particular drugs can be more closely related to the number of approved indications than to the number of products. In contrast, pharmaceutical industry spending on research and development has expanded greatly in the past few decades. From total spending of less than $5 billion in 1970, these outlays increased to $30 billion by 2002. There has thus been an increasing discrepancy between the relatively stable number of new drugs approved and the increasing number of dollars spent on R&D to discover new drugs. The result, of course, has been declining research productivities in terms of the numbers of new products introduced, and also increasing costs for new drugs.

Berndt, Cockburn, and Grepin (2005) employ the number of medical indications to measure pharmaceutical innovation. A substantial share of industry research and development expenditures, estimated at between 25% and 30%, is directed toward finding new indications for existing products.

Berndt et al. use the term "*incremental innovation*" to describe these efforts. For the three therapeutic areas they examined, the number of FDA approvals for new indications increased substantially in the past decade. In addition, the greater number of approved indications has led to increased utilizations of the drugs concerned. On that basis, they maintain that reported declines in pharmaceutical research productivity are overstated.

An important feature of recent trends in pharmaceutical innovation is that they have accompanied the increasing disintegration of the research process. As noted earlier, an increasing share of pharmaceutical research is carried out in small biotechnology companies that deal with one or a small number of products. With increasing frequency, the major drug companies enter the process only at the development and testing phases. What seems clear, however, is that this new structure has not led to increased productivity or lower costs, at least in terms of the number of new products introduced, although it may have influenced the therapeutic properties of the new drugs. The shift of drug research to a more science-based mode has thus been associated with a substantial increase in research costs. What is unclear is whether these higher costs reflect the increased requirements of the science- based process or the effects of a more vertically disintegrated structure in which higher costs are borne or higher margins charged by participating firms.

The reverse side of this same picture is, of course, the higher research costs of developing new drugs. There is a continuing literature on this question, which began with the 1979 paper by Hansen. Building on that foundation is the major study by DiMasi, Hansen, and Grabowski (1991). From a sample of 93 self-originated new chemical entities (NCEs) introduced by 12 companies in the 1970s and 1980s, they report mean cash outlays of $114 million per approved product (1987 dollars) and fully capitalized costs of $231 million. Because the R&D process is so lengthy, expenditures were just under half of total costs. Kettler (1999) updated DiMasi et al.'s estimates to 1997 values, based on the GDP implicit price deflator. Her resulting estimate is $312 million. Because project-level data were available only for development and testing costs, DiMasi et al.'s estimates depended also on parameters derived from other sources. These included (1) an estimated success rate of 23% at which investigational NCEs gain approval, (2) an estimated ratio of 55.7% between preclinical and total R&D costs, (3) an estimated lag structure of 98.9 months between the initiation of clinical testing and NDA approval, and (4) a discount rate of 9%. All of these factors influenced their cost estimates.

Finding an appropriate discount rate is particularly important. Although the 9% rate used by DiMasi and colleagues may be appropriate for private firms making investment decisions, this rate may be much higher than is appropriate for public decision making. Fuchs and Zeckhauser (1987) argue that as long as future citizens are given equal weight to current ones, "the value of life-years to future generations should be discounted at the time-value-of-money rate". And Viscusi (1995) observes: "many cost-effectiveness studies currently use a real rate of discount of 5%,... [and] real rates of return of 3%, or even less, are more consistent with U.S. economic performance in the past decade". At lower discount rates, total research costs per new drug are much lower. More recently, DiMasi, Hansen, and Grabowski (2003) employ a similar methodology to provide updated estimates of research costs. They examine development expenditures for a sample of 68 randomly selected new drugs introduced by 10 leading pharmaceutical companies during the 1990s. These firms accounted for 42% of industry R&D expenditures. They then apply a real discount rate of 11% to capitalize costs to the point of marketing approval, which is a substantially higher rate than the 9% discount rate used earlier.

While their previous study estimated R&D expenditures per new drug at $231 million in 1987 dollars, their more recent one provides an estimate of $802 million in 2000 dollars. These figures indicate sharply higher costs for new product development. From this vantage point as well, the growth of a science-based research effort has not reduced research costs but led to higher ones.

Efficiency of Pharmaceutical Research

There are various perspectives from which to evaluate the efficiency of pharmaceutical research. One is whether the optimal amount of research is being conducted. Too many or too few resources could be allocated to this purpose. A second dimension is whether this research is carried out in the most effective manner so that output is maximized for given levels of input. In this section I consider both of these dimensions; the first is termed allocative efficiency, and the second is termed technical efficiency. On the allocative efficiency of pharmaceutical research, there are theoretical reasons why there could be either under- or overinvestment in research. On the one hand, research activities, and particularly basic research, generate substantial positive externalities in that their total benefits to society exceed those accruing to the particular firm. As a result, firms do not incorporate their full measure of benefits when making their investment decisions. On the other hand, there is more recent economic literature on racing behavior as applied to research activities. An important conclusion is that in a "winner take all" situation, there can be overinvestment in research activities. The reason is that the prospective gains may be less than the aggregate amount of the investment undertaken to achieve these gains.

The authors first review the available theoretical literature on rivalrous research and emphasize its "winner take all" feature. In the case of pharmaceutical research, the firm completing the invention and receiving the patent wins the race. It gains most of the benefits from this research while others receive much lower returns on their investment. Although this picture is not always correct when applied to the pharmaceutical industry, it is largely so since the first and second entrants into a particular therapeutic market generally capture most of the net returns. Furthermore, firms understand that others are competing for the same prizes, and set their research strategies in anticipation of rival investment.

Cockburn and Henderson construct a data set to test the implications of this behavior. These data included the spending and output levels of individual research programs gathered from the internal records of 10 large pharmaceutical companies. Applying these data to an underlying model, they report that R&D investment is only weakly correlated across firms, but that R&D outcomes are positively correlated with the firm's own research productivity. Although "me-too" investment occurs occasionally, it is not a major characteristic of this industry. In their judgment, "a better characterization... is that investment decisions are driven by the heterogeneous capabilities of the firm, by adjustment costs, and by the evolution of technological opportunity". Although strategic considerations may play some role, they argue that such factors do not drive investment decisions. Cockburn and Henderson also note: "there are some grounds for believing that the entry of additional firms into the pharmaceutical research 'race' is not unambiguously welfare-destroying. Competing projects are better described as complements rather than substitutes, and there are significant spillovers of knowledge across firms". They conclude that rivalrous research activity is not the dominant factor behind the decision to invest in pharmaceutical research.

An alternate approach is not to examine variations in pharmaceutical research spending among firms but rather to consider the trends over time in total industry spending. Scherer (2001) employs this approach. His goal is to explain the long-term trend in real research spending, which had increased between 1962 and 1996 at a mean annual rate of 7.5% per year. In contrast, the growth rate of gross margins was 4.23% per year. Rather than comparing these two series directly, Scherer computes the deviations of each series from its best-fitting linear trend. He finds a high correlation between these two sets of deviations and concludes that "the similarity of trend deviation patterns suggest that there was indeed cyclical co-movement in pharmaceutical industry growth margins and R&D outlays". He goes on to explain: "As profit opportunities expand, [pharmaceutical] companies compete to exploit them by increasing R&D investments, and perhaps also promotional costs, until the increase in costs dissipate most, if not all, supranormal profit returns". Consistent evidence is provided by Giaccotto, Santerre, and Vernon (2005), who estimate the influence of real drug prices on R&D intensity. Since drug prices are directly related to industry revenues, this study offers a similar picture of the process by which research spending is determined. These authors report "a 10% rise in the growth of real drug prices is associated with nearly a 6% increase in growth of R&D intensity". What both these studies suggest is not an investment model at all, but rather one that employs available internally generated funds specifically for research and development purposes.

Where uncertainty levels are high, this process has the advantage of ensuring that all available funds are used for research purposes. What it does not demonstrate, nor could it do so, is whether this allocation process leads to an excess or insufficient spending on pharmaceutical research. What we observe is that spending has increased strongly in recent decades. New resources have flowed into the process by which new drugs are discovered, and there are no indications that promising avenues of research are neglected. On this point, Grabowski and Vernon (1990, 1994) estimate rates of return from investment in pharmaceutical research and development, and report values slightly higher than the associated cost of capital. In their latter study they conclude: "the estimated mean return on pharmaceutical industry new chemical entity (NCE) introductions for the first half of the 1980s was 11.1% compared with the estimated (real) cost of capital of 10.5% over the same period". This finding also suggests that one is unlikely to find major unexploited opportunities. Still, without determining a social optimum, one cannot make firm conclusions about the sufficiency of resources directed toward these activities.

On the question of technical efficiency, results are also mixed. The productivity of pharmaceutical research funds has receded sharply in recent years, at least when measured by the number of new chemical entities introduced; and the cost of discovering and developing these products has correspondingly increased. The promise of a science-based research process has not led to the greater efficiency that was projected by its early proponents. As Cockburn (2004) emphasizes, there are pluses and minuses to the process of disintegration of pharmaceutical research. One cannot conclude that the new structure of pharmaceutical research is the source of the higher costs and fewer products per research dollar that we observe. However, as Cockburn also suggests, "there is a genuine possibility... that the restructuring of the pharmaceutical industry will ultimately prove quite costly in terms of reduced productivity". Whether or not this concern is justified is unclear at this time.

23

EXPLORATORY DEVELOPMENT

The term *exploratory development* (ED) can be defined as "the first part of clinical drug development in which tolerability, pharmacokinetics and pharmacodynamic activity are defined in man and in which an early indication of therapeutic efficacy is often obtained". A *new active substance* (NAS) can be defined as "an unlicensed new chemical or biological entity with activity in biological systems whose therapeutic potential is under investigation". The overall aim of ED should be to select appropriate NASs for *full development* (FD) and to reject those that will not make useful medicines, as early as possible.

ED begins with the identification of critical questions about a NAS. Starting with preparation for the first administration to humans, studies in ED should be designed to provide answers to these questions. A small number of clinical pharmacology studies that have been well designed and conducted should go a long way to describing the profile of the drug, in particular providing information on the "*critical success factors*".

From the outset of ED, we aim to learn about the human pharmacology of a NAS. Every attempt should be made to establish, as soon as possible, the range of drug doses that produce the desired effect, and the relationships between dose, plasma concentration and the magnitude of desired and undesired effects. If successful, much time and resource can be saved later in development because it should be possible to enter clinical trials with the clinically effective dose range. The ratio of doses producing a particular undesired effect to that of the desired effect can be determined to provide a preliminary assessment of the therapeutic index. It is inappropriate to consider the incidence of adverse events without reference to the dose of drug, plasma concentrations and their variability and both magnitude and variability of desired effects.

The terms *proof of principle* and *proof of concept* are used more or less synonymously and pertain to the criteria that must be fulfilled in human studies before a NAS can be considered to be a candidate for development to licence. These are particularly useful terms when applied to a drug thought to act by a novel mechanism of action. They are perhaps less appropriate when the biological principle is well established and the critical issues relate to a number of properties of a particular NAS.

The *desired profile* of a drug is usually easy to define since it is generic, i.e. good efficacy, high oral bioavailability, once-daily dosing, low incidence of adverse reactions in the therapeutic range, no serious adverse reactions etc., but drugs only occasionally turn out to fulfil such promise. From the point of view of drug development, it is more demanding but of much greater value to define the *minimum acceptable profile* (MAP), concentrating particularly on the critical success factors. Then, by comparing the actual profile, as revealed by ED, with the MAP, decisions can be made about the future of a project, i.e. whether it is worth taking from ED into FD. The intention is that the findings in ED will predict the benefit:risk ratio that will be established in FD. FD should thus be a confirmation of the findings of ED, hopefully with few surprises and a low risk of failure late in development.

It is insufficient to define the MAP simply in terms of "the drug works and seems to be safe". Thus, the acceptable benefit:risk ratio will depend greatly on the seriousness of the target disease and the availability of other treatments. For an agent that works by a novel mechanism of action and could be the first in class for treatment of a life-threatening disease the MAP will be quite different from that of a "me too" for a non-serious condition. For the former, demonstration of clinical benefit despite troublesome side-effects might be acceptable, whereas for the latter success might perhaps depend on demonstration of a single advantageous property of the compound over its competitors, such as greater oral bioavailability or a longer duration of action. To summarise, whilst there is always considerable uncertainty in ED and no decision will be infallible, the risk of selecting the wrong compounds for development can be minimised by identifying critical success factors and an MAP that will provide the basis for go/no-go decisions.

The term *Phase I* refers to studies in healthy volunteers or patients to determine the safety and tolerability, pharmacodynamic effects and the pharmacokinetics of a NAS. The term is often used to imply studies performed in healthy volunteers, but early evaluation of cytotoxics and many other drugs is performed in patients. Conversely, healthy volunteer studies are often performed throughout the drug development process. For example, studies of drug interactions and pharmacokinetics of new formulations are frequently conducted at a late stage in drug development, while clinical pharmacology studies to support new indications and other line extensions may be performed years after the first licence is granted. *Phase II* refers to studies in patients with the target disease to determine tolerability, pharmacokinetics, with, if possible, preliminary evidence of the dose-response relationship (Phase IIa) and efficacy (Phase IIb). Thus, Phase I and at least part of Phase IIa and IIb are encompassed by ED. These terms provide a useful shorthand but are ambiguous and do not capture the exploratory nature of early drug development. They also suggest that the process is linear, whereas in practice the phases of drug development are often not well demarcated and different activities run concurrently.

Planning Exploratory Development

Need for a Regulatory Strategy

If the purpose of ED is to generate data on which to base decisions about future development, the strategy for future registration of the drug needs to be well defined. It may seem premature to be discussing regulatory matters before the drug has been administered to humans, but the plan for ED may look quite different depending on the target profile. Even if the design of the first one or two studies might not be affected, the data these studies generate will certainly be critical in deciding whether to continue or stop development, or change direction. For example, a molecule that has been shown to have both anticonvulsant and antinociceptive activity in animal models might be developed as an antiepileptic, an analgesic or both.

The plan for ED will look quite different for these indications, and the MAP of pharmacokinetics and tolerability will probably differ substantially. Similarly, a molecule that is active in animal models of diabetes and obesity might be developed for either indication, or both. Again, the ED plan of studies and desired or acceptable outcomes will depend on the chosen indication. The strategy may seem relatively straightforward for an antibiotic with a long half-life in animals that would, if translated to man, give it a clinically meaningful advantage over the competitors. However, even this needs careful definition of the MAP in terms of pharmacokinetics, spectrum of bacterial sensitivity, target diseases, tolerability and safety profiles by different routes of administration. There also has to be a clear understanding of the likely development times needed to achieve registration for different indications by different routes of administration and the impact on the drug's market potential.

Devising the Plan

The timeline should of course be as short as possible and it may be possible to conduct some studies in parallel or at least with a stagger rather than sequentially; however, this must not be at the expense of the safety of the study subjects. Often there is no choice but to wait for the results of one study before starting the next. On the other hand, predefining the core data required for decision making, and making arrangements for rapid quality control and database lock, can substantially reduce the delays between studies.

The ED plan should lead to one or more *decision milestones* at which an agreed body of information will be provided in a defined time. The plan may consist of as few as one or two studies in healthy volunteers which will deliver in 6-9 months or it may involve a complex series of studies in healthy volunteers and patients, which might take a couple of years. Whatever is appropriate, the information available at the decision milestones should enable the company to compare the actual profile with the previously agreed MAP. The company will then be in a position to make a well-founded decision on whether to continue development with a much reduced risk of failure or whether to stop and concentrate precious resources elsewhere.

The first study commonly involves single ascending doses and the second study might involve repeated administration, but the specific study objectives must be tailored to the strategic goals and provide clear information that will define the profile. For example, if it is critical that the absorption of an antiarrhythmic drug is not affected by prior ingestion of food, the effect of food on the bioavailability of the drug should be an objective that can be easily evaluated in the first study in humans. Or, if an antimigraine drug must be effective in doses that are devoid of sedative activity, tests of cognition and sedation, as well as spontaneous adverse event reporting, should be included in the first and subsequent studies. And, to take one of the examples mentioned above, the patient population, objectives and endpoints of the first study in patients for a drug targeted at diabetes will be quite different from those for a drug targeted at obesity, even if some of the patients may have both conditions.

Presentation of the Plan

An overview of the project plan, with timeline and delineated critical path, may be conveniently presented as a Gantt chart. A decision tree is another visual aid which can serve to clarify the critical information required for each milestone decision. Although the ED plan should be carefully thought out and well defined, it must be recognised that it is not written in tablets of stone. The very scientific nature of ED means that there will be new, often unexpected, findings. Results of one or two doses administered to humans may show that assumptions were wrong and that the plan must be changed accordingly. For example, if a drug or one of its major metabolites is found to have a much longer half-life than predicted by preclinical studies, this is likely to affect not only the design of present and future studies but also the acceptable tolerability and safety profile, and perhaps the commercial potential of the drug either favourably or adversely. The plan may have to be revised to take into account these considerations. Planning is therefore essential, but execution of the plan needs to be flexible and the plan may have to be modified considerably, even if the overall goals remain unchanged.

Requirements for Administration of an NAS to Humans

Evidence of Primary Pharmacodynamic Activity

Pharmacodynamics can be defined as "the action of a drug on molecular or cellular targets or on the whole organism". The decision to proceed with preclinical development of a compound should only be made after thorough characterisation of its pharmacodynamics in terms of dose–concentration–response relationships *in vitro* and *in vivo* in animals. The commitment to take a compound into man should not be taken lightly since very considerable resources are required to meet the demands of the safe and ethical administration of a NAS to humans. No pharmaceutical company can afford to waste precious resources on projects that have little chance of success. By contrast, the cost of thorough evaluation of the mode of action and pharmacodynamic effects of a substance in relation to its desired therapeutic target is small. This is the scientific basis for all rational drug development today and is the information required for the design of the first human pharmacology studies. It does not, however, preclude the possibility of serendipitous discoveries, which have played such an important part in drug discovery in the past.

Secondary Pharmacodynamic Activity and Safety Pharmacology

Characterisation of the activity of primary interest must be accompanied by an equally thorough evaluation of the pharmacology of the compound at other receptors and in other systems. Secondary pharmacodynamic activity refers to the pharmacology of a substance not related to its desired therapeutic target. Studies of secondary pharmacodynamic activity may reveal desired or undesired properties. For example, a substance may be found to have the desired effect at sites or in systems other than the one first considered. On the other hand, non-selectivity may imply that the doses producing the desired therapeutic effect are likely to be accompanied by adverse effects. In addition to this secondary pharmacodynamic activity, a package of so-called safety pharmacology studies should be completed. As well as *in vitro* and *ex vivo* testing, these studies will generally include parenteral administration of high single doses of the compound and any major active metabolites to rodent and non-rodent species. These studies are at least as important as the formal toxicity studies for the initial selection of dosage in man. Such a safety package is not appropriate for biotechnology products. A much reduced package may also be required for substances to be applied topically, which do, however, require specific studies of local irritancy, phototoxicity and photosensitivity.

Pharmacokinetics and Drug Metabolism

The physical properties and pharmacokinetic profile, with data on absorption, distribution, metabolism and excretion (ADME) in animals, form an essential part of the drug selection process since the desired pharmacokinetic profile should be defined *ab initio*. For example, if it is decided that a potential new antihypertensive is to have a half-life in humans of at least 15 hours to permit once-daily administration, there really is no point in developing a compound that has a maximum half-life of 45 minutes in larger mammals. A potential antiarrhythmic, which is likely to have a low therapeutic index, requires consistent bioavailability; therefore, a compound that undergoes extensive first-pass metabolism or is absorbed poorly and inconsistently in animals is unlikely to be worth developing as an oral therapy to be taken over long periods. The potential value of a NAS that is metabolised primarily by an enzyme exhibiting polymorphism in the general population such as CYP2D6 needs to be carefully considered. Potent enzyme induction is another serious disadvantage which should be tested for in animals, and inhibition of cloned cytochrome P450 isozymes should be tested as part of a routine screen, since drug interactions with concomitant medications may be critical to the value of a new therapy.

The pharmacokinetics of a drug in rodents, dogs and primates are certainly of some predictive value to humans, although there can often be surprises. Not surprisingly, if there is good agreement between species, it is likely that humans will handle the drug in a similar fashion. Conversely, if the major clearance mechanism, metabolic or renal elimination of unchanged drug or metabolite profile differ greatly between species, it is far more difficult to predict the pharmacokinetics in humans. Reliable predictions about metabolic clearance in humans can often be made using cloned human metabolic enzymes, human hepatocytes, microsomes or, if available, whole-liver slices.

When a compound undergoes metabolism, the pharmacokinetics of major metabolites, particularly those that have pharmacological activity or are responsible for toxicities, should be examined. A long half-life of a metabolite may result in accumulation long after the concentration of the parent molecule has reached steady state. Much of the evaluation of the pharmacokinetics and the rates and routes of metabolism will be studied in animals using radiolabelled drug, but should be supported by "cold" assays.

Toxicology

Physicians and other clinical scientists responsible for ED are unlikely to be expert in toxicology but they must be familiar with the preclinical safety requirements for human studies in general and with the detailed toxicology of the NAS under consideration. *The final responsibility for the decision whether and how to conduct the first study in man lies with the physician.* Toxicity findings that give cause for concern should always be discussed with the toxicologist even if they are considered to be unrelated to the drug. Explanation may suffice but if reassurance is inadequate, additional studies may be needed or it might be necessary to limit exposure in man until further information becomes available.

It should be appreciated that the objective of the toxicologist is to identify target organ toxicity whereas that of the clinical pharmacologist is to minimise risk and avoid significant toxic effects. Thus, the clinical pharmacologist needs to know:

1. The organs in which toxicity was demonstrated and any abnormalities in laboratory tests
2. The maximum no observed adverse effect dose level (NOAEL)
3. The toxicokinetics, in particular the peak concentrations (C_{max}) and exposure (AUC) to parent drug and any major metabolites at the NOAEL and at toxic doses in the animal species tested.

This information may affect selection criteria for the study population and the choice of tests in addition to routine safety monitoring, and will certainly determine the starting dose, range of doses, maximum exposure and dose increments to be studied. Pharmacokinetics in man may be quite different from those in animal species so that plasma and, if possible, tissue concentrations are generally more important than dose. One exception to this may be hepatotoxicity resulting from exposure of the liver to portal blood drug concentrations, when the oral dose administered to the animals may be more relevant than the systemic plasma concentrations, which reflect first-pass metabolism as well as absorption.

Before administration of a NAS to man, a mutagenicity test in bacterial cells (Ames test), with and without metabolic activation, and tests for chromosomal aberrations in mammalian cells should be negative. Any positive or equivocal results will require additional tests to be performed before proceeding to man. Studies of embryo/fetal toxicity should be performed before administration of a NAS to women of reproductive potential. Segment I and Segment III reproductive toxicology and carcinogenicity studies are not required at this stage of development.

An additional consideration is the safety assessment of agents that will be used for challenge stimuli in the evaluation of pharmacodynamics. In some cases, there is a long history of uneventful clinical use of tests, for example bronchial challenge with histamine and methacholine. If used in a similar manner, there may be no need to consider performing safety studies in animals prior to their application in ED. On the other hand, the use of agents which are much less well established and which have an unproven safety record must raise the question of whether toxicology and pharmacological safety assessments should be performed in animals.

Pharmaceutical Formulations

The size and quality of the batch of bulk chemical or biological material that will be formulated for the first study in man are critical to the expeditious transfer from animals to man. Wherever possible, the same batch that has been used for toxicology should be used for the human studies. This avoids difficulties in attributing toxicity findings to different impurities or different proportions of the same impurities that are frequently encountered in early batches. Although the batch size may be limited, the amount of material required for the initial human studies is generally small compared with that used for toxicology.

It is always difficult to provide the pharmacist with sufficient information to facilitate manufacture of an optimal formulation. The dose range of interest is not known, and careful consideration should be given to selection of unit doses that will provide the greatest flexibility. Good communication is essential and adequate lead time must be allowed. Compounds with poor absorption are difficult to formulate and may take considerable time and resources. Repeated *in vitro* and *in vivo* testing in animals may be required before a satisfactory formulation is found.

The need for placebos generally from the first human study onwards typically involves manufacture of dummy capsules or tablets, and if oral solutions or suspensions are to be used, these must be matched as closely as possible for taste, colour and appearance.

Consideration must also be given to agents that are intended to be used for challenge stimuli. Some may be available commercially for use in humans, others may not and considerable work may have to done to obtain raw material of sufficient purity and stability, followed by development and manufacture of an appropriate formulation.

All formulations for administration to humans must be prepared in compliance with good manufacturing practice (GMP) and the certificates of analysis must be provided. The new European Clinical Trials Directive requires that details of the formulations be provided to and approved by regulatory authorities and a "qualified person" at the investigator site(s). This will apply to healthy volunteer as well as patient studies.

Transfer from Preclinical to Clinical

Collaboration

The establishment of good working relationships between the preclinical scientists (chemists, immunologists, pharmacologists, toxicologists, drug metabolism, etc.) and the clinical scientists responsible for ED is of enormous value. This is sometimes hard to achieve when the different groups are separated geographically or a molecule is licensed in from another company or academic institution. However, it should be recognised that at this stage, the preclinical scientists generally have far more knowledge about the compound and of the related science than do the clinical scientists, and their contribution to the ED plan can be extremely valuable. On the other hand, the clinical pharmacologist has an important role to play in assessing the preclinical data. Consideration of the ED plan may reveal that studies additional to those planned may be required. Review of the toxicity, safety pharmacology and metabolism data acquired to date may raise concerns and indicate that further work is necessary.

Close co-operation for a year or more before the first administration to humans is likely to lead to a smooth transfer of the compound and the rapid movement of a compound out of preclinical into man. This lead time can be used to devise the ED plan, design the first studies and, when appropriate, to select and develop methodologies which will contribute to the drug's evaluation in man. This may include validation of pharmacodynamic measures to be used in the clinical pharmacology unit, assessment of various imaging techniques, development of bioanalytical methods for biomarkers, the drug and metabolites. Not infrequently, the assays that were perfectly adequate to support preclinical work are insufficiently sensitive, specific or accurate to quantify the comparatively low concentrations in humans. At the very least, assays require validation in human plasma and urine.

Preparation of the Clinical Investigator's Brochure

The rate-limiting step, which usually defines when a NAS can be transferred to clinical, is the subacute (usually four week) toxicology. While reports of these studies are being written, preparation of the key documents required for the first study in humans can begin. When the toxicology reports are available, and providing thorough review is supportive of proceeding to man, the documentation can be completed. In addition to the protocol, and information for volunteers, with consent form, the clinical investigator's brochure (CIB) needs to be prepared. It is usual for each of the preclinical disciplines to contribute sections to this document, but the clinical scientists need to ensure that the document is appropriate for a largely clinical readership. The outline content and format of the CIB is provided in a guideline published by the International Conference on Harmonisation (ICH).

It should always be remembered that the CIB is not a promotional document aimed at presenting the NAS in its best light; on the contrary, it is intended to inform investigators and ethics ommittees about every aspect of the drug, to enable them to make wise judgements in the interest of study subjects, be they healthy volunteers or patients. The CIB is necessarily a summary, but less than full disclosure of important information about the drug, whatever the source, is not acceptable and all documents should be referenced and made available on request.

The first edition of this important document will of course contain no clinical information, but the next edition should be produced immediately after completion of the first study in humans, with a summary of the findings. The principal investigator must become fully familiar with the CIB when the protocol is being developed and, once finalised, both editions of the CIB should be submitted to the relevant independent ethics committee (IEC).

Aspects of the First Protocol and Ethics Review

A protocol for the first and other early studies with a NAS in man is similar to those for later studies in healthy volunteers and patients but has some particular features which are worth special consideration. The protocol should be written to satisfy not only the needs of regulatory authorities and personnel who will be involved in conduct of the study but also to facilitate the work of the IEC, which bears considerable responsibility in such cases. The nature of the scientific material contained in the protocol is often complex, highly specialised and quite unlike most protocols for clinical trials handled by such committees.

The emphasis is essentially on safety rather than ethics, although of course a study that does not minimise risk is also unethical. As well as a summary of the preclinical information, some comment and interpretation about its significance should be provided. The choice of starting dose and increments for dose escalation should be justified. The number of subjects and amount of data that will form the basis for a decision to escalate should be clearly stated, as should the criteria for stopping the escalation.

The clinical procedures that will be undertaken, and intended doses may need to be revised after review of the first results. The protocol should therefore be written with some flexibility so that, for example, within a defined dose range, adjustments of dose can be made. Similarly, whilst the minimum interval between doses should be explicit, there should be an option to increase the proposed interval if the half-life is longer than expected. There should be some flexibility in timing of blood samples and urine collections, which may need to be changed in light of pharmacokinetic and pharmacodynamic data generated during the study. Although the maximum number of samples and total blood volume to be sampled should be unchanged. On the other hand, the IEC cannot and should not be expected to give *carte blanche*. Therefore the basis for decisions and alternatives should be detailed carefully.

When the IEC meets to review the protocol it is advisable for a senior toxicologist to be present to answer questions if required. Of course members of the committee may have access to any other company documents such as toxicology reports if they desire. Pharmaceutical companies frequently establish a committee of senior management to authorise the first study of a NAS in humans, the review and approval generally being a prerequisite for submission to the external IEC. However, the clinician responsible for the first study in humans must be personally satisfied that the preclinical data relating to efficacy and safety justify administration to man. A useful test is for the physician and other responsible personnel to ask themselves: "Would I be prepared to volunteer for this study and would I be happy for a loved-one to do so?".

Studies in Healthy Volunteers

What is a Healthy (Non-patient) Volunteer?

In the report of the Royal College of Physicians on studies in healthy volunteers a healthy volunteer is described as "an individual who is not known to suffer any significant illness relevant to the proposed study, who should be within the ordinary range of body measurements such as weight, and whose mental state is such that he is able to understand and give valid consent to the study". In the Association of the British Pharmaceutical Industry (ABPI) guidelines for medical experiments in non-patient human volunteers it is stressed that the individual cannot be expected to derive therapeutic benefit from the proposed study. While these descriptions are correct, I would suggest that words like "relevant to the proposed study" are too ambiguous and the definition should state unequivocally that a healthy volunteer must indeed be in good health. Perhaps a more satisfactory definition of a healthy or "non-patient" volunteer (the word "human" is superfluous) is as follows: "An individual who is in good general health, not having any mental or physical disorder requiring regular or frequent medication and who is able to give valid informed consent to participation in a study". Thus, a healthy young man taking an antibiotic for acne does not qualify, but a woman taking an oral contraceptive does (unless specifically excluded by the protocol). Similarly, a migraine or hayfever sufferer who takes daily prophylactic medication is excluded but one who takes medication only at the time of infrequent acute attacks is acceptable in principle. Obviously individuals will not be able to participate if suffering from an acute attack or if they have taken medication within a period defined in the protocol.

Even with this somewhat stricter definition, there is room for disgression. A sportsman who takes an occasional puff of a bronchodilator for exercise- induced asthma but is otherwise asymptomatic may be considered eligible by some. Individuals who have undergone surgery for a congenital condition and are in excellent health may or may not be suitable. Thus, an asymptomatic patient with a hip prosthesis who is taking no medication may be acceptable whereas an equally healthy individual with a prosthetic heart valve should be excluded from a study involving a cannula because of the risk, however remote, of endocarditis. Clearly, whatever definition of a healthy volunteer is used, sensible clinical judgement is still required.

The advent of healthy volunteer studies has also revealed findings which are generally thought to be pathological but in fact are not associated with any adverse prognosis. For example, short runs of non-sustained ventricular tachycardia were found in 2% of healthy individuals with normal hearts on 24-hour ambulatory ECG monitoring. Microscopic haematuria is also a common finding. Epileptiform activity on EEG is found in subjects with no history of epilepsy. In addition, laboratory values will frequently fall outside the "normal" range for the laboratory simply on the grounds of probability because of the statistical criteria used to define the normal range.

Although not of direct relevance to screening, it should also be recognised that some of the procedures to which a volunteer may be subjected can affect test results. Perhaps the most important example of such findings is the rise in transaminases that occur in some subjects resident in a clinical pharmacology unit for a week or more, possibly because of dietary factors. The importance of a placebo group to help distinguish between effects resulting from active drug and procedural-related abnormalities cannot be over emphasised.

Healthy volunteers can be of either sex, although early studies are mostly confined to men because results of reproductive toxicity are generally not available at the time. Companies are not usually prepared to incur the cost of a reproductive toxicology package before there is some confidence that the compound is a reasonable candidate for development. In the absence of such data, medicolegal and ethical considerations relating to the risk of causing embryo/fetal damage have deterred companies from including women in the first studies in humans. Men are also frequently favoured for later studies because of concerns over the inability to detect very early pregnancy, and the possibility that the menstrual cycle or oral contraceptives may affect drug metabolism. Concerns that the results from studies conducted mainly in men may not be representative of both sexes are rarely justified because, unlike in the rat, there are few important sex-related differences in drug metabolism in humans.

For legal reasons, the lower age limit for volunteers is generally 18 years. The first studies with a new candidate drug are usually conducted in young healthy volunteers with an upper age limit of 35-40 years. The lower age limit for the elderly is usually 65 years but when specifically addressing tolerability, pharmacokinetics and pharmacodynamics in the elderly, a representative population should certainly include many subjects in their 70s or older.

Why Use Healthy Volunteers?

The decision to use healthy volunteers, a particular patient population or a combination of the two should be based on ethical, safety, scientific and practical grounds. Some drugs are too toxic or produce effects that would be unacceptable in healthy volunteers. These include cytotoxic agents, neuromuscular blocking drugs, anaesthetics and most biological response modifiers such as monoclonal antibodies, growth factors and interleukins. On the other hand, physicians responsible for patient care are, rightly, conservative about exposing their patients to unknown risks. Thus, asthmatics, who have hyperreactive airways, are far more likely to develop serious impairment of respiratory function because of bronchoconstriction from an inhaled material, drug or vehicle, than are healthy volunteers. An elderly patient with an acute stroke is far more susceptible to the sedative effects of a NAS than is a young healthy subject. Furthermore, the appropriate dose range to be studied can frequently be established in healthy subjects using biomarkers so that exposure of patients to excessively high (or low) doses can be avoided. Of course this does not imply that less caution is required when dosing healthy volunteers, simply that the risks may be considerably reduced in this population.

In addition to the greater risk in patients, results in patients are frequently confounded by the effects of disease, concomitant medication, age and other variables. By contrast, healthy subjects are much more homogeneous and subjects are studied under standardised conditions. It is sometimes argued that healthy volunteers are not representative of the patient population and therefore that the studies are of less relevance. This argument fails to take into account the study objectives; some questions about a drug are much more easily answered by deliberately excluding sources of variation.

In addition to the scientific benefit to be gained from studies in healthy volunteers, there are a number of practical advantages.

1. Healthy volunteers can generally be recruited much more rapidly than patients.
2. Healthy volunteers are generally much more willing and able than patients to make themselves available on scheduled study days so that groups of subjects can be studied together, thereby expediting completion of the study and enabling staff and laboratories to be used efficiently.
3. Clinical pharmacology studies are frequently very intensive, with a tight schedule of complex measurements, often requiring training and a high degree of co-operation from subjects. Young healthy volunteers are more suited to this type of study.

In summary, studies in healthy volunteers have become an integral part of the drug development process because they are capable of rapidly providing a large amount of data which is not confounded by other variables and which can thereby expedite the subsequent evaluation of the drug in patients.

Regulatory Position

At the time of writing, the conduct of studies in non-patient volunteers in the UK is not regulated by the Medicines Act (1968). Similarly, studies in non-patient volunteers in the Netherlands, Belgium and some other European countries do not require regulatory approval. This situation is about to change, as the EU Directive issued in 2001 will require to be implemented in all European countries by 2004. All healthy volunteer studies will then require regulatory approval in addition to that of an ethics committee. The Directive, with which all member states must comply, makes no distinction between healthy volunteer studies and clinical trials in patients who may benefit from treatment. However, the precise details of documentation required for authorisation of healthy volunteer studies may vary from country to country; it is possible that the application in the UK will be somewhat less detailed than the current Clinical Trials Exemption.

Source of Healthy Volunteers

The majority of healthy volunteer studies are conducted by contract research organisations, which recruit subjects from the general public by advertising and word of mouth. The composition of the volunteer database depends to some extent on the location, some being comprised mainly of students or the local residential population, others, particularly in large cities, having a preponderance of backpackers and temporary workers. The source of volunteers does have implications for safety, motivation and withdrawal rates. The more itinerant volunteers may not be available for follow up and little is known about their medical background. Whilst the "*professional volunteer*" is wholly inappropriate, a stable population of volunteers who understand what is involved, are well motivated and who have long-term medical screening records is highly desirable.

A few large pharmaceutical companies, mainly in Europe, run their own clinical pharmacology facilities, sometimes using company employees as volunteers. Such individuals often make excellent study subjects, being highly motivated and well informed, with medical screening records going back over several years. However, in such circumstances, it is essential that adequate safeguards and procedures are in place to ensure that performance reviews, career progression and other employment issues are quite separate from volunteer activities.

The chance of mishap occurring in a volunteer study is increased when little or nothing is known about the volunteers. The information that can be provided by the individual's general practitioner (GP) is vital to ensure that he/she is in good health. Another concern is that a volunteer may fail to disclose that they have recently participated in another trial or indeed may be currently doing so. To deal with this problem, attempts are being made to establish national, and possibly international, databases that will facilitate cross-checking of volunteer participation.

Facilities and Staff

The minimum standards for the facilities in which clinical pharmacology studies should be conducted are described in the ABPI guidelines. Clearly, the same standards should apply to pharmaceutical companies, academic units and contract research organisations. In the UK, the Medicines Control Agency has instituted inspection of facilities and procedures, and a system of certification will be implemented.

Provision of adequate competent medical staff is essential for the safe and ethical conduct of studies in humans. Decisions about whether a volunteer fulfils the entry criteria for a healthy subject or should be withdrawn from a study, how to respond to an unexpected adverse event and when to discontinue a study can prove challenging to the most experienced physician. Similarly, research nurses need many organisational and other skills over and above those that they acquired during their basic clinical training. Scientific staff must be competent in the techniques that will provide the essential data. All must be properly briefed about what will be required of them during the course of a study, and must be fully familiar with local standard operating procedures (SOPs) in compliance with good clinical practice (GCP).

Non-clinical as well as clinical staff involved in conducting studies in humans, should be trained in *basic life support*, with regular updates, preferably every six months, and medical and nursing staff should also receive training in *advanced life support*. Training records should be kept for each member of staff and practice emergency call sessions should be run frequently. Staff development is a subject beyond the scope of this text but it is worth emphasising the value of offering training for clinical research nurses in the medical and scientific aspects of their work, as well as expecting them to learn on the job under supervision. Motivation and performance will be greatly enhanced by staff who understand something of the science behind the compound being tested and the medical as well as commercial rationale for its development.

Recruitment Procedures

Detailed written information, which generally constitutes part of the consent form, should not be provided to potential volunteers until ethics approval has been obtained. Most importantly, the information should be provided in clear non-technical language. A copy of the study schedule and an oral explanation should complement the written information. Volunteers should be given every opportunity to ask questions and to obtain additional information. They should be encouraged to contact the study physician about any symptoms, however trivial, that occur between study occasions, particularly if they wish to take medication such as analgesics, decongestants or antihistamines. A cooling off period of at least 24 hours should be allowed after provision of information to allow the volunteer to consider and have the opportunity to discuss with their partner, family or friends. Therefore, medical screening should not be arranged to follow immediately after information sessions.

If volunteers are required to give specimens for genotyping for drug metabolising enzymes or for proteins that might be involved in pharmacodynamic responses, a separate consent form should be provided for this purpose. If it is intended that a DNA sample be stored for future analysis, consent should be requested and it should be made clear that all data will be held in a format which will make it impossible to link the data to an identifiable individual. Subjects should be free to refuse or withdraw consent independent of their consent to participation in the study. In the event of a withdrawal, any samples taken should be destroyed.

The size of the honorarium should reflect the amount of *inconvenience* that the study causes to the participant, and not the perceived risk. It is best decided by relatively disinterested parties, such as a medical director in consultation with a senior research nurse or head of clinical pharmacology. The sum must be submitted for ethics committee approval with the protocol and is non-negotiable.

It should be a precondition of acceptance of a volunteer into a study that he or she is registered with a GP and that permission is given to contact the GP to inform them of the study and to seek confirmation that their patient is suitable to participate. Although communication about a patient between physicians is always confidential, the GP is not bound to disclose personal information and may recommend that their patient does not participate, without having to give a specific reason.

Good Clinical Practice

However, it is emphasised that the standards required of large clinical trials in patients apply equally to small clinical pharmacological studies in healthy subjects. Studies should be conducted in accordance with SOPs. Many SOPs will resemble those pertaining to later phase clinical trials, but some will be specific to healthy volunteer studies. Details of procedures not covered by SOPs should be specified in the protocol. Studies must be monitored by the sponsor or a representative; the monitor should not be one of the investigators so that monitoring visits and assessments can maintain objectivity.

Adverse Reactions in Volunteer Studies

There are no accurate data that provide a comprehensive picture of the extent of healthy volunteer studies and hence of the incidence of adverse reactions. However, surveys and clinical series have been published from time to time. In 1984 the ABPI requested information from its member companies on their activities in this area. Of the 43 companies that responded, 28 conducted in-house studies and 41 commissioned external work. In the in-house studies, there were 18,671 subject exposures to drugs. There were no deaths or life-threatening suspected reactions. The incidence of serious suspected reactions that might have been attributable to drug was 0·27 per 1000 subject exposures. Of the 8733 subject exposures in external studies, there was one death on which the inquest reported an open verdict and no life-threatening suspected reactions. The incidence of suspected serious reactions was 0·91 per 1000 subject exposures.

In another survey conducted by the clinical section of the British Pharmacological Society over a one-year period from 1986 to 1987, 8163 healthy volunteers received drugs for research purposes. Potentially life-threatening adverse effects were reported in 0·04% and moderately severe adverse effects in 0·55%, with no lasting sequelae. The three severe reactions were skin irritation and rash requiring hospitalisation, anaphylactic shock after an oral vaccine, and perforation of a duodenal ulcer after multiple-dose non-steroidal anti-inflammatory drug; all made a complete recovery. The results were similar to those reported in the earlier ABPI survey and the authors concluded that the risk involved in these studies is very small and that most of the moderately severe reactions are of the predictable kind, generally being attributable to the known pharmacological activity of the drug.

In a much larger survey of 93,399 subjects participating in non-therapeutic research in the USA, 37 subjects were reported to be temporarily disabled and one to be permanently disabled. The latter was due to a stroke occurring three days after investigation, and its attributability is unknown.

In a report of two five-year periods in a single centre in France, the incidence of adverse events in 1015 healthy volunteers was 13·7% in subjects receiving active drug and 7·9% in those receiving placebo. Headache, diarrhoea and dyspepsia occurred in more than ten per thousand. Three percent of adverse events were rated severe but there were no deaths or life-threatening events. Some events such as vasovagal attacks were related to procedures rather than treatment.

All these studies indicate that the incidence of serious adverse events in such studies is very low and is comparable with the normal hazards of everyday life. Nevertheless, it must always be remembered that the volunteer is placing his/her welfare in the trust of the research physician, who therefore bears an enormous responsibility.

Insurance and Compensation

These topics are covered at some length in the Report of the Royal College of Physicians and the ABPI guidelines. Essentially, the company must undertake to pay compensation to any volunteer who has suffered bodily injury as the result of participating in a study, without having to prove negligence or that a test drug or procedure failed to fulfil a reasonable expectation of safety. This contractual agreement should be stated in the consent form that the volunteer signs. Ethics committees should ensure that arrangements for such "no-fault" compensation are in place. Regarding personal insurance, companies will not normally exclude cover for accidents occurring as the result of research, but volunteers are advised to seek clarification on this from their insurers, particularly when taking out a new policy.

Study Objectives in Exploratory Development

The first and subsequent studies of a NAS in humans should aim to obtain dose–concentration–response relationships for desired and undesired effects. These objectives may be summarised as follows:

To investigate over a range of doses

1. Tolerability and safety
2. Pharmacokinetics
3. Pharmacodynamic activity.

Tolerability and Safety

The word *tolerability* is perhaps a little clumsy but it describes accurately what is assessed, namely how well the drug is tolerated by those to whom it is administered. This last qualification is necessary because there are many instances in which a drug is better tolerated or less well tolerated by young healthy volunteers than by patients. For example, anxiolytics and tricyclic antidepressants are usually far better tolerated by patients with depression than by healthy volunteers. However, healthy volunteer studies generally provide useful information about tolerability even if it may under- or overestimate tolerability in patients. Many adverse reactions will be directly related to the known pharmacological activity of the drug and are therefore predictable.

The investigation of tolerability must cover a number of doses thought to be in the range required for therapeutic benefit. The relevance of these data can only be interpreted when they are related to plasma concentrations and, when appropriate, measurements of pharmacodynamic activity. Adverse reactions occurring at ten times the therapeutic dose may not pose a problem; conversely, the absence of adverse reactions at one-tenth the therapeutic dose is of little relevance and, if misinterpreted, may give unfounded confidence. This may seem obvious but has important implications for study design that are frequently ignored.

Tolerability should not be confused with the term *tolerance* which describes the diminution in effects of a drug on prolonged exposure. Tolerance may be due to increased clearance because of autoinduction of the enzymes that metabolise the drug, such as occurs with some antiepileptic drugs, for example carbamazepine. Tolerance may also result from altered pharmacodynamics, which is common with drugs acting on the CNS.

Tolerability should also be distinguished from safety. A drug that causes mild sedation may be safe except to individuals undertaking certain activities that are affected adversely by sedation, for example driving a car. On the other hand, a drug may be tolerated well in the short to medium term but may cause elevation of liver transaminases, suggesting that it is hepatotoxic. Similarly, a drug may be tolerated extremely well by healthy volunteers and by the vast majority of patients but may cause prolongation of the QT interval on ECG, which poses a significant risk of cardiac arrhythmias in susceptible patients. A preliminary assessment of safety may be obtained in repeat-dose studies in exploratory studies in healthy volunteers and patients, but it should be recognised that the chances of detecting an uncommon serious adverse event are remote because of the relatively small number of subjects exposed.

Pharmacokinetics

The pharmacokinetic information that can be obtained from the first study in man is dependent on the route of administration. When a drug is given intravenously, its bioavailability is 100%, and *clearance* and *volume of distribution* can be obtained in addition to *half-life*. Over a range of doses it can be established whether the area under the plasma concentration–time curve (AUC) increases in proportion to the dose and hence whether the kinetic parameters are independent of dose. When a drug is administered orally, the half-life can still be determined, but only the apparent volume of distribution and clearance can be calculated because bioavailability is unknown. However, if the maximum concentration (C_{max}) and AUC increase proportionately with dose, and the half-life is constant, it can usually be assumed that clearance is independent of dose. If, on the other hand, the AUC does not increase in proportion to the dose, this could be the result of a change in bioavailability, clearance, or both.

In addition to the pharmacokinetics of the drug, the first study in man can provide important information about its metabolites. If assay methodology has been developed, metabolites in plasma can be detected and the AUCs and half-lives determined. Further information can be obtained from assaying urine for drug and, if possible, metabolites. Renal clearance can be calculated over time intervals and the ratio of renal to systemic clearance calculated so that the relative importance of renal and metabolic clearance can be assessed. The relative proportions of parent compound and identifiable metabolites will give an important, albeit incomplete, picture of how the drug is excreted in urine. The total amount of parent compound and metabolites measured in urine will give a minimum value for bioavailability of the drug. Early administration by both intravenous and oral routes can be extremely useful to ascertain the bioavailability and, if low, whether this is because of poor absorption or high first-pass metabolism.

It is a great mistake to think that the information obtained from such a study of pharmacokinetics is mainly the concern of pharmacokineticists. Pharmacokinetic data are essential for making rational decisions about the future development of a compound. At the simplest level, a half-life that is so short that the drug would have to be administered six times a day in order to maintain therapeutic benefit may be a good enough reason to discontinue development. A drug that has to be administered in very large doses to achieve adequate plasma concentrations, or fails to reach them at all because of poor or saturable absorption, is obviously unattractive. Large variability in bioavailability because of inconsistent absorption or extensive first-pass metabolism might constitute another reason for stopping development. Saturation

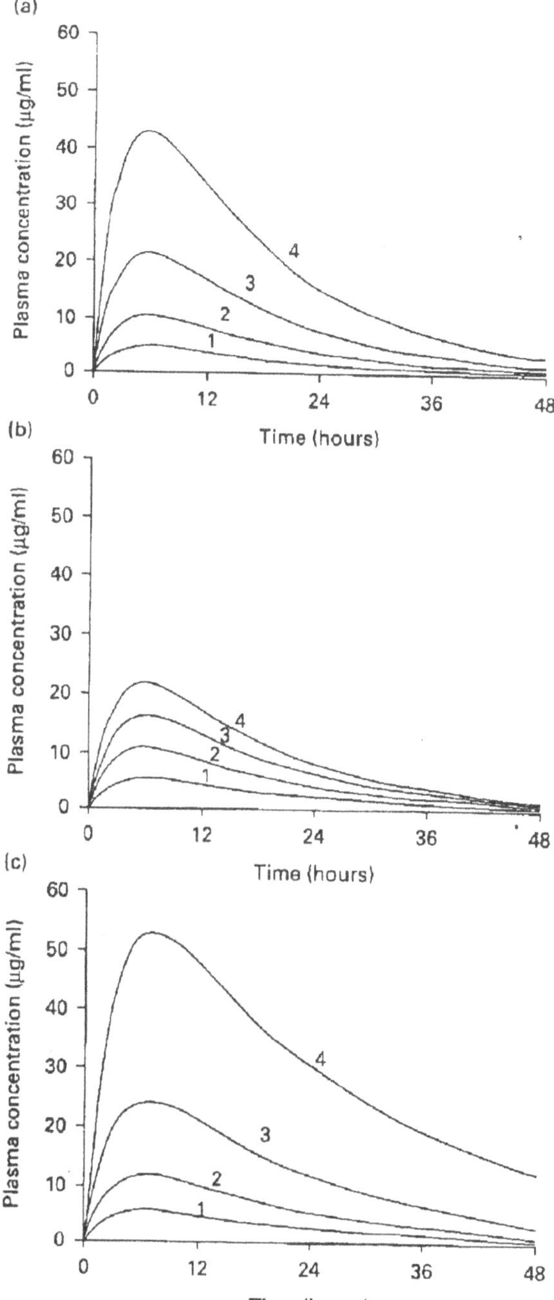

Fig. 23.1. Plasma concentration profiles after doubling doses showing (a) proportional increase with dose, (b) less than proportional increase with dose, (c) greater than proportional increase with dose.

of clearance, mechanisms which, at the very least, will make dosing complicated, could result in unacceptable toxicity. The presence of a large number of metabolites may be undesirable, particularly if not all of them were detectable in the animal species used for toxicology so that additional toxicity studies might be required to support further work in humans.

At the end of the first study in man, the pharmacokinetic profile should be compared with that desired for the compound. If reality compares unfavourably with the ideal, the unpleasant decision to discontinue development may have to be taken. Even if single-dose pharmacokinetics are acceptable, a further assessment will need to be made after repeat-dose administration of the drug since this may reveal plasma concentrations which do not match the predictions from single doses. For example, saturation of elimination resulting in higher than predicted steady-state concentrations, with associated toxicity, may make dosing too difficult for practical purposes. Conversely, autoinduction of metabolic enzymes, with resultant increased clearance, may occur, making it necessary to increase the dose over a period of weeks and also rendering the drug susceptible to interactions with other drugs and disease. Another consideration may be the accumulation of a metabolite that has a much longer half-life than that of the parent compound and which was perhaps undetectable after single doses.

However, none of the reasons given for stopping development is applicable to all drugs. Thus, a short plasma half-life may be perfectly acceptable when the effect of the drug persists long after the drug has gone, for example the effect of aspirin on platelet cyclooxygenase, or when only brief exposure is are needed to obtain therapeutic benefit, for example penicillin in pneumococcal pneumonia. Saturation of metabolism at high doses may be irrelevant if much lower doses are required for therapeutic benefit. Low bioavailability may not constitute a problem if the therapeutic index is high, as for example with propranolol. The presence of multiple metabolites does not necessarily contraindicate proceeding; many useful lipophilic drugs undergo extensive metabolism. A persistent active metabolite may actually convert a drug that would have been unattractive into a very useful one; that, after all, is the principle of prodrugs. The point is that rational decisions can only be made if the information is actively sought and then matched against the desired profile.

Pharmacokinetics may also form the basis of a decision on the choice of compound from a series for development. It is not uncommon for a company to take three or four compounds of a series as far as the first study in man and to choose for development the compound that is most attractive from the pharmacokinetic point of view. Similarly, the development of achiral compounds rather than racemic mixtures is generally preferred and it may be necessary to establish whether stereo-selective metabolism occurs in man and, if so, which enantiomer has the more desirable profile.

From the pharmacokinetics of single doses it is possible to simulate the expected accumulation and concentrations on reaching steady state that will occur on repeat dosing. However, it cannot be assumed that these predictions will hold, and repeat dosing studies in ED should generally include a comparison of pharmacokinetic profiles after the first dose and then at steady state, preferably after dosing for at least ten days. An increase in clearance because of autoinduction will result in lower C_{max} and AUC and a shorter half-life than predicted. Conversely, saturation of metabolic enzymes at steady state may result in higher than predicted plasma drug concentrations. Accumulation of metabolites that were only present in low, perhaps undetectable, concentrations after single doses may be observed after repeat dosing.

Pharmacodynamics

The third major objective of ED studies in man is to evaluate pharmacodynamic effects that may serve as biomarkers. A *biomarker* is "a characteristic that is objectively measured and evaluated as an indicator of a normal physiological process, pathogenic process or pharmacological response to a therapeutic intervention". Such measures may be biomarkers of the desired effect of the drug (i.e. efficacy) or of undesired effects (i.e. toxicity). When a biomarker is not merely a measure of pharmacodynamic effect but is intended to substitute for a clinical endpoint, it may be called a *surrogate endpoint*. The implication is that extensive study of the biomarker has generated sufficient confidence that linkage to a clinical endpoint has been established. A *clinical endpoint* is defined as "a characteristic or variable that measures how a patient feels, functions or survives". When the validity of a surrogate endpoint is widely accepted, it may replace a clinical endpoint for registration purposes.

As mentioned in the introduction, decisions in ED will often depend on the dose–response curves for desired and undesired effects and hence predictions about benefit: risk. It may be just as important to assess undesired as well as desired effects: such information can again be used as the basis for decisions on future development. For example, the decision to develop a new histamine H_1 antagonist, will depend on assessments of the dose–response curves for sedation and effect on the QT interval of the ECG, as well as demonstration of the dose–response for antagonism of weals and flares to intradermal histamine, or histamine bronchial challenge.

The use of imaging techniques such as ultrasound scanning, positron emission tomography (PET), single positron emission computed tomography (SPECT), magnetic resonance imaging (MRI), including functional MRI, in later phase clinical development is becoming well established and a number of drugs have been approved on the basis of radiological surrogate endpoints. The use of these techniques in early evaluation of drugs is less well established but imaging of cerebral opioid, 5-hydroxytryptamine (5HT; serotonin) $5HT_{1A}$, $5HT_2$, dopmaine D_2, muscarinic, nicotinic and other receptors, monoamine oxidase (MAO) B and other enzymes using specific ligands holds great promise. Measurement of receptor occupancy, for example, may prove a rapid and relatively simple means of selecting one or more doses for inclusion in clinical trials. This is likely to be of enormous value for trials of treatment of diseases in which group sizes can be extremely large, such as stroke and dementia. Whenever possible, investigations of pharmacokinetics should be combined with pharmacodynamic measures to establish the relationship between concentration and effect. Such relationships can be handled very simply or with modelling so that predictions can be made.

The limitations of the use of biomarkers in healthy volunteers must be recognised. For example, although there have been attempts to simulate migraine headache in volunteers, to date none of these models can be considered adequate to serve as a surrogate endpoint with which to assess the effect of a new putative antimigraine drug. Patients with migraine are not difficult to recruit and are usually healthy apart from their migraine. In this case it may be more appropriate to establish tolerability and pharmacokinetics in healthy volunteers and then to select a maximum well tolerated dose with which to perform a small *"proof of principle"* clinical trial in patients. This will need to be followed by larger trials to establish the dose–response relationship. Promising attempts have been made to develop models of acute anxiety in volunteers but there is no reliable biomarker of depression, and for conditions such as acute stroke the proof of principle currently requires very large clinical trials, a very expensive and lengthy development with a high risk of failure.

The value of biomarkers to establish the dose- and concentration response curves at the earliest stage of drug development cannot be overestimated. However, it should be recognised that the utility of any biomarker depends at least in part on the expertise of the experimentalists. Long before the study takes place a decision will need to be made about where the study will be placed and who precisely will perform the measurements. Whether assaying the concentrations of a hormone, performing respiratory function tests or measuring receptor occupancy with a PET ligand, adequate time must be allowed to assess the quality of data produced by a potential investigator or, if appropriate, whether to develop the technique in-house or in collaboration with an academic centre or contract research organisation. Choice of an investigator must also take into account logistic concerns such as availability of suitable subjects, capability of staff and access to particular equipment. All developmental methodology work must take place before its application to assessment of a NAS so that results are sufficiently reliable as a basis for decisions about the NAS.

Even if a technique is well established and the methodology has been used many times by the chosen investigator, it is usually worth including an active comparator in such studies. First and foremost, this acts as a verum - it is a concurrent control which verifies that the technique is capable of producing a positive result in that study, thereby avoiding the false negative conclusion. In addition, it will provide a measure with which the magnitude, duration and quality of responses obtained with the NAS can be compared (i.e. a bioassay). The main exception to the use of an active comparator is the first study in humans in which formal statistical comparisons are rarely appropriate and the emphasis is on safety.

Design of First Study in Humans

The first study of a NAS in man will inevitably involve an escalating-dose design, usually with single doses, although in oncology, repeat dosing is more appropriate for ethical reasons. The choice of starting dose, increments, range and interval between occasions, number of subjects and use of placebo all need to be considered. Paramount is the safety of the subjects.

Choice of Dose Range

Factors that must be taken into account in selecting the dose range to be studied include the following.

1. Maximum concentration (C_{max}) and exposure ($AUC_{steady\ state}$) in toxicity studies at NOAEL using the most sensitive species, based on the concentrations of drug unbound to plasma proteins, for which substantial corrections may be necessary if plasma protein binding in one or more species is above 95%
2. The nature and severity of toxicity seen in animals - some findings are of more serious consequence than others
3. The range of doses and plasma concentrations that exhibited pharmacodynamic effects in animals, the nature of the effects, and the slope of the dose-response curve
4. The comparative disposition in different species and predicted exposure in humans, with particular attention to the presence of active metabolites with long half-lives
5. The range of doses and number of increments likely to be required in man.

Knowledge of the concentration-response relationship and the nature of the pharmacodynamic responses and toxicity in animals are the only sound basis for deciding on the starting dose and dosage increments to be used in man. This information needs to be interpreted and applied using common sense; application of formulae is not appropriate.

Magnitude of Dose Increments

It is quite usual to escalate the doses by doubling, which is consistent with the linear relationship between logarithm of the dose and response. However, if the slope of the dose-response curve is steep, doubling increments may be excessive, and for some drugs the relationship between dose (rather than log dose) and response is linear. Sometimes, it is preferred to start with a very low dose, examine the pharmacokinetics and then increase the dose 4-5 fold if appropriate. Once into the expected therapeutic range, increments should not generally be greater than doubling. Even when all this has been considered, the doses scheduled are only tentative and they may well need to be modified in the light of the first experience in man.

Should We Dose to Toxicity?

The choice of the top dose in a dose-escalating study may be difficult. The view is often expressed that dosing should continue to "toxicity", that is that the dose should be escalated until intolerable adverse effects are experienced by one or more volunteers. Although an adequate definition is lacking, this suggests that the maximum tolerated dose (MTD) will be one increment below that toxic dose. There are certainly some drugs for which the therapeutic index is expected to be low and the putative therapeutic dose will be close to that which can just be tolerated. However, deliberate production of serious adverse events is always unacceptable in healthy volunteers and usually unacceptable in patients, an exception in the latter case being haematological toxicity with cytotoxic chemotherapy. Therefore, for most ED studies of drugs with a low therapeutic index, it is of much greater relevance to determine a dose which produces some mild non-serious effects. The term *minimum intolerated dose* (MID) has been applied to patients, and although the dose may be different, the term can equally be applied to healthy subjects. Examples of effects that determine the MID may be sedation, flushing, headache, loose stools or a small change in heart rate or blood pressure. Of no less importance is the dose below the MID, which may be defined as the *maximum well tolerated dose* (MWTD). The MWTD is frequently used as the top dose in subsequent ED dose-range finding studies in healthy volunteers and patients.

The "*dosing to toxicity*" approach was adopted because investigators did not take the trouble to measure pharmacodynamic effects or even follow plasma drug concentrations during the course of a study. Many drugs have a reasonably high therapeutic index and for these it should be perfectly possible to stop the escalation at a predefined pharmacodynamic endpoint such as maximum inhibition of a target enzyme. For an anti-infective agent devoid of pharmacological effects and with a high therapeutic index, it is usually unjustifiable to continue dose-escalation beyond a particular plasma concentration that is greatly in excess of that predicted to be of therapeutic benefit from *in vitro* and perhaps *in vivo* animal studies.

Number of Doses for Individual Subjects and Interval between Doses

For reasons that have little to do with science, it has been traditional in the US to dose individual subjects just once, with a new cohort of subjects recruited for each dose level. In Europe first administration studies have typically involved dosing individuals at several if not all dose levels tested in a study.

If the number of dose increments expected is to be no greater than six, the study can be conducted with a single group of volunteers, or with two groups dosed on alternate occasions. Such a design enables a set of pharmacokinetic as well as dynamic data to be obtained for each individual over a range of doses. Since intra-individual variation is generally much less than interindividual variation, it should be possible to make meaningful comparisons of pharmacokinetic parameters at each dose to establish whether the pharmacokinetics are independent of dose. With respect to pharmacodynamics, it is often possible to plot a dose-concentration-response for each individual.

An alternating group design is certainly preferred if the half-life of the drug or a metabolite is more than about 24 hours. Thus, the first cohort might receive dose levels 1, 3 and 5 (or placebo) and the second cohort dose levels 2, 4 and 6. This allows individual subjects to be dosed with a longer interval between doses, say two weeks, with dose escalation in the alternate cohort on the intervening weeks. However, drugs (or metabolites) with very long half-lives are best studied using a new cohort of volunteers for each dose.

Situations may arise when the dose range that has to be studied is very wide and the number of increments required to cover the range is large. It may then be advisable to use successive cohorts of volunteers so that the first cohort might receive dose levels 1 to 4, the second dose levels 4 to 7, and so on. Note that each cohort is introduced at the top dose level received by the preceding cohort, the overlap being necessary to avoid exposure of a naive subject to what might be a high dose.

Whichever design is preferred, the interval between dose escalations should be determined on grounds of safety, not convenience or availability of subjects. For drugs with half-lives of two or three hours it may theoretically be possible to study the subjects two or three times in one week and thereby conclude the study quickly. However, analytical laboratories can rarely support such a short turnaround time and there is a limit to the time in which data can be collated and reviewed. Failure to obtain, scrutinise and evaluate all the data puts volunteers at unnecessary risk, as does inadequate time for follow up safety assessments of subjects. For drugs or metabolites with long half-lives, clinical assessment and blood sampling for pharmacokinetics and clinical pathology may have to continue for many days or weeks before it is prudent to dose escalate, whether in the same or different individuals.

Use of Placebo

In general, studies in ED should be placebo controlled, an exception being some pharmacokinetic studies, for example bioavailability. In a dose- escalating design, it is obviously not possible to randomise or balance the order of doses, and there may be insufficient power to subject pharmacodynamic endpoints to statistical analysis; however, the advantages of a placebo group outweigh the disadvantages. It is not uncommon for a large number of trivial symptoms to be reported by volunteers and it may only be possible to interpret the significance of these when the incidence in the placebo and treated groups is compared. Substantial changes in vital signs such as heart rate and blood pressure occur in the course of a day, and a placebo is invaluable in distinguishing drug-induced effects from others. Similarly, it is not uncommon for some external factor such as an influenza epidemic, food poisoning, caffeine withdrawal or even a change in the weather to affect a study. Frequently, minor elevation of liver transaminases or lymphocytosis occur as the result of intercurrent viral infections. Liver transaminases also tend to rise with prolonged periods of incarceration in a study unit, probably because of diet, lack of exercise, or other lifestyle factors. A placebo group can be invaluable in deciding whether the problem is likely to be drug related.

Blinding

As far as possible, the study should be conducted under *double-blind* conditions. Sometimes, pharmacological effects, desired or undesired, tend to unblind the study but even in these circumstances the identity of treatment will be unknown to subjects and observers at the time of dosing and before onset of effects, thereby minimising bias. Specified personnel, such as the pharmacist, bioanalyst and pharmacokineticist, may require to know the treatment allocation code but this should not compromise the blinding of all other study personnel.

Parallel Groups or Crossover

If subjects are to receive more than one dose level of active drug, there are a number of ways in which subjects can be allocated to active drug (A) or placebo (P) but essentially they fall into two approaches.

1. Subjects are randomised to receive either A or P throughout the study, i.e. *parallel groups.*
2. Subjects are randomised to receive A or P on different occasions in a *crossover* design.

The pros of a parallel group design can be summarised as follows:

1. The design is simple and robust.
2. No doses are omitted so the full dose–response and linearity of pharmacokinetics can be established within individuals.

The cons of a parallel group design can be summarised as follows:

1. It can be very difficult to maintain the blind through the study because as soon as pharmacodynamic effects are observed both subjects and investigators will know whether an individual has been allocated to the active or placebo group for the remainder of the study.
2. Subjects cannot serve as their own placebo controls for intrasubject comparisons of pharmacodynamic effects, including adverse events.

3. Large variability in intersubject data may obscure meaningful comparisons unless large cohort sizes are used.
4. Only a proportion of subjects participating in the study receive active drug.

The pros of a crossover design are as follows:

1. Maximum information is obtained from a comparatively small number of subjects.
2. Randomisation to A and P is different on every study day, therefore it is comparatively easy to maintain the blind throughout the study.
3. Intrasubject variability in pharmacodynamics is generally much smaller than intersubject variability, allowing meaningful comparisons with placebo.

The disadvantage of a crossover design is that individual subjects skip a dose level when they receive placebo so that no pharmacokinetic data are available for this subject/occasion and the subject is exposed to a large dose increment on the next occasion. This disadvantage can be avoided by administering every dose of A to each subject and in addition each subject receives placebo on one randomised occasion. The problem with this modification is that after the first occasion, subjects are at different dose levels on any particular study day, making it difficult to obtain data from adequate numbers of subjects before dose escalation without using large cohorts.

Size of Cohorts

The number of subjects per cohort needed for the initial study depends on several factors. If a well established pharmacodynamic measurement is to be used as an endpoint, it should be possible to calculate the number required to demonstrate significant differences from placebo by means of a power calculation based on variances in a previous study using this technique. However, analysis of the study is often limited to descriptive statistics such as mean and standard deviation, or even just recording the number of reports of a particular symptom, so that a formal power calculation is often inappropriate. There must be a balance between the minimum number on which it is reasonable to base decisions about dose escalation and the number of individuals it is reasonable to expose to a NAS for the first time. To take the extremes, it is unwise to make decisions about tolerability and pharmacokinetics based on data from one or two subjects, although there are advocates of such a minimalist approach. Conversely, it is not justifiable to administer a single dose level to, say, 50 subjects at this early stage of ED. There is no simple answer to this, but in general the number lies between six and 20 subjects.

Minimising Risk

The principle governing all studies in humans is that of "minimal risk", so that a healthy volunteer leaves a study in as good health as when he/she entered it. The Royal College of Physicians has stated that, "A risk greater than minimal is not acceptable in a healthy volunteer study". A healthy volunteer stands to gain nothing directly from a new medication and the risk should therefore be negligible but it can never be reduced to zero. One must never be deluded into believing that a NAS is going to be "safe". If all the toxicity studies are reassuring and the molecule belongs to a well- known class that has an exemplary safety record, the NAS must still be treated with the greatest respect. Some of the ways in which risk can be minimised are mentioned below.

A comprehensive knowledge of all the preclinical information about a compound is an essential requirement for the safe conduct of the first study in man. Toxicology, metabolism, pharmacokinetics and pharmacodynamics are all important despite their limited predictive power for man. As explained above, the study design must take the findings into account.

The most carefully designed study and the most ethical protocol do not guarantee safety. A study that is not prepared and executed properly is likely to put volunteers at unnecessary risk. There must be sufficient staff to cover all practical aspects of the study. At least one nurse and a doctor should be present for dosing and for a specified period afterwards, usually at least a few hours. All staff should be thoroughly briefed by the investigator, the case report forms checked against the schedule, and every member of staff should know precisely what he/she will be doing during the course of a study day. The detailed schedule for each study day must also be optimal. For example, the design may require administration of intravenous infusions to six volunteers. It may be perfectly feasible to perform these on a single day but it is inadvisable to start all the infusions simultaneously. Drug-related adverse reactions would be likely to occur at the same time in all the subjects, which could be very difficult to manage and put subjects at unnecessary risk. Indeed, it may be wise to stop the study after the first significant adverse reaction has been seen and reconsider the dose, speed of administration or whether to proceed at all. For orally administered drugs with expected pharmacodynamic effects, it is wise to study two or three lead volunteers on one day before the remaining subjects receive the same dose on another day, or to keep the number of subjects studied at one time to no more than six, at least two of whom will receive placebo.

It should be noted that pharmacokinetic data are included, which places a strain on the bioanalysts and laboratory facilities. However, with proper planning and adequate development time, preliminary but reasonably reliable data can usually be obtained within two or three days of receiving samples. Knowledge of maximum concentrations, dose proportionality of AUC and half-lives of the parent molecule and major metabolites greatly adds to making rational decisions about adverse events, times for sampling and measurements, the appropriate next dosage increment and the interval that should be allowed between study occasions.

Adverse events should be tabulated for easy inspection but the case report form should be available and all laboratory data such as blood counts, renal function and liver function tests should be inspected closely. The absence of obvious adverse events does not mean that all is well, and careful scrutiny of data by an experienced physician can often spot problems before they become troublesome. Not infrequently one or more volunteers become unwell during the course of a study, usually due to intercurrent viral infections, and decisions about postponement of study days, subject withdrawal follow up can be made during these meetings. Data that are missing because of non-attendance of volunteers, for whatever reason, may lead to a delay in the study, with postponement of dose-escalation until they have caught up.

The review requires that all the data be collated for presentation, which is a useful discipline. An opportunity is also provided for practical problems to be discussed and acted upon. All decisions should be documented, and any significant modifications to the protocol will have to be put before the IEC before proceeding. The volunteers also need to be updated about any changes to the schedule and adverse events as the study unfolds. As always, a volunteer must be free to withdraw from a study at any stage.

The decision to halt a dose escalation is not always straightforward. There may have been adverse events that are not serious but which are disliked by the volunteers. While decisions about the future of a study must always be in the hands of the physicians, the investigator must listen carefully to the volunteers and nurses. When hitherto sensible and well motivated volunteers begin to adopt a negative attitude to a study for whatever reason, it is usually time to stop.

Subsequent Studies in Healthy Volunteers

The limitations of the first day study in man should be recognised. Even if the study has achieved all its objectives in terms of tolerability, pharmacokinetics and pharmacodynamics, the data will only be of a preliminary nature. It is then necessary to re-examine the provisional plan of exploratory studies, reconsider priorities and which data require early verification in carefully designed, controlled studies. The design of subsequent studies cannot be discussed in detail here but the underlying principle is that the design must reflect the primary objectives, and these in turn are determined by the critical questions driving the ED plan.

Multiple Doses

Frequently information on tolerability and safety, and pharmacokinetics of multiple or repeat-dosing for up to 14 days is the highest priority. A placebo-controlled, parallel-groups, dose-escalating design is generally appropriate, with each cohort receiving a single dose level or placebo for the defined duration. Typically, such a study would involve three or four dose levels, selected on the basis of results of the first study. If three dose levels were chosen to be studied, cohorts of 12 subjects might be randomised 9:3 A:P so that at the end of the study nine subjects will have received each dose level and nine will have received placebo. If biomarkers are to be employed to assess the relationships between dose, concentration and response, consideration should be given to use of a positive control as well. Plasma pharmacokinetic profiles should generally be obtained with the first dose and at the end of the dosing period.

Pharmacodynamics

Study of single-dose pharmacodynamics of desired or adverse effects in healthy volunteers is best done using double-blind crossover designs, typically with three or four dose levels, placebo and active controls, randomised and balanced for order according to Latin squares. For studies in patients, multiple-limb crossover designs are less appropriate but crossover studies with single doses of A versus P are certainly feasible, and of course parallel groups, single or repeat dosing are commonly employed designs.

Studies in the Elderly

For a drug that will be used commonly in the elderly, it is important to obtain early information about tolerability and pharmacokinetics in this age group. Since glomerular filtration rate declines with age, exposure to drug is likely to be greatly increased in the elderly if the drug is eliminated primarily by the kidney. In the case of a high extraction drug, impairment of cardiac output in the elderly is likely to increase exposure because of reduced first-pass metabolism. Single- and multiple-dose studies in healthy elderly volunteers can provide extremely valuable information prior to exposure of patients in this age group, who are inevitably a vulnerable group and in whom many factors may confound results.

Drug and Food Interactions

If a drug is to be tested in patients who will inevitably be receiving other medications with which the NAS is likely to interact, it may be important to design drug interaction studies in healthy volunteers early in ED. Repeat dosing of one or both drugs to achieve steady-state concentrations is often appropriate. Potential interactions with drugs used commonly by the elderly, such as digoxin, antihypertensives and warfarin, need not be studied in the elderly but some of these studies may need to be done before exposing patients in clinical trials.

A preliminary assessment of the effect of food on pharmacokinetics can generally be studied in a single-dose, two-arm, randomised, crossover design. Preliminary information can often be obtained by including a "fed" occasion in the first, dose-escalating study. This will be inadequate for registration, which requires an adequately powered study performed with the final formulation, but the information should be sufficient to indicate whether there is need for restrictions on dosing relative to meals in repeat- dose studies in healthy volunteers and patient clinical trials.

Radiolabelled Studies

Critical features of metabolism frequently require administration of radiolabelled material to man during ED. Such studies generally involve administration of single doses, with subsequent collection of excreta as well as blood sampling until virtually all drug has been eliminated. The clinical phase of such studies is generally not complex, but preparation for the study, with synthesis of the radioactive molecule and development of "cold" assays of metabolites as well as parent molecule, may take many months. Such studies also require submission of applications with detailed dosage and radioactive exposure calculations for authorisation by external bodies such as the Administration of Radioactive Substances Advisory Committee (ARSAC) in the UK.

Studies in Patients

The ED plan will enumerate which studies are to be performed in healthy volunteers and which in patients. As the first studies progress, the information generated needs to be constantly evaluated while still blinded, and of course on unblinding after database lock at the end of each study. The decision to proceed to the patient population should take into account how well the studies have actually achieved their objectives.

The first consideration, as always, will be safety; information that can be obtained more safely in healthy subjects, which may subsequently reduce risk to patients, should prompt a debate on whether it is wise to progress according to plan or whether an additional study should be performed in healthy subjects. Another option that may be considered is to proceed with the planned study in patients but to admit them to hospital or a clinical investigation unit for all or part of the dosing period. However, this might not be feasible because suitable facilities and staff are not available or because the anticipated rate of patient recruitment might be considered unacceptably slow.

Perhaps the most frequent problem at this stage of ED is that the dose range of interest has not been adequately defined. If this can only be achieved in the target patient population there is no point in doing more studies in healthy subjects. If, on the other hand, an additional study using an established biomarker in healthy subjects would clarify the dose range of interest, thereby avoiding under- or overdosing and reducing the number of dose levels that need be examined in the patient population, this option should be considered. Whilst competition demands that drug development should proceed at a fast pace, companies frequently waste time in development because they fail to maximise the information they can obtain in ED. A delay of a few months to obtain critical data in ED may save a year or two of development time later on. The use of biomarkers and surrogate endpoints in patients is well established in virtually all therapeutic areas. After all, blood pressure has been used as a surrogate for cardiovascular risk for many decades.

An important qualification must be made. While a biomarker may be of proven value in establishing whether a drug has the desired effect in patients or healthy volunteers and for evaluation of the dose–response relationship, a biomarker may not be a surrogate for the clinical endpoint. Thus, suppression of testosterone after an initial rise will give an almost immediate endpoint for the effect of gonadotrophin-releasing hormone analogues in prostate cancer but the relationship breaks down later in the disease. Measures of blood glucose control are vital for establishing dose–response in early studies of new agents for type 2 diabetes but they are not surrogates for the complications of the disease, despite the proven relationship between glycaemic control and complications. Bone mineral density is inversely related to fracture rates in osteoporosis and is an end point for efficacy, but for regulatory purposes vertebral fracture rates constitute the primary outcome variable. An important exception is mRNA viral load in HIV-positive patients, which is accepted by regulatory authorities as a surrogate for a delay in progression to AIDS and survival. Such a conservative approach may sometimes seem to place unnecessary demands on the pharmaceutical industry but there is precedent. Suppression of ventricular extrasystoles seemed at one time to be an obvious marker of efficacy of type Ic antiarrhythmic agents. The complete failure of this "surrogate" to predict the incidence of sudden death in patients with heart disease justifies the extremely cautious position of regulatory authorities in accepting surrogate endpoints for registration purposes. An interesting aspect of the use of biomarkers as surrogates is exemplified by the statins, which lower serum low-density lipoprotein cholesterol. It has recently been shown that their contribution to improved prognosis in patients with cardiovascular disease is not entirely due to lowering of cholesterol and may be related to anti-inflammatory activity. Thus, the apparently obvious surrogate turns out to be an inadequate biomarker for predicting outcome. Of course, it is not always necessary to rely on biomarkers for rapid evaluation of dose-response relationships in ED. Thus, efficacy of new drugs is readily demonstrated in terms of the clinical endpoint for diseases such as migraine, inflammatory pain, asthma, psoriasis, glaucoma and many others.

Outcomes of Exploratory Development

As discussed in the introduction, results of ED are intended to give a clear indication that the drug is a serious candidate for full development to product licence, or that it is not viable and development should be stopped forthwith. Sometimes it takes a little longer before the picture becomes clear but the aim should be to make a go/no-go decision at the earliest opportunity. Overall, results of ED should impact on both the project itself and on the research programme from which additional compounds are actively being sought. A more successful outcome of ED will usually commit the company to proceed with full development, usually on an international basis. If ED has achieved its objectives it should be possible to make use of the pharmacodynamic and pharmacokinetic information obtained to optimise the design of subsequent pivotal clinical trials. In particular, it should be possible to use dosage regimens that are rational and justifiable on scientific as well as commercial grounds. Active research programmes should proceed with the search for follow-up compounds.

INDEX